EVIDENCE-BASED ENDOCRINOLOGY

Second Edition

EVIDENCE-BASED ENDOCRINOLOGY

Second Edition

EDITORS

Pauline M. Camacho, MD, FACE
Director, Loyola University Osteoporosis and Metabolic
    Bone Disease Center
Associate Professor of Medicine
Division of Endocrinology and Metabolism
Department of Medicine
Loyola University Chicago Stritch School of Medicine
Chicago, Illinois

Hossein Gharib, MD, MACP, MACE
Professor of Medicine
Division of Endocrinology, Metabolism, and Nutrition
Department of Medicine
Mayo Clinic College of Medicine
Rochester, Minnesota
Past President, American Association of Clinical
    Endocrinologists

Glen W. Sizemore, MD, FACE
Professor of Medicine Emeritus
Division of Endocrinology and Metabolism
Department of Medicine
Loyola University Chicago Stritch School of Medicine
Chicago, Illinois

Lippincott Williams & Wilkins
a Wolters Kluwer business
Philadelphia · Baltimore · New York · London
Buenos Aires · Hong Kong · Sydney · Tokyo

Executive Editor: Charles W. Mitchell
Managing Editor: Lisa Kairis
Developmental Editor: Grace R. Caputo, Dovetail Content Solutions
Project Manager: Jennifer Harper
Senior Manufacturing Manager: Benjamin Rivera
Marketing Manager: Angela Panetta
Design Coordinator: Terry Mallon
Production Services: Nesbitt Graphics, Inc.
Printer: R.R. Donnelley, Crawfordsville

© 2007 by **LIPPINCOTT WILLIAMS & WILKINS, a Wolters Kluwer business**
530 Walnut Street
Philadelphia, PA 19106 USA
LWW.com

Printed in the USA

Library of Congress Cataloging-in-Publication Data

Evidence-based endocrinology / editors, Pauline M. Camacho, Hossein
  Gharib, Glen W. Sizemore. -- 2nd ed.
    p. ; cm.
  Includes bibliographical references and index.
  ISBN-13: 978-0-7817-7154-2
  ISBN-10: 0-7817-7154-4
    1. Endocrinology--Handbooks, manuals, etc. 2. Evidence-based
medicine--Handbooks, manuals, etc. 3. Endocrine glands--Diseases
--Handbooks, manuals, etc.   I. Camacho, Pauline M. II. Gharib,
Hossein, 1940-   . III. Sizemore, Glen W.
    [DNLM: 1. Endocrine System Diseases--Handbooks. 2. Endocrine
System Diseases--Practice Guideline. 3. Endocrine System Diseases
--Review. 4. Cost-Benefit Analysis--methods--Handbooks. 5. Cost-
Benefit Analysis--methods--Practice Guideline. 6. Cost-Benefit
Analysis--methods--Review. 7. Evidence-Based Medicine--methods
--Handbooks. 8. Evidence-Based Medicine--methods--Practice
Guideline. 9. Evidence-Based Medicine--methods--Review.
10. Treatment Outcome--Handbooks. 11. Treatment Outcome
--Practice Guideline. 12. Treatment Outcome--Review.
WK 39 E95 2007]
RC649.E95 2007   616.4--dc22   2006025686

Care has been taken to confirm the accuracy of the information presented and to describe generally accepted practices. However, the authors, editors, and publisher are not responsible for errors or omissions or for any consequences from application of the information in this book and make no warranty, expressed or implied, with respect to the currency, completeness, or accuracy of the contents of the publication. Application of this information in a particular situation remains the professional responsibility of the practitioner.

The authors, editors, and publisher have exerted every effort to ensure that drug selection and dosage set forth in this text are in accordance with current recommendations and practice at the time of publication. However, in view of ongoing research, changes in government regulations, and the constant flow of information relating to drug therapy and drug reactions, the reader is urged to check the package insert for each drug for any change in indications and dosage and for added warnings and precautions. This is particularly important when the recommended agent is a new or infrequently used drug.

Some drugs and medical devices presented in this publication have Food and Drug Administration (FDA) clearance for limited use in restricted research settings. It is the responsibility of the health care provider to ascertain the FDA status of each drug or device planned for use in their clinical practice.

To purchase additional copies of this book, call our customer service department at (800) 638-3030 or fax orders to (301) 223-2320. International customers should call (301) 223-2300.

Visit Lippincott Williams & Wilkins on the Internet: at LWW.com. Lippincott Williams & Wilkins customer service representatives are available from 8:30 am to 6 pm, EST.

10 9 8 7 6 5 4 3

The book is dedicated to our spouses—
Francis, Minoo, and Juliet; our families;
the teachers who inspired us; and our
fellows, who taught us so much.

Acknowledgments

We thank our contributors for their diligence in maintaining focus on their areas of endocrine expertise. Their participation made the editing of this work both fun and exciting. We hope readers will enjoy their efforts and those of the exceedingly helpful and patient professionals at Lippincott Williams & Wilkins. Our special thanks to Acquisitions Editor Lisa McAllister and Developmental Editor Grace R. Caputo of Dovetail Content Solutions. Without their help, this book would not exist.

Contents

10. Carcinoid Tumors 243

*Nathan J. O'Dorisio, M. Sue O'Dorisio, and
Thomas M. O'Dorisio*

11. Paraneoplastic Endocrine Syndromes 249

Subhash Kukreja

12. Genetics 261

Peter Kopp

Contributors

Haitham S. Abu-Lebdeh, MD, MSc
Assistant Professor of Medicine
Mayo Clinic College of Medicine
Rochester, Minnesota

Consultant
Department of Medicine
St. Mary's Hospital
Rochester, Minnesota

Francis Q. Almeda, MD, FACC, FSCAI
Assistant Professor of Medicine
Section of Cardiology
Rush University Medical Center
Chicago, Illinois

Interventional Cardiologist
Section of Cardiology
Ingalls Memorial Hospital
Harvey, Illinois

Elise M. Brett, MD
Assistant Clinical Professor of Medicine
Division of Endocrinology, Diabetes and Bone Disease
Mount Sinai School of Medicine
New York, New York

Attending Physician
Division of Endocrinology, Diabetes and Bone Disease
Mount Sinai Hospital
New York, New York

Pauline M. Camacho, MD, FACE
Associate Professor of Medicine
Department of Medicine
Loyola University Chicago Stritch School of Medicine
Maywood, Illinois

Director
Loyola University Osteoporosis and Metabolic Bone Disease Center
Maywood, Illinois

M. Regina Castro, MD
Assistant Professor of Medicine
Department of Endocrinology
Mayo Clinic College of Medicine

Senior Associate Consultant
Division of Endocrinology
Mayo Clinic
Rochester, Minnesota

Gerald A. Charnogursky, MD
Assistant Professor of Medicine
Department of Medicine
Loyola University Chicago Stritch School of Medicine
Maywood, Illinois

Rhoda H. Cobin, MD
Clinical Professor of Medicine
Division of Endocrinology
Mount Sinai School of Medicine
New York, New York

Co-Chief
Endocrine Clinic
Mount Sinai Hospital
New York, New York

Steven A. DeJong, MD
Professor of Surgery
Department of Surgery
Loyola University Chicago Stritch School of Medicine
Maywood, Illinois

Vice Chair of Clinical Affairs and Chief of General Surgery
Department of Surgery
Loyola University Chicago Stritch School of Medicine
Maywood, Illinois

Mary Ann Emanuele, MD
Professor of Medicine
Department of Medicine
Loyola University Chicago Stritch School of Medicine
Maywood, Illinois

Nicholas V. Emanuele, MD
Professor of Medicine
Department of Medicine
Loyola University Chicago Stritch School of Medicine
Maywood, Illinois

Dana Z. Erickson, MD
Assistant Professor of Medicine
Division of Endocrinology, Diabetes, Metabolism, and Nutrition
Mayo Clinic College of Medicine
Rochester, Minnesota

Hossein Gharib, MD, MACP, MACE
Professor of Medicine
Mayo Clinic College of Medicine
Rochester, Minnesota
Past President
American Association of Clinical Endocrinologists

Tiffany A. Karas, MD
Attending Physician
Department of Internal Medicine
Delnor Community Hospital
Geneva, Illinois

Peter Kopp, MD
Associate Professor of Medicine
Associate Division Chief for Education
Division of Endocrinology, Metabolism and Molecular Medicine
Northwestern University
Feinberg School of Medicine
Chicago, Illinois

Subhash C. Kukreja, MD
Professor of Medicine
University of Illinois at Chicago

Chief, Medical Service
Jesse Brown VA Medical Center
Chicago, Illinois

Jeffery I. Mechanick, MD
Associate Clinical Professor
Division of Endocrinology, Diabetes, and Bone Disease
Mount Sinai School of Medicine
New York, New York

Director of Metabolic Support
The Mount Sinai Hospital
New York, New York

Fadi Nadhan, MD
Assistant Professor of Medicine
Department of Medicine
Loyola University Chicago Stritch School of Medicine
Maywood, Illinois

M. Sue O'Dorisio, MD
Professor of Pediatrics
Department of Pediatrics
University of Iowa
Iowa City, Iowa

Nathan J. O'Dorisio, MD
Assistant Professor
Department of Internal Medicine
Ohio State University
Columbus, Ohio

Assistant Director
Division of Hospital Medicine
University Hospital
Columbus, Ohio

Thomas M. O'Dorisio, MD
Professor of Medicine
Department of Internal Medicine
University of Iowa Carver College of Medicine
Iowa City, Iowa

Professor of Medicine
Department of Internal Medicine
University of Iowa Hospitals and Clinics
Iowa City, Iowa

Stephanie Painter, MD
Division of Endocrinology and Metabolism
Loyola University Chicago Stritch School of Medicine
Maywood, Illinois

Steven Petak, MD, JD, FACE, FCLM
Associate
Texas Institute for Reproductive Medicine and Endocrinology
Houston, Texas

Shailesh U. Pitale, MD, DNB, DAB, FACE
Consultant Endocrinologist
Diabetes and Hormone Center
Shriman Complex
Nagpur, India

Glen Sizemore, MD
Emeritus Professor of Medicine
Department of Medicine
Loyola University of Chicago Stritch School of Medicine
Maywood, Illinois

Preface

In 2004, we asked, "Why is there no evidence-based handbook in endocrinology?" Clearly, endocrine disorders lend themselves to evidence-based medicine. They encompass large patient populations: an estimated 14 million persons have diabetes mellitus, an estimated 44 million have osteoporosis or low bone mineral density, and 127 million U.S. citizens are overweight. These diseases are associated with high morbidity and mortality rates, a considerable social price, and high treatment costs.

The endocrine literature is huge and can be overwhelmingly so to a busy clinician. For some disease states, large controlled studies of quantifiable treatment regimens with quantifiable results have been undertaken and published; for other disorders, no such trials are found in the literature, but case studies or small trials of drug therapies or diagnostic measures are available. In the contemporary health care environment, some physicians treating endocrine patients may have little specialized training or experience in endocrine disease and only minimal appreciation of the quality of its vast literature. A manual encapsulating the best available evidence-based information in endocrinology was needed. We therefore set out to publish the first concise handbook that contained the latest clinical trials and evidence. We were gratified that the book was very well received in the United States and internationally, and the readers' feedback was most rewarding.

Given the rapidity and extent of new developments in endocrinology, another edition of the book was warranted. In the second edition of *Evidence-Based Endocrinology*, we have added a new chapter on genetics and expanded chapters on lipids, obesity, and nutrition. All chapters received a fresh look from the authors, and hundreds of new references were added. Diabetes and osteoporosis are perhaps the most rapidly growing fields, and the authors present a comprehensive update of new therapies for these diseases. Finally, a minor but notable change has been the omission of the possessive ending on eponyms, in keeping with the prevailing trend in healthcare publications.

Why should clinicians benefit from this book? At its most basic, it frees them from having to find and digest the huge volume of endocrine literature. The latest and best publications have been sought out and summarized here. At its most useful, *Evidence-Based Endocrinology* may improve diagnosis and treatment of endocrine disorders. Applying a modification of the McMaster criteria (see Introduction), the contributors have critically assessed and graded studies, assisting the readers in quickly evaluating the articles that have led to practice recommendations. This should allow them to apply the latest and, it is hoped, the best science to the diagnostic and therapeutic aspects of their practice.

The text is organized into the traditional clinical areas in endocrinology—hypothalamic–pituitary, thyroid, adrenal, metabolic bone, reproductive, diabetes, lipid disorders, obesity and nutrition, unusual endocrine malignancies, and genetics. Within this framework, our goals were multiple. First, we wished to present a concise, reference-based handbook to students, residents, physicians who provide primary care, and specialists who seek information about endocrine management. Second, we used a modification of the McMaster grading system to evaluate the quality of the references and provide practice recommendations based on summarized and graded references chosen by knowledgeable authors. Third, where possible, we wanted to provide estimates of the cost-effectiveness of clinical choices. With the limited studies available to date in some areas, the final goal has been the most elusive.

It is our hope that readers find the second edition of *Evidence-Based Endocrinology* to be a worthwhile addition to office libraries, to medical reference areas, and, as primarily intended, to the pockets of their lab coats.

Pauline M. Camacho, MD, FACE
Hossein Gharib, MD, MACP, MACE
Glen W. Sizemore, MD, FACE

Introduction

In the early years of medicine, patient management was generally based on oral or written strategies gleaned from the interpretation of existing literature or first-hand observation of patients. The results were handed down from "seasoned" or senior authorities to their juniors. Although not uniformly difficult, this form of education certainly had problems. It suffered from the empiric attitudes of some clinicians and their lack of ability or failure to assess current, "best" literature; a bias inherent in the overweighting of the results of limited observations in few patients; often a lack of systematic outcome observation, with failure to include measurements of benefit or harm to patients; and a lack of formal rules to evaluate clinical evidence.

To improve the diagnostic and therapeutic decisions offered in *Evidence-Based Endocrinology*, we have used summarized, graded references based on modifications of the McMaster classification [1]. The evidence-based effort to improve patient care began in the late 1980s at McMaster University [2] and was founded on two ideas: that more emphasis could be placed on the benefits and risks of therapy and that it was best for patients to use the top therapies from pyramids of research information that contained methodologically weak work at the base to outstanding results at the peak. This latter idea recognized that we could separate gold from junk in medical studies [3] and that some results are more certain than others. Although the classification recognizes that validity exists for an initial, intuitive, observational case report or a case–control study, it gives greater weight to placebo-controlled, randomized, double-blind clinical trials.

The grades used in the McMaster classification are 1A, 1B, 1C+, 1C, 2A, 2B, and 2C (Table 1). A grade 1 recommendation suggests that the benefits clearly outweigh harms and cost, whereas grade 2 indicates a weaker recommendation (Table 2). The letter part of the grade denotes the quality of the study. The A grade is given to randomized controlled trials with consistent results. Grade B is applied to randomized trials with less consistent results. Grade C is given to observational studies or the generalization of randomized trial results from one group of patients to a different group. Grade C+ is given to observational studies with compelling results.

The McMaster classification was developed for therapeutic information only. In clinical practice guidelines, recommendations and evidence are usually graded separately. In this book, however, we have asked authors to grade the references and the implied recommendations together. We have also modified its use to include studies of diagnostic tests and, more generally, to use it as a grading system for most types of medical literature. Because many areas remain somewhat controversial, authors have been given broad latitude after reviewing literature in their area to make judgments based on their interpretation of all evidence.

REFERENCES

1. Montori VM, Schunemann HJ, Guyatt GH. What is evidence-based medicine? Endocrinol Clin 2002;31:521–526.
2. Evidence-Based Medicine Working Group. Evidence-based medicine: a new approach to teaching the practice of medicine. JAMA 1992;268:2420–2425.
3. Brody JM. Separating gold from junk in medical studies. New York Times, October 22, 2002.

Table 1.   McMaster Approach to Grades of Recommendation

Grade[a]	Clarity of Risk/Benefit	Methodologic Strength of Supporting Evidence	Implications
1A	Clear	RCTs without important limitations	Strong recommendation, can apply to most patients in most circumstances without reservation
1B	Clear	RCTs with important limitations (inconsistent results, methodological laws[b])	Strong recommendation, likely to apply to most patients
1C+	Clear	No RCTs but RCT results can be unequivocally extrapolated, or overwhelming evidence from observation studies exists	Strong recommendation, can apply to most patients in most circumstances
1C	Clear	Observational studies	Intermediate-strength recommendation; may change when stronger evidence available
2A	Unclear	RCTs without important limitations	Intermediate-strength recommendation; best action may differ depending on circumstances of patients' or societal values
2B	Unclear	RCTs with important limitations (inconsistent results, methodological flaws)	Weak recommendation; alternative approaches likely to be better for some patients under some circumstances
2C	Unclear	Observational studies	Very weak recommendation; other alternatives may be equally reasonable

RCTs = randomized controlled trials.

[a] The following considerations will bear on whether the recommendation is grade 1 or 2: the magnitude and precision of the treatment effect, patients' risk of the target event being prevented, the nature of the benefit, and the magnitude of the risk associated with treatment, variability in patient preferences, variability in regional resource availability and health care practices, and cost considerations. Inevitably, weighing these considerations involves subjective judgment. Also, since studies in categories B and C may be flawed, it is likely that most recommendations in these classes will be grade 2.

[b] These situations include RCTs with both lack of binding and subjective outcomes, where the risk of bias in measurement of outcomes is high, and with large loss to follow-up.

(After Montori VM, Schunemann HJ, Guyatt GH. What is evidence-based medicine? Endocrinol Clin 2002;31:521–526.)

Table 2. Factors That May Weaken a Recommendation to Treat, Changing Grade 1 to Grade 2

Less serious outcome
Smaller treatment effect
Imprecise estimate of treatment effect
Lower risk of target event
Higher risk of therapy
Higher costs
Varying values

(After Montori VM, Schunemann HJ, Guyatt GH. What is evidence-based medicine? Endocrinol Clin 2002;31:521–526.)

Hypothalamic–Pituitary Disorders

Gerald A. Charnogursky, Tiffany A. Karas,
Nicholas V. Emanuele, Mary Ann Emanuele, and
Fadi Nabhan

EVALUATION OF THE HYPOTHALAMIC–PITUITARY AXIS
Mary Ann Emanuele and Nicholas Emanuele

Proper sample collection and transport, including timing and condition (e.g., fasting, stress, sleep, posture, and drugs), are of primary importance in the evaluation of all hormone levels [1], and the responsible laboratory should be consulted before obtaining a sample. Basal evaluation should consist of trophic and target hormone levels (Table 1.1). Although both radioimmunoassay (RIA) and immunoradiometric assay (IRMA) measure hormone concentrations, IRMAs are usually more rapid, more specific, and more sensitive than RIAs. Binding proteins, precursors, and metabolites may interfere with both assays and can produce spuriously high or low values. Further evaluation depends on the clinical question of hypofunctioning or hyperfunctioning of the suspected endocrine gland. Stimulatory tests provide insight into cases of hypofunction, whereas suppression tests are best for cases of hyperfunction.

Growth Hormone

Deficiency

Insulin-induced hypoglycemia is the test used as the standard criterion for growth hormone (GH) deficiency [2]. After an overnight fast, baseline glucose, GH, and cortisol levels are determined. Intravenous regular insulin is then given i.v. push (0.1–0.15 U/kg), and glucose, GH, and cortisol levels are measured again 30, 60, and 90 minutes after the initial bolus. If no clinical evidence of hypoglycemia (e.g., tachycardia and sweating) is found after 45 minutes, a repeated bolus of insulin should be given, and sampling repeated. Adequate hypoglycemia occurs when the blood glucose decreases to less than 40 mg/dl. Normally, GH levels should increase to more than 5 mg/L. Ischemic heart disease, cardiac conduction disorders, and epilepsy are contraindications to the test. Other stimulatory tests include the administration of

Table 1.1.   Pituitary and Target Hormones

Pituitary Hormone	Target Gland	Feedback Hormone
Growth hormone (GH)	Liver, bone, adipocytes, and other tissues	IGF-1
Luteinizing hormone (LH)	Gonad	Testosterone (men) Estradiol (women)
Follicle-stimulating hormone (FSH)	Gonad	Testosterone (men) Estradiol (women)
Thyrotropin (TSH)	Thyroid	T4, T3
Corticotropin (ACTH)	Adrenal	Cortisol
Prolactin	Breast	Unknown

GH-releasing factor, arginine, L-Dopa, or glucagon. GH-releasing factor (1 μg/kg/i.v.) is injected, and blood obtained at 0, 15, 30, and 60 minutes for GH levels. Peak GH levels occur at 15 to 30 minutes and range from 10 to more than 50 ng/ml in normal young adults. Arginine hydrochloride (0.5 μg/kg body weight in normal saline) is administered i.v. over a 30-minute period. GH peak occurs at 45 to 60 minutes. Levodopa (500 mg if weight is >30 kg; 250 mg if weight is 15–30 kg, and 125 mg if >15 kg) is given orally. Transient nausea is common. Peak GH response usually occurs between 45 and 90 minutes. Glucagon, 1 mg, is given intramuscularly, and peak GH response occurs 2 to 3 hours later.

Growth Hormone Excess
Basal levels of GH are not very useful, whereas elevated levels of insulin-like growth factor 1 (IGF-1) indicate excess GH. In addition, IGF-binding protein-3 (IGFBP-3) is increased in association with acromegaly.

The oral glucose tolerance test is useful. Glucose (75 g) is given after an overnight fast. Serum GH is measured at 30-minute intervals for 150 minutes. In normal individuals, GH values are suppressed below 0.5 mg/L. In patients with acromegaly, this suppression does not occur, and a paradoxical increase in GH levels may occur.

Gonadotropins
Deficiency
Gonadotropin deficiency can usually be diagnosed by measuring basal serum values of luteinizing hormone (LH), follicle-stimulating hormone (FSH), and concomitant gonadal steroids (free testosterone in men and estradiol in women). A low free testosterone or estradiol concentration in association with low or inappropriately normal levels of gonadotropins is suggestive of hypothalamic–pituitary dysfunction. Usually, dynamic tests are not needed for the diagnosis. In men, serum testosterone has a diurnal variation and is higher in the early morning; therefore it must be drawn at 8 a.m.

Excess
Gonadotropin excess is extremely rare and is discussed in the section on pituitary tumors.

Thyrotropin
Deficiency
A low or inappropriately normal TSH level associated with low serum free thyroxine (T4) suggests TSH deficiency. Current sensitive TSH assays have eliminated the need for dynamic testing with thyrotropin-releasing hormone (TRH) stimulation.

Excess
TSH excess states are extremely rare and are discussed in the section on pituitary tumors.

Adrenocorticotropic Hormone

Deficiency

Deficiency of adrenocorticotropic hormone (ACTH) is diagnosed when screening levels of cortisol and ACTH are low, prompting use of the insulin-induced hypoglycemia challenge test. In situations of normal ACTH reserve, the serum cortisol increases to above 20 mg/dl. In addition, a low random cortisol level in the presence of normal response to exogenous ACTH indicates ACTH deficiency.

The corticotropin-releasing hormone (CRH) stimulation test is used to distinguish between hypothalamic and pituitary causes of hypoadrenalism. An intravenous bolus of synthetic ovine CRH (1 mg/kg body weight) is injected after the patient fasts for a minimum of 4 hours. Blood samples are collected 15 and 0 minutes before and 5, 10, 15, 30, 45, 60, 90, and 120 minutes after CRH injection for ACTH and cortisol. Normal response is documented when plasma ACTH increases by at least 35% and/or the serum cortisol increases by at least 20% [3]. A decreased plasma ACTH level and serum cortisol responses to CRH are noted in patients with primary pituitary ACTH deficiency. Those with hypothalamic disease have exaggerated and prolonged plasma ACTH response and a subnormal cortisol response.

The metyrapone test is also used to determine the ACTH reserve. Metyrapone blocks synthesis of cortisol by blocking 11β-hydroxylase, which in turn stimulates ACTH production. This ACTH increase leads to an increase in the precursor of cortisol, 11-deoxycortisol, thus testing the ACTH reserve. Metyrapone is given orally in the dose of 750 mg every 4 hours for 24 hours. In unaffected patients, it suppresses the 8 a.m. cortisol level to less than 7 mg/dl and increases the serum 11-deoxycortisol to at least 10 mg/dl. Hydrocortisone, 100 mg, should be given intravenously to reverse the cortisol deficiency after the 8 a.m. samples are taken. In patients with hypothalamic or pituitary disease, the serum 11-deoxycortisol level is less than 10 mg/dl.

ACTH Excess

Tests for Cushing syndrome are described in a subsequent section of this chapter.

Posterior Pituitary

Deficiency

Polyuria exceeding 2 L/day could be due to diabetes insipidus (DI). Glucocorticoid deficiency, if associated, may prevent polyuria from occurring, given that it reduces free water clearance by the glomeruli, which may obscure symptomatic DI. Hence the clinician should evaluate anterior pituitary function completely and replace corticosteroid before evaluating the patient for DI.

The water-deprivation test is useful. The patient need not be fasting, but water is the only fluid allowed. He or she should also avoid smoking. After emptying the bladder, the patient is weighed, and water consumption is not allowed until the test is completed. Urine osmolality, total volume, and weight are measured every hour. The test is continued until the patient's weight falls by 3%, until there is hypotension, or until osmolality does not change by more than 30 mOsm between two samples. Urine osmolality that exceeds 500 mOsm/kg is the normal response. At the end of the test, 2 mg of arginine vasopressin is given intravenously. Patients with central DI (CDI) have a concentration of urine after vasopressin injection.

IMAGING OF THE HYPOTHALAMIC–PITUITARY SYSTEM
Mary Ann Emanuele and Nicholas Emanuele

Radiologic Imaging Techniques

Magnetic resonance imaging (MRI) usually provides the best visualization of the hypothalamic–pituitary anatomy, followed by high-resolution coronal computed tomography (CT) with 1.5-mm sections through the pituitary. Even though both are equally effective in identifying large pituitary tumors, MRI is superior in defining the relation to surrounding structures. It is more accurate in identifying small lesions [4], especially after administration of gadolinium diethylenetriamine pentaacetic acid (Gd-DTPA). In patients with surgically proven microadenomas, MRI visualized all lesions, whereas CT scan revealed only half these lesions [5]. Although both imaging modalities were equivalent in detecting macroadenomas, bony invasion, and displacement of the pituitary stalk, MRI was more sensitive in defining the extrasellar extent of the adenomas and in detecting cavernous sinus invasion. CT is superior to MRI in demonstrating cortical bone, often critical in the case of pituitary adenomas causing erosion of the sellar floor. Cerebral angiography may be required before surgical intervention, but it has no place in the initial evaluation.

A pituitary microadenoma ($\leq$10 mm) seen on an MRI scan is round and hypointense to the normal gland on T1-weighted images, with higher signals seen on T2-weighted scans. The infundibulum may deviate away from the tumor. Macroadenomas tend to have signal characteristics similar to those of the normal gland, but they may contain cystic or hemorrhagic areas. Intravenous administration of Gd-DTPA enhances the MRI of the normal pituitary maximally after approximately 30 minutes; adenomas enhance more slowly, and the enhancement persists longer. Gd-DTPA and coronal images increase the probability of identifying small lesions.

MRI may also identify nonpituitary intrasellar masses (e.g., meningioma or internal carotid artery aneurysm). Hemorrhage into the brain, and presumably into a pituitary tumor, has a characteristic appearance, which depends on the age of the hemorrhage and the degree of disruption of the blood–brain barrier [6]. An acute hemorrhage that occurred less than a week before, consisting of deoxyhemoglobin, is isointense with the gland on T1-weighted images and has low signal intensity on T2-weighted images. A subacute hemorrhage, between 1 and 4 weeks old, contains methemoglobin that forms from the periphery to the central region and is of high signal intensity on both T1- and T2-weighted images. A hemorrhage older than 4 weeks produces a homogeneously high signal on both T1- and T2-weighted images; hemosiderin appears as a ring around the hemorrhage and is of low signal intensity on these images [6].

Octreotide

Octreotide, a somatostatin analogue, is used to detect the presence of tissues expressing somatostatin receptors. Octreotide scanning may be used to detect both pituitary and ectopic neuroendocrine tumors expressing these receptors. It provides both a visual image and a physiologic measure. Increased uptake on an octreotide scan predicts the success of medical therapy with somatostatin analogues. However, given that these receptors are expressed by normal endocrine tissue, a positive result may not represent the location of a tumor. Despite the high incidence of false-positive results, it can be helpful when coupled with an abnormal CT or MRI result.

PITUITARY TUMORS
Mary Ann Emanuele and Nicholas Emanuele

Etiology

Besides pituitary adenoma, the differential diagnosis of a pituitary mass includes pituitary hyperplasia, lymphocytic hypophysitis, granulomatous hypophysitis, sarcoidosis, pituitary abscess, craniopharyngioma, Rathke cleft cyst, pars intermedia cyst, colloid cyst, arachnoid cyst, empty sella, teratoma, hamartoma, astrocytoma, aneurysm, histiocytosis X, chordoma, melanoma, and metastatic carcinoma [7]. Pituitary adenoma is the most common finding. In the case of hormone-secreting tumors with associated clinical syndromes, an appropriate hormone assessment will determine the best initial treatment and the need for further therapy. Surgical, pharmacologic, and radiotherapeutic treatments are available for hormone-secreting pituitary tumors. These same modalities are useful for nonsecreting adenomas and for nonpituitary intrasellar masses, which require the same investigation as tumors arising from pituitary cells [7].

Epidemiology

The increased sensitivity of endocrine tests and imaging procedures has improved the diagnosis of pituitary tumors. The prevalence of pituitary adenomas in an unselected autopsy series is as high as 20% to 25% [7]. Routine endocrine testing can also disclose hormone abnormalities and lead to the diagnosis of pituitary tumors. It is important to remember, however, that most pituitary tumors are microadenomas, and many are nonfunctioning. Researchers anticipate that the prevalence of clinically significant pituitary tumors in the general population will continue to increase.

Pathophysiology

Electron microscopy, immunohistochemistry, in situ hybridization for measurement of mRNA, and assessment of cell proliferation markers (such as MIB-1 by light microscopy) may be useful in predicting biologic behavior and tumor aggressiveness. The mutated form of p53, a tumor-suppressor gene, also can be examined; it can be an indicator of rapid growth. In marked contrast to other tumors, pituitary adenomas are less vascular than the normal pituitary gland, suggesting that inhibitors of angiogenesis may play an important role in their behavior [8].

Diagnosis

Subsequent sections of this chapter discuss the diagnosis of hyperprolactinemia, acromegaly, and Cushing disease. TSH-producing pituitary tumors are first seen with classic signs and symptoms of thyrotoxicosis, elevated T3 and T4 levels, and an elevated or inappropriately normal TSH level. A sellar mass without excess target hormone production or without elevated prolactin, GH, ACTH, or TSH levels indicates a nonfunctional pituitary adenoma. The alpha subunit, which is common to FSH, LH, and TSH and has no metabolic activity (the beta subunit of these glycoproteins is unique and confers specificity to the hormone) can be elevated. If initially high, this level can be followed up as a marker of tumor recurrence.

Treatment

Tumor type, function, and size determine therapy for pituitary tumors. Initial evaluation should determine the presence and type of hormone hypersecretion, any hormonal deficiencies and the need for replacement therapy, the presence of any visual abnormalities, and the presence of extrasellar extension. Therapeutic interventions include medical therapy, transsphenoidal or frontal surgery, and radiotherapy. Dopamine agonists effectively treat most types of prolactin-secreting tumors. Transsphenoidal surgery is indicated in most patients with tumors that secrete GH, ACTH, and TSH and with large nonfunctional tumors. Medical therapy with somatostatin analogues alone or in combination with dopamine agonists should be undertaken in patients with persistent elevations of GH and IGF-1. Radiotherapy can benefit patients with significant residual tumor in whom medical therapy has been unsuccessful. Ideally, excess levels of pituitary hormones normalize, and the hypothalamic–pituitary-target-organ responses, both stimulatory and inhibitory, are restored. Other goals of therapy are relief of headaches, reversal of visual loss, and recovery of pituitary function.

Because most pituitary tumors are benign, the results of surgery are usually gratifying, particularly in patients with suprasellar extension and visual abnormalities. Improvement in visual field abnormalities occurs in 80% of such patients; progression of visual disturbance is arrested in 16%, whereas visual deterioration occurs in 4%. The results of surgery depend on the experience and expertise of the surgeon, the size of the tumor, invasion of bone or dura, and previous therapy. Prevention of recurrence and avoidance of DI are perhaps the most challenging goals of pituitary tumor surgery. Finally, surgery provides the opportunity for a complete histopathologic characterization of the lesion. A tissue diagnosis is desirable, because the differential diagnosis of sellar masses is wide, and some lesions appear as pseudoprolactinomas (hyperprolactinemia secondary to pituitary stalk compression or hypothalamic damage that leads to interference with dopaminergic inhibition of pro-lactin secretion).

The complications of pituitary surgery in a large series are few. Mortality rates of 0.86%, 0.27%, and 2.5% have been reported in patients with macroadenomas, mi-croadenomas, and macroadenomas previously treated with other modalities, respec-tively [9–13]. For patients with previous treatment or macroadenomas, visual loss oc-curred in 2.5% and 0.1%, leakage of cerebrospinal fluid in 5.7% and 1.3%, stroke or vascular injury in 1.3% and 0.2%, meningitis or abscess in 1.3% and 0.1%, and oculo-motor palsy in 0.6% and 0.1%, respectively. Incidence of postoperative hypopitu-itarism is about 3% in patients with microadenomas, and this increases slightly with size and invasiveness of the tumor. The background rate of pituitary tumor recur-rence is about 1% to 2% per year in patients treated with surgery alone [9,10]; postop-erative external pituitary irradiation reduces this level. More recent studies have em-phasized the effectiveness of administering radiotherapy after initial surgery to reduce the risk of tumor regrowth [13].

Radiation

Radiation therapy to a pituitary tumor usually prevents further tumor growth; it eventually reduces hormone hypersecretion. However, prompt reduction in either tumor size or hormone hypersecretion is rare. Reduction in hormone hypersecretion may occur within 3 to 6 months of therapy, but attainment of normal values usually requires at least 5 and often 10 years. Finally, hypopituitarism, either total or partial, is a risk and may occur at any time after treatment. In one study, half the patients treated with conventional supervoltage radiation developed hypopituitarism within 26 months of therapy [13]. In another series, at least one third of patients had pitu-itary deficiencies within 2 to 3 years. The incidence of hypopituitarism increases with length of follow-up, necessitating life-long monitoring of patients, with appropriate hormone measurements and dynamic studies. Other complications of radiotherapy include damage to the optic chiasm, the optic nerves, and cranial nerves, with conse-quent visual loss or ophthalmoplegia, vascular damage causing cerebral ischemia, seizures, and development of a pituitary or brain malignancy. Loss of cognition is less well documented.

The different types of radiotherapy include conventional supervoltage teletherapy, implantation of radioactive stereotactic radiosurgery by using a linear accelerator, alpha particles, or proton beam therapy, and single high-dose focused stereotactic ra-diation (gamma knife). The type of radiation treatment administered must be indi-vidualized according to the tumor size and location (proximity to the optic chiasm and cavernous sinus) and the availability of the radiation source. Most commonly, conven-tional supervoltage therapy is provided 5 days per week for 4 to 5 weeks. This type of treatment may be used in patients with large or small pituitary tumors. Alpha-parti-cle or proton-beam radiotherapy can be used to treat small tumors only and requires a cyclotron for the energy source, thus limiting availability. Focused radiation from a gamma knife (e.g., radiosurgery) decreases the risk of damage to the hypothalamus and other brain structures and can be given effectively as a single dose.

In most studies, relatively few patients have progression of disease after radiother-apy, but the recurrence rate despite radiation therapy in one series was 10%. Cur-rently, pituitary radiation is most often recommended for patients with residual dis-ease after surgery and patients who cannot undergo surgical resection.

Postoperative radiotherapy for nonsecreting tumors is also an option if consider-able residual tumor or evidence of tumor growth is found on follow-up MRI [12–15]. Evaluation and treatment of hypopituitarism are important parts of the management of all patients with pituitary tumors. Development of new medical therapies, such as GH antagonists, as well as refinements of surgical, radiotherapy, and imaging tech-niques should continue to improve future management of pituitary tumors.

Response of pituitary tumors to medical, surgical, and radiation therapy varies de-pending on etiology and is discussed in succeeding sections.

HYPOPITUITARISM

Mary Ann Emanuele and Nicholas Emanuele

Pathophysiology

Total or partial hypopituitarism may occur in patients with pituitary adenomas, parasellar disease, or hypophysitis; after pituitary surgery or radiation (including head and neck radiation for malignancy); or after head injury. Pituitary apoplexy resulting from a bleed into an existing adenoma is also commonly associated with hypopituitarism. This also can occur in the postpartum setting when the pituitary is markedly enlarged, after a complicated delivery with a large amount of bleeding and hypotension. In a recent retrospective chart review of patients with classic pituitary apoplexy over a 20-year period, approximately 90% of the patients had permanent hypopituitarism, independent of whether they underwent surgical decompression [16]. Deficiency of any or all of the six major hormones (LH, FSH, GH, thyrotropin, corticotropin, and prolactin) can occur. The most common symptom is hypogonadism due to LH and FSH deficiency. Classically, pituitary hormones decline in the following order: gonadotropins (LH, FSH), GH, thyrotropin, and corticotropin [17]. However, some patients have isolated corticotropin or thyrotropin deficiency. Prolactin deficiency is uncommon except with pituitary infarction.

Diagnosis

Classification and Clinical Findings

Growth Hormone Deficiency

Deficiency of GH may be a factor in the increased mortality rate found in patients with hypopituitarism who receive replacement hormones other than GH [18]. This risk is predominantly in the form of cardiovascular disease [19]. Symptoms of GH deficiency in adults include decreased muscle strength, lower exercise tolerance, and diminished sense of physical and psychological well-being (e.g., less energy, emotional lability, sense of social isolation, and diminished libido). GH deficiency allows increased total body fat and produces an abnormal distribution of fat. Bone density, particularly in the lumbar spine, is reduced in some patients with adult-onset GH deficiency. Levels of serum low-density-lipoprotein (LDL) cholesterol may be increased, whereas high-density-lipoprotein (HDL) cholesterol remains normal.

Gonadotropin Deficiency

Gonadotropin deficiency results from either a pituitary defect or a deficiency of hypothalamic gonadotropin-releasing hormone (GnRH) stimulation. Etiologies include hypothalamic disease, disease of the pituitary stalk, or a functional abnormality such as occurs in association with hyperprolactinemia, cortisol excess, anorexia nervosa, secondary adrenal insufficiency, or secondary hypothyroidism. Gonadotropin deficiency often occurs early in the course of hypopituitarism. It causes delayed or arrested puberty in adolescents and causes infertility, menstrual disorders, or amenorrhea in women. Hypoestrogenemia is often associated with lack of libido and dyspareunia. Long-standing estrogen deficiency produces breast atrophy and osteopenia. In men, hypogonadism may remain undiagnosed because the syndrome develops slowly, and the findings of diminished libido and impotence may be attributed to aging. Beard growth and muscle mass may be reduced, and osteopenia may develop. Hypogonadism is often diagnosed retrospectively after the patient exhibits the symptoms of a mass lesion.

Thyrotropin Deficiency

Secondary hypothyroidism usually occurs relatively late in the course of hypopituitarism and is characterized by malaise, weight gain, lack of energy, cold intolerance, and constipation. The degree of hypothyroidism depends on the duration of TSH deficiency.

Corticotropin Deficiency

Secondary adrenal failure may occur as an isolated deficiency, as a result of corticotropin-releasing hormone (CRH) deficiency, or in the course of the development of panhypopituitarism. The symptoms are essentially the same as those of primary adrenal insufficiency, but they differ in several respects.

First, secondary adrenal insufficiency results from lack of ACTH stimulation of the adrenal; therefore only adrenal steroids under predominant ACTH regulation (cortisol and adrenal androgens) are affected. Mineralocorticoid secretion, primarily regulated by renin and angiotensin, is preserved, although it may be suboptimal. Thus electrolytes may be normal, in contrast to primary adrenal insufficiency. The usual symptoms are malaise, loss of energy, anorexia, weight loss, postural hypotension, orthostatic dizziness, and sometimes headache. Women tend to lose pubic and axillary hair because, in women, the adrenal represents a major source of androgen. They also have decreased libido. Beard and body hair are preserved in men unless gonadotropin deficiency coexists.

Second, in contrast to patients with primary adrenal insufficiency, who may have abnormal tanning, these patients have a pale and sometimes slightly sallow complexion. Patients with secondary or tertiary cortisol deficiency tend to have milder symptoms than do those with primary adrenal insufficiency. Severe cortisol deficiency may result in hypoglycemia and hyponatremia; hyperkalemia usually occurs only with coexisting aldosterone deficiency. These patients, particularly those with panhypopituitarism, may deteriorate gradually, but a relatively trivial illness may precipitate vascular collapse, coma, or hypoglycemia. Adrenal insufficiency, regardless of the cause, is a medical emergency.

Laboratory Findings

Serum Growth Hormone
Growth hormone is secreted in a pulsatile fashion, and values in a normal individual may vary from undetectable (during an interpulse interval) to more than 40 mg/L. GH secretion is affected by food ingestion; it is suppressed by hyperglycemia and stimulated by amino acids and hypoglycemia. Slow-wave sleep is also associated with increased GH secretion. For these reasons, a random serum GH measurement is of limited value. IGF-1 is a more reliable screening test for GH deficiency. If one suspects GH deficiency, a stimulation test is required. Provocative tests of GH secretion include insulin-induced hypoglycemia, GH-releasing factor, arginine, levodopa, or glucagon administration.

Serum Luteinizing Hormone and Follicle-Stimulating Hormone
Serum LH and FSH are also secreted in a pulsatile fashion. In men, the levels of these hormones, despite pulsatile secretion, fall within a fairly narrow range; therefore marked abnormalities of secretion are easily diagnosed from a pool of three blood samples drawn at 20-minute intervals. The values should be interpreted with the clinical findings, simultaneous testosterone level, and possibly semen analysis. In women, marked changes in gonadotropin secretion occur during different phases of the menstrual cycle. Measurement of serum LH and FSH in a woman who is not taking oral contraceptives and who has regular menstrual cycles is usually not useful. Documentation of a normal menstrual cycle and normal luteal-phase serum progesterone level excludes significant gonadotropin dysfunction. In amenorrheic, nonpregnant women, measurement of serum LH and FSH, estradiol, and prolactin levels can provide insight into the cause of hypogonadism. Primary ovarian failure occurs with increased LH and FSH, whereas hypogonadism due to pituitary or hypothalamic causes has low estradiol and low or inappropriately normal LH and FSH levels.

Serum Thyrotropin
Sensitive IRMAs make it possible to distinguish among low, normal, and high levels of thyrotropin. If the thyrotropin concentration is normal in association with normal serum thyroid hormone levels, the patient is euthyroid and does not require further testing. If the serum thyroid hormone levels are low and the thyrotropin level is normal (but inappropriately low for the prevailing thyroid hormone levels) or is low, the patient has secondary or tertiary hypothyroidism. In the past, distinguishing pitu-

itary and hypothalamic failure could be attempted by administering TRH, but TRH is no longer available.

Plasma Corticotropin

Measurement of corticotropin is required only in the evaluation of adrenal failure or Cushing syndrome. The short plasma half-life of corticotropin requires that samples be collected in a cold syringe, placed in a tube containing ethylenediaminetetraacetic acid, centrifuged quickly at 4°C, and stored immediately in a freezer. ACTH is secreted in a pulsatile fashion with a circadian rhythm and at increased levels during stress. Therefore ACTH results must be interpreted with knowledge of time of sample collection, whether the patient was under stress, and whether exogenous synthetic glucocorticoids were previously administered. A simultaneously obtained plasma cortisol sample is necessary to interpret the appropriateness of the plasma corticotropin level. An 8 a.m. cortisol value between 10 and 20 mg/dl effectively excludes adrenal insufficiency, although patients with secondary or tertiary cortisol deficiency may have low-normal plasma cortisol levels. If clinical suspicion is high, further evaluation with insulin hypoglycemia testing should probably be pursued.

Serum Prolactin

Clinically, measurement of a random serum prolactin level is useful if the level is undetectable or markedly elevated. An undetectable level may suggest hypopituitarism. Although prolactin concentrations vary during the day, being lower in the afternoon, the time of sampling is usually not critical. Similarly, changes in prolactin secretion can occur with eating; however, the magnitude of the change is small and not clinically significant.

Combined Anterior Pituitary Test

Simultaneous administration of three hypothalamic releasing hormones and measurement of the response of target pituitary hormone concentrations permits assessment of pituitary reserve in an ambulatory care setting. The combined anterior pituitary test is a tool in suspected pituitary dysfunction. Patients receiving long-term hormone replacement therapy may also be reassessed after hormone withdrawal to determine the extent of hypopituitarism. This test is particularly useful in assessing pituitary function after pituitary surgery or radiation. The three hypothalamic hormones, GHRH (1 μg/kg body weight), CRH (1 mg/kg body weight), and GnRH (100 mg) are administered intravenously (sequentially) over a 20-second period. Corticotropin, cortisol, LH, FSH, GH, and prolactin levels are measured at −30, 0, 15, 30, 60, 90, and 120 minutes. Results must be interpreted in light of the baseline levels of the target-gland hormones. Normal responses are as follows:

- GH increases by fivefold to 10-fold.
- LH increases by two- to threefold.
- FSH minimally increases.
- ACTH increases 2 to 4 times at 30 minutes.
- Cortisol peaks at more than 20 mg/dl.

Baseline samples are obtained at 8 a.m. for cortisol, T4, estradiol (amenorrheic women), testosterone (men), and IGF-I.

Pituitary reserve is likely to be normal if the pituitary hormone response is normal in the setting of an appropriate peripheral target hormone level. The combined anterior pituitary test is useful for amplifying subtle abnormalities. Deficient response to a hypothalamic hormone may result from absent or dysfunctional pituitary cells or from increased negative feedback by the peripheral hormone. An absent or a diminished pituitary response may also be due to insufficient priming because of insufficient exposure to the hypothalamic hormone, as in isolated gonadotropin deficiency, usually the result of GnRH deficiency. Administration of CRH may also be useful in distinguishing between ectopic ACTH production and Cushing disease (see later discussion). A deficient GH response to GHRH makes a diagnosis of GH deficiency likely.

Insulin Tolerance Test

The insulin tolerance test is widely used to determine ACTH and GH reserves. Clinical manifestations of hypoglycemia and a plasma glucose level less than 40 mg/dl are required for the interpretation of ACTH and GH levels. If these two criteria are fulfilled, the plasma cortisol level should exceed 20 mg/dl, and the GH level should exceed 5 mg/L. If these levels are not achieved, ACTH or GH deficiencies, or both, are likely.

Treatment

Hormone replacement is possible for all the target-organ hormones (e.g., cortisol, thyroxine, estrogen, testosterone) and some of the pituitary hormones (e.g., gonadotropins, GH). Replacement must be tailored to the individual hormone deficiency, and, if possible, it should not be instituted until the hypothalamic–pituitary–target organ axis has been assessed. For example, thyroid hormone replacement before institution of glucocorticoid therapy in a patient with cortisol deficiency may precipitate adrenal crisis.

Growth Hormone

Growth hormone is most often given as a daily subcutaneous injection at bedtime. The recommended starting dose for adults is 0.006 mg/kg/day with a maximal dose of 0.0125 mg/kg/day. Dosage adjustment is based on the clinical response and the achievement of an appropriate serum IGF-1 level for unaffected patients matched for age and gender. Optimal GH replacement is most appropriately achieved by dose titration, with individual tailoring of GH dose for each patient to achieve a normal serum IGF-1 level [19]. Use of GH replacement titrated against serum IGF-1 is not associated with an obvious early increase in the rate of hypothalamic or pituitary tumor recurrence if pituitary radiation is given postoperatively. GH replacement partially reverses the abnormalities; specifically, it increases lean body mass, decreases fat mass (particularly abdominal fat), increases bone density, and increases serum HDL levels [17,21]. Improvement in exercise tolerance, muscle strength, psychosocial assessments, and mortality related to cardiovascular disease have all been observed in adults with hypopituitarism that has been ameliorated with use of GH [21]. Finally, one open clinical trial assessing carotid artery intimal wall thickness (IWT) in GH-deficient adults demonstrated a potent inhibitory effect of 1-year GH replacement on IWT progression, which was maintained after 2 years [19]. The rapid effect of GH replacement on IWT may indicate a beneficial effect of GH treatment on the vascular system. The most common side effects of GH include fluid retention, carpal tunnel syndrome, and arthralgia; these side effects are usually dose related and disappear with dose reduction [20,22]. The contraindications for GH use include malignancy and diabetic retinopathy.

Gonadal Steroids

Testosterone

Testosterone replacement for hypogonadal men can be administered intramuscularly, 200 mg every 2 weeks or 300 mg every 3 weeks; through a transdermal route in the form of a gel, a patch, or hand cream; or via a buccal preparation. The patch may be placed on the back, chest, abdomen, thighs, or upper arms. Transdermal testosterone is the preferred method of replacement, because it provides continuous absorption of the amount of testosterone normally secreted by the testes (~6 mg/day), and it is more physiologic in its action than are the intramuscular injections. Advantages of transdermal testosterone administration include avoidance of wide fluctuations in serum testosterone concentrations and avoidance of intramuscular injection. Men older than 40 years should have measurement of prostate-specific antigen and a prostate examination before beginning testosterone replacement and periodically thereafter. Complete blood counts should also be assessed at baseline and periodically, because testosterone can cause erythrocytosis. Hepatotoxicity is rare, but it is prudent to follow liver-function tests.

Estrogen

Estrogen replacement therapy is given to hypogonadal women to reduce the risk of osteoporosis, to improve the woman's sense of well-being, and to maintain or promote feminization. Calcium supplementation is usually necessary to provide the recommended amount of elemental calcium (1.0–1.5 g/day). If the uterus has not been removed, estrogens are administered cyclically or continuously with appropriate progesterone. One such regimen consists of conjugated estrogens at 0.625 mg/day for 3 weeks, together with medroxyprogesterone acetate at 5 or 10 mg/day for the last 7 or 10 days. Withdrawal menses should occur within a few days of stopping the medications during the fourth week of the cycle. If avoidance of withdrawal bleeding is desired, conjugated estrogens with medroxyprogesterone acetate can be given daily throughout the month. A combined conjugated estrogen and medroxyprogesterone preparation is available. A regular pelvic examination, Papanicolaou's smear, and mammography are necessary for adequate follow-up.

Gonadotropins

Gonadotropins and GnRH are administered to initiate puberty and to restore fertility. Regimens are beyond the scope of this review.

Thyroid Hormone

This deficiency is treated with levothyroxine; the oral dose usually ranges from 0.075 to 0.15 mg once daily, or 1.67 µg/kg body weight. The dose is adjusted according to the clinical response, and the serum free thyroxine (free T4) values should be in the middle to upper part of the normal range. Measurement of serum TSH is of no value in assessing a response to levothyroxine in patients with hypothalamic–pituitary disease.

Cortisol

Cortisol deficiency is usually treated by oral administration of 20 mg hydrocortisone on awakening and 10 mg at 6 p.m. This is the simplest way to simulate the circadian rhythm of cortisol secretion. Some patients require an additional 5 mg at midday or early afternoon, and others, particularly physically small patients, may require a lower dose. Other glucocorticoids may be used—either cortisone acetate, 25 mg in the morning and 12.5 mg in the early evening; prednisone, 5 mg on awakening and 2.5 mg at 6 p.m.; or dexamethasone, 0.5 mg on awakening. The appropriate replacement dosage and dose adjustments are determined clinically. Dose adjustment is made on the basis of symptoms. Overreplacement causes Cushing syndrome and accelerates bone loss. During stress (whether psychological or physical), fever, and illness, the dose is usually doubled or increased to an equivalent of 20 mg hydrocortisone every 6 to 8 hours, depending on the severity of stress. If parenteral administration is required, 100 mg hydrocortisone is given by continuous intravenous infusion every 8 hours. Alternatively, dexamethasone is given intravenously or intramuscularly at a dose of 1 mg every 12 hours; this regimen is frequently used in patients undergoing surgery. The patient should be instructed to increase the oral dose during times of illness, and if vomiting occurs, a prepared syringe of dexamethasone, 4 mg, should be available for self-intramuscular injection.

Medical Alert Bracelet

Every patient receiving adrenal or posterior pituitary replacement therapy should wear an identifying necklace or bracelet to alert caregivers in the event of medical emergency.

DISORDERS OF THE PROLACTIN SYSTEM
Fadi Nabhan

Etiology

The major causes of hyperprolactinemia are listed in Table 1.2. Prolactinoma is a prolactin-producing pituitary adenoma and is the main focus of this review.

Table 1.2.   Causes of Hyperprolactinemia

Physiologic	Drugs
Pregnancy	Neuroleptics (e.g., haloperidol)
Lactation	Dopamine receptor blockers
Pathologic	(e.g., metoclopramide)
Hypothalamic-pituitary disorders	Antidepressants (e.g., imipramine)
Tumors	Antihypertensives (e.g., α-methyldopa)
Craniopharyngioma	Estrogens
Glioma	Opiates
Hamartoma	Neurogenic
Microadenoma	Spinal cord lesions
Macroadenoma	Chest wall lesions
Metastatic cancer	Breast stimulation
Germinoma	Miscellaneous
Meningioma	Primary hypothyroidism
Infiltrative disorders	Chronic renal failure
Sarcoidosis	Cirrhosis
Giant cell granuloma	Stress (physical, psychological)
Eosinophilic granuloma	Idiopathic
Lymphocytic hypophysitis	
Other	
Cranial radiation	
Pseudotumor cerebri	
Pituitary stalk section (trauma)	
Empty sella	

Pathophysiology

Chronic hyperprolactinemia causes hypogonadism through a negative effect on the secretion of GnRH, which leads to reduction of LH and FSH and gonadal hormone production. This leads to amenorrhea/oligomenorrhea in women, impotence, and decreased libido in men and infertility in both genders. It can also lead to decreased bone mineral density in both genders [23]. Hyperprolactinemia can also cause galactorrhea, mainly in women. In cases of prolactinomas, mass effects such as headache, visual field defects, decreased visual acuity, and ophthalmoplegia can be seen.

Epidemiology

The prevalence of hyperprolactinemia is about 15% in anovulatory women. This increases to 43% if they also have galactorrhea [24]. Prolactinoma accounts for 40% of pituitary tumors, with 90% of them being microadenomas. Macroadenomas are more commonly seen in men and postmenopausal women [23]. The prevalence of medication-induced hyperprolactinemia varies between medications. In one study on patients with schizophrenia taking typical and atypical antipsychotics, the prevalence was between 67% and 70% [25].

Diagnosis

If an elevated serum prolactin level is detected, pregnancy, the use of medications that increase prolactin, and primary hypothyroidism must be ruled out. When this is done, an MRI of the sellar region should be done. If the patient is taking a medication known to cause hyperprolactinemia, it is still essential to rule out a coincident prolactinoma. This can be done if the prolactin level is normalized after stopping the medication or switching to another one that does not cause hyperprolactinemia. If this is not possible, an imaging of the pituitary is indicated [26]. The level of hyperprolactinemia correlates with the size of the prolactinoma. When one encounters a patient with a pituitary macroadenoma associated with only a mild elevation in prolactin level, one should suspect either a non–prolactin-producing tumor causing hyperprolactinemia through pituitary stalk compression or a prolactinoma in which the prolactin level, although very elevated, is artificially low due to the assay used. This artifact, called the *hook effect*, can be avoided by dilution of the serum [23]. Elevation of bioinactive macroprolactin can cause hyperprolactinemia. The prevalence of this macroprolactinemia is about 10% [27]. Macroprolactinemia does not cause symptoms and signs of hyperprolactinemia. Its clinical relevance is mainly avoiding expensive workup of hyperprolactinemia and a delay in the diagnosis of the patient's presenting symptoms by inappropriately relating them to the macroprolactinemia [28].

Treatment

The goals of therapy in hyperprolactinemia are reduction of tumor size if the cause is a prolactinoma and the correction of the hyperprolactinemia to treat the gonadal dysfunction and the galactorrhea. In both cases of microadenoma and macroadenoma, medical therapy is preferred. Dopamine-receptor agonists normalize prolactin and decrease the size of the tumor in a significant number of patients. The two used dopamine-receptor agonists approved for treatment of hyperprolactinemia in the United States are bromocriptine [29] and cabergoline [30,31]. Bromocriptine, an ergot derivative, binds and stimulates the dopaminergic neurons and pituitary dopamine receptors. The therapy is initiated with a low dose (1.25 mg) once a day at bedtime and then titrated to twice a day and then further titrated over several weeks to achieve a normal prolactin level. The usual dose of bromocriptine is 5 to 7.5 mg per day in divided doses. The most common side effects of bromocriptine are nausea and orthostatic hypotension. The side effects can be minimized by vaginal administration of the drug [32]. Cabergoline is another ergot derivative that is more specific than bromocriptine in targeting the dopamine receptors in the pituitary and hence has fewer systemic side effects. It is also more effective [30,31]. It is started at a dose of 0.25 mg once or twice weekly and titrated up to achieve a normal prolactin level. Repeated imaging of the pituitary is usually done in 6 months to determine response to therapy.

It is appropriate to elect to observe and monitor without normalization of the hyperprolactinemia in a patient with a microadenoma and regular menses [23]. It is probably safe to discontinue medical therapy in patients whose serum prolactin levels normalize and have no evidence of tumor or the tumor has decreased in size by 50% without involving the optic chiasm [33]. However, careful monitoring with prolactin level and pituitary imaging is required, as prolactin may increase in a substantial number of patients.

Surgery is indicated in patients with medical treatment failure or signs or symptoms of local compression after a failure of a trial of medication. If pressure symptoms are found and surgery is contraindicated, radiation therapy may be given.

In the case of medication-induced hyperprolactinemia, stopping the medication if possible or switching to another that does not cause hyperprolactinemia should be considered after careful consultation with prescribing physician. If this is not possible, then treatment either with gonadal steroid replacement to treat hypogonadism or rarely with dopamine agonist can be entertained. Giving dopamine agonist to psychiatric patients who have medication-induced hyperprolactinemia must be carefully considered, as it may worsen the underlying psychiatric condition [26].

Pregnancy and Hyperprolactinemia

It is possible that a prolactinoma may enlarge in pregnancy. In pregnant women with prolactinoma who have not been treated with surgery or radiation, 1% to 5% of microadenomas and 23% of macroadenomas will have clinically significant growth during pregnancy [34]. Surgical debulking of a macroadenoma with suprasellar extension before pregnancy to prevent growth during pregnancy is debatable and should be individualized and discussed with each patient [34]. Patients with macroadenomas should have visual field assessment during pregnancy. If the tumor grows, the options of treatment are either medication with dopamine agonists or surgery. Generally, use of dopamine agonists should be discontinued immediately when pregnancy is diagnosed, and then use during the rest of pregnancy should be avoided if possible. However, if necessary, both bromocriptine and cabergoline [35,36] have been reported to be safe in pregnancy, but more data are available on the use of bromocriptine, and therefore it is preferred.

ACROMEGALY
Gerald A. Charnogursky and Tiffany A. Karas

Definition
Prolonged excessive secretion of GH results in acromegaly. GH causes hepatic production of IGF-1, which over the years leads to overgrowth of bone, soft tissues, and internal organs, and thus contributes to left ventricular hypertrophy, cardiomyopathy, sleep apnea, and diabetes mellitus. Pituitary gigantism occurs when GH excess begins before epiphyseal fusion in childhood.

Etiology
Pituitary somatotroph adenomas secreting GH cause 98% of cases of acromegaly. Approximately 60% of these adenomas secrete exclusively GH, with 25% secreting both GH and prolactin (PRL). Ectopic GH secreted by neoplasms of the pancreas, the lung, and the ovary account for fewer than 1% of cases. Rarely, excess GHRH from hypothalamic hamartomas and ganglioneuromas and peripheral lesions including bronchial carcinoid, pancreatic islet cell tumors, small cell lung cancer, adrenal adenoma, medullary thyroid carcinoma, and pheochromocytoma can cause acromegaly [37].

Epidemiology
The incidence of acromegaly is approximately 3 to 4 per million population. The disease is most commonly diagnosed in the fifth decade. Because of gradual onset of symptoms, GH excess has usually been present for 7 years before diagnosis.

Pathophysiology and Clinical Presentation
Prolonged excesses of GH and IGF-1 cause acral changes including enlarged hands and feet as well as coarsened facial features. Joint cartilages and synovial tissues hypertrophy, leading to arthritis and arthralgias.

Cardiac function is frequently impaired, first seen as left ventricular hypertrophy with diastolic dysfunction and dysrhythmias. Systemic hypertension magnifies the cardiac dysfunction. Obstructive and central sleep apnea occur in more than 50% of patients. GH contributes to insulin resistance; glucose intolerance and diabetes are commonly seen.

Most GH-secreting pituitary lesions are macroadenomas. These tumors can present with mass effects such as headache, impaired peripheral vision, and cranial nerve palsies. Patients can also have loss of other pituitary trophic hormones such as FSH, LH, TSH, and ACTH.

Diagnosis
The major diagnostic criteria are elevation of IGF-1 and nonsuppressibility of GH in response to oral glucose loads. Random GH levels are often misleading because of the pulsatile nature of GH secretion and because of its short plasma half-life.

IGF-1, produced by the liver, reflects GH secretion during the past day. IGF-1 is a stable, integrated assessment of GH activity. IGF-1 levels vary with age and gender. IGF-1 ranges are highest in teenagers and lowest in adults older than 55 years. IGF-1 is lowered by systemic illnesses including malnutrition, renal failure, and liver failure.

Unaffected patients will have GH levels less than 2 ng/ml (e.g., RIA) or less than 1 ng/ml (immunoradiometric or chemiluminescent assay) 2 hours after a 75-g oral glucose load.

MRI of the pituitary is recommended after GH hypersecretion has been documented. If the MRI does not reveal a lesion, rare syndromes of ectopic GH- or GNRH-secreting lesions should be considered. GNRH levels should then be obtained. Chest and abdominal imaging assist in localizing ectopic sources of GH production.

Treatment

The therapy for acromegaly now commonly involves a combination of transsphenoidal surgery, radiotherapy, and pharmacologic agents [38]. The goals of therapy for acromegaly include normalization of age- and gender-adjusted IGF-1, GH less than 1 ng/ml (immunoradiometric or chemiluminescent assay) after glucose load, and alleviation of mass effect [39]. The correction of GH excess will reduce clinical signs and may also improve cardiac function, sleep disorders, and glucose intolerance. If untreated, mortality accelerates largely from cardiovascular disease and cancer. Effective treatment leading to prolonged normalization of GH and IGF-1 can reduce these mortality rates [38].

Neurosurgery

Given that the likelihood of postoperative normalization of IGF-1 and GH in large invasive macroadenomas is generally 50% or less, medical therapy remains the primary approach. Transsphenoidal resection is the treatment of choice for suitable microadenomas and macroadenomas, as well as for macroadenomas that are causing visual disturbances.

Surgical cure rates reach 70% to 90% [40,41]. However, criteria for cure and duration of follow-up do vary, which makes comparison of studies difficult. Cure rates have increased over time as imaging and surgical techniques have improved. General pituitary surgical outcomes tend to be better with surgeons and centers with higher case volumes [42].

Somatostatin Analogues

Somatostatin, or somatotrophin release–inhibiting factor, is the physiologic inhibitor of GH. Octreotide is a synthetic analogue of somatostatin that is available in both short-acting and depot preparations. A second long-acting analogue, lanreotide, is available in Europe. These agents are most commonly used in patients who do not achieve normal IGF-1 and GH levels postoperatively. Primary octreotide therapy should be considered in patients in whom surgical cure is unlikely [43]. The depot octreotide preparation has also been shown to normalize IGF-1 in 73% and GH in 69%, whether given as primary therapy or as postoperative adjunctive therapy [44]. Preoperative octreotide can decrease tumor size and improve clinical symptoms and cardiopulmonary function before surgery. A systematic literature review of tumor shrinkage with somatostatin analogues revealed that 36.6% of treated patients showed a significant decrease in tumor volume, averaging 19.4% [45]. Results of clinical studies with preoperative octreotide have not shown consistent improvement in surgical outcomes [46,47]. Because microadenomas can have 90% cure rates with expert neurosurgeons, it may be difficult to show further improvement with preoperative somatostatin analogues. Preoperative therapy controlling IGF-1 and GH may improve cure rates in macroadenomas, in which general cure rates are approximately 50% [48].

Radiation Therapy

External beam fractionated radiation therapy controls tumor growth, but it is not likely to achieve normalization of IGF-1 or GH. Levels of these hormones decline gradually after at least 10 years [49]. Loss of pituitary trophic hormones is a late consequence of radiation therapy. Stereotactic radiosurgery (e.g., gamma knife) can lower IGF-1 and GH more rapidly with less chance of hypopituitarism [50].

Dopamine Agonists

Cabergoline and bromocriptine rarely normalize IGF-1 or GH levels when used as primary therapy [51]. These agents have been used as additive therapy when surgery, radiation, and octreotide do not normalize hormone levels. Dopamine agonists are more likely to lower IGF-1 and GH in somatotroph adenomas cosecreting prolactin.

Growth Hormone Receptor Antagonist

Pegvisomant is a genetically engineered analogue of GH that binds to the GH receptor and prevents production of IGF-1. Pegvisomant normalizes IGF-1 in more than 89% of cases [52,53]. GH levels increase with this agent, and tumor size should be monitored. The agent is given by daily s.c. injection in patients uncontrolled by or intolerant to octreotide [54].

CUSHING DISEASE
Fadi Nabhan

Etiology and Pathogenesis

Cushing syndrome (CS), due to increased pituitary ACTH secretion by a pituitary tumor, is called Cushing disease (CD). It is rare, but it is the most common cause of CS and is caused usually by a benign pituitary microadenoma [55]. Excessive ACTH can also result from ectopic ACTH secretion (EAS). All other etiologies leading to CS are discussed in Chapter 3.

Diagnosis

Clinical Manifestations

This is reviewed in Chapter 3. Overall, the onset of symptoms is usually insidious and gradually progressive over 2 to 10 years before the diagnosis. An important difference between CD and adrenal causes of CS is hyperpigmentation, which is seen in CD when the ACTH level is increased.

Laboratory Findings

After establishing the diagnosis of CS, which is detailed in Chapter 3, the next step is to determine whether CS is ACTH dependent or not. Plasma ACTH less than 5 to 10 pg/mL (depending on the assay) at 09:00 a.m. is indicative of an ACTH-independent etiology, whereas a level greater than 20 pg/ml is indicative of an ACTH-dependent etiology. A level between 10 and 20 pg/ml is indeterminate but usually indicates an ACTH-dependent etiology [56,57]. In this indeterminate case, measurement of ACTH after a CRH stimulation test can be helpful. ACTH does not change appreciably in ACTH-independent cases. The criteria for this test, however, are not well defined [56]. After establishing ACTH dependence, the source of ACTH should be determined. The most commonly used test for that purpose is the high-dose dexamethasone suppression test (HDDST). It relies on the concept that high-dose dexamethasone can suppress ACTH in CD but not in EAS. It can be done either by giving 2 mg dexamethasone every 6 hours for 2 days in eight doses and measuring 24-hour urinary free cortisol (UFC) and 17-hydroxysteroids before and then on the second day or by giving 8 mg oral dexamethasone overnight at 11 p.m. and measuring cortisol at 08:30 before and at 09:00 after dexamethasone. A decrease of 24-hour UFC by more than 90%, and of 24-hour urinary 17-hydroxycorticosteroids by more than 69% identify patients with CD with a sensitivity of 79% and a specificity of 100%. In the overnight HDDST, a decrease of plasma cortisol by more than 68% indicates CD with a sensitivity of 71% and specificity close to 100% [58]. Limitations of this test include the facts that some benign tumors with EAS can suppress with HDDST and that some pituitary macroadenomas may not. Another test used to differentiate between CD and EAS is the CRH stimulation test, which depends on the concept that pituitary adenoma in

CD exhibits more CRH receptors than tumors with EAS. It is performed by administering an ovine or human CRH as an i.v. injection at a dose of 1 µg/kg body weight, or a total dose of 100 µg. ACTH and cortisol are measured at baseline and then at 15-minute intervals for 2 hours after the injection. The criteria consistent with CD vary considerably between different studies. One used the increase from baseline in peak plasma cortisol of 14% or more and peak plasma ACTH of 105% or more after the administration of human CRH. The sensitivity was 70% and the specificity of 100% for the increase in ACTH, while the sensitivity was 85% and the specificity was 100% for the increase in cortisol [59]. This test is not well standardized mainly for the cutoff values of ACTH and cortisol, and therefore its use is limited [57].

Pituitary MRI should be done in patients with CD. It is positive between 50% and 70% of cases. A pituitary tumor larger than 6 mm with biochemical testing indicating CD may be sufficient to confirm the diagnosis. However, 10% of unaffected patients may be identified as having pituitary adenoma by MRI scans [60]. Therefore if the results are not confirmatory, bilateral inferior petrosal sinus sampling (BIPSS) should be done. This procedure requires placement of catheters in the left and right inferior petrosal sinuses and measuring ACTH simultaneously from both sinuses and peripherally before and after CRH stimulation. A baseline (without, for instance, CRH) ratio of petrosal sinus to peripheral vein ACTH of 2.0 or higher and a post-CRH above 3.0 confirms CD with sensitivities of 95% and 100%, respectively, and 100% specificity for both [61]. A gradient between right and left petrosal sinus (>1.4) helps in lateralization of the lesion [61]. It is debatable whether the BIPSS should be done routinely because pituitary incidentalomas are common. An alternative to the BIPSS is the jugular vein sampling, which is less invasive and has shown promising results [62].

The most common tumors causing EAS are neuroendocrine and are intrathoracic. Localization of the tumor is frequently unsuccessful [9]. Localization methods include imaging of neck, chest, and abdomen with CT scan and/or MRI and somatostatin analogue. A combination of these studies is frequently recommended for successful localization [63].

Treatment
The primary therapy for CD is microadenomectomy by transsphenoidal approach [64,65]. The criteria for cure are debatable. One study recommended criteria of cure as basal or dexamethasone-suppressed plasma cortisol level of 5 g/dl or less within the first week after surgery [65]. The initial cure rate is about 86% in microadenomas and 65% in macroadenomas, with worse prognosis in patients with extensive suprasellar extension [64,65]. Those successfully treated with surgery will frequently require glucocorticoid replacement for up to year or more. Persistent disease after surgery is associated with increased long-term mortality [65]. Recurrence rates vary depending on defining criteria for cure, and all patients should be evaluated annually for recurrence. One study revealed a long-term cure rate of 67% [66].

Persistent disease can be treated with reoperation or with radiation therapy, by using conventional fractionated radiotherapy or stereotactic focused radiation. With radiation therapy, cure is usually delayed, as is hypopituitarism, the main side effect [67]. Patients who do not respond to surgery or radiation are treated by medical means [68] (discussed in Chapter 3) or surgical adrenalectomy. Treatment of EAS is treatment of the underlying tumor. Medical or surgical adrenalectomy also is indicated in patients with incurable or nonlocalized tumors.

DIABETES INSIPIDUS
Gerald A. Charnogursky and Tiffany A. Karas

Definition
Diabetes insipidus (DI) produces hypotonic polyuria; the cause of this is either deficient secretion of arginine vasopressin—central diabetes insipidus (CDI)—or resistance to the action of this hormone—nephrogenic diabetes insipidus (NDI). Primary polydipsia results from inhibition of AVP release due to excess fluid intake.

Etiology

Central Diabetes Insipidus

Most cases of CDI fall into one of three categories: head trauma or neurosurgery; primary or metastatic pituitary neoplasms or granulomatous diseases (e.g., sarcoidosis, histiocytosis X); or idiopathic, which may be related to autoimmune destruction of AVP, producing hypothalamic nuclei [69]. Less common etiologies include mutations of genes involved in the production of AVP, infections of the central nervous system, hypoxic encephalopathy, or CNS vascular accidents (e.g., Sheehan syndrome).

Nephrogenic Diabetes Insipidus

Hereditary NDI is caused by X-linked transmission of a deficient V2 receptor for AVP and also an autosomal dominant defect in the aquaporin-2 gene. Many drugs, including lithium, antibiotics (e.g., demeclocycline), antifungals, and antineoplastics, can cause acquired NDI, which usually resolves with discontinuation of the agent; however, long-term lithium therapy tends to cause irreversible NDI [70]. Persistent hypercalcemia (>11 mg/dl) and severe hypokalemia (<3 mEq/L) can also cause resistance to the action of AVP, with this NDI resolving with correction of the metabolic abnormalities.

Gestational diabetes insipidus is an unusual polyuric condition caused by increased placental vasopressinase activity, which resolves postpartum.

Pathophysiology

AVP is produced in the supraoptic and paraventricular nuclei of the hypothalamus. It travels down the pituitary stalk for storage in the posterior pituitary. AVP decreases urine flow by increasing reabsorption of solute free water in the distal and collecting tubules of the kidney. AVP binds to the tubular V2 receptors, leading to production of cyclic adenosine monophosphate, which increases tubular permeability to water by perforating the luminal surface with water channels made of aquaporin-2 [70,71].

Hypothalamic osmoreceptors and baroreceptors in the carotids, the atria, and the aorta regulate the secretion of AVP.

Diagnosis

Urine volume exceeding 50 mL/kg/day with 24-hour urine osmolality of 300 mOsm or less is suggests DI. One must rule out uncontrolled diabetes mellitus; however, this situation usually has a higher urine osmolality owing to glycosuria.

The clinical history helps distinguish among CDI, NDI, and primary polydipsia.

Trauma or pituitary neoplasm increases the suspicion for CDI, whereas a family history or onset in childhood suggests NDI. One commonly sees a history of psychiatric disturbances in association with primary polydipsia. Thirst can be affected directly by the psychiatric problems or by the medications used in treatment. The serum sodium is normal or slightly elevated in CDI and NDI, so long as thirst is intact and water is available. In primary polydipsia, sodium may be low as a result of water overload.

Water-deprivation testing may be required to differentiate these conditions. Water is withheld, and the patient's weight, blood sodium, and urine and plasma osmolalities are closely monitored. The patient is given exogenous AVP once urine osmolalities have been stable for several determinations. After the patient has achieved a plasma osmolality that exceeds 295 mOsm, exogenous AVP does not further increase urine osmolality in unaffected patients. Normal patients and patients with primary polydipsia have increases in urine osmolality less than 9%. In CDI, urine osmolality increases exceed 50%. With partial AVP deficiency, patients show a lesser increase. Patients with NDI do not increase urine osmolality above plasma osmolality in response to AVP.

Pituitary imaging in DI is discussed in the earlier section on imaging of the hypothalamic–pituitary axis.

Treatment

Central Diabetes Insipidus

Desmopressin (DDAVP) is a synthetic modification of AVP that has prolonged antidiuretic activity without vasopressive effects. DDAVP is available by injection form, nasal spray, and tablets. The bioavailability of DDAVP tablets is approximately 5% that of the nasal spray. The patient can also become water intoxicated with DDAVP, so that dosage must be periodically reassessed. The usual starting dose of DDAVP is 1 mg orally twice daily. This is titrated based on clinical symptoms or urinary specific gravity measurements.

Other agents that increase AVP secretion (e.g., clofibrate) or action (e.g., chlorpropamide, indapamide, carbamazepine) are less effective, and their use is limited.

Nephrogenic Diabetes Insipidus

Desmopressin, even in supraphysiologic doses, has a limited response because NDI is caused by resistance to AVP. Treatment of acquired metabolic and pharmacologic causes can decrease urinary volume in NDI and usually lead to resolution of this acquired NDI. Thiazide diuretics may decrease urine volume by causing mild volume depletion. In conjunction with a low-salt diet, thiazides increase proximal tubular absorption of sodium and water, leading to decreased water delivery to the collecting tubule where AVP action occurs. Nonsteroidal antiinflammatory drugs decrease renal prostaglandins and thus augment AVP action, decreasing urine volume in NDI.

SYNDROME OF INAPPROPRIATE ANTIDIURETIC HORMONE SECRETION

Nicholas Emanuele and Mary Ann Emanuele

The syndrome of inappropriate antidiuretic hormone secretion (SIADH) is a constellation of findings that result from imbalance of water in relation to sodium. It is a dilutional, euvolemic hyponatremia.

Etiology

SIADH can arise from several disease states and pharmacotherapies. They may be categorized into six main categories, as shown in Table 1.3. Those arising from the central nervous system cause SIADH by increasing ADH secretion through the body's physiologic pathway. Carcinomas that are causative usually produce ADH themselves, regardless of the hypothalamic–pituitary axis, as part of the paraneoplastic syndrome. Small cell lung carcinoma is the most common oncologic cause of SIADH [72,73]. In a study by Comis et al. [74], at least 46% of patients with small cell lung cancer had elevated ADH levels. Another cause of SIADH that is becoming increasingly more prevalent is acquired immunodeficiency syndrome (AIDS). Up to 25% of hospitalized patients with AIDS have possible SIADH [75].

Epidemiology

The epidemiology of SIADH can be extrapolated from that of hyponatremia. SIADH can occur in anyone with any of the precipitators already suggested, but the elderly, the hospitalized, and residents of chronic care facilities are at greatest risk.

Pathophysiology

The path toward SIADH begins when a water imbalance occurs; the body receives more water than it excretes. If a patient has excess ADH, he or she is unable to excrete the additional amount of water. The intracellular and extracellular fluid volumes increase subsequently, and the concentration of sodium decreases, leading to hyponatremia. This elevated level of fluid is detected by the renal juxtaglomerular cells, and the level of renin and aldosterone decreases. Depressed levels of these substances increase sodium excretion, which prevents fluid overload but also perpetuates the low sodium concentration.

Table 1.3.   Causes of Syndrome of Inappropriate Secretion of Antidiuretic Hormone

Central nervous system
   Stroke (hemorrhagic or ischemic)
   Hemorrhage
   Neoplasm
   Infection
   Hydrocephalus
   After transsphenoidal hypophysectomy
   Schizophrenia
   Lupus
   Acute intermittent porphyria
Carcinoma
   Small cell lung carcinoma
   Pharyngeal carcinoma, thymoma
   Pancreatic carcinoma
   Bladder carcinoma
   Lymphoma, sarcoma
   Others: prostate, duodenal, ovarian, mesothelioma
Pulmonary
   Infections (pneumonia, abscess, tuberculosis)
   Bronchiectasis
   Mechanical ventilation
Medication related
   Psychiatric: antipsychotics, tricyclics, selective serotonin receptor
      inhibitors, carbamazepine
   Neurologic: narcotics, ecstasy
   ACE inhibitors
   Oncologic: vincristine, vinblastine, cyclophosphamide
   Endocrine: oxytocin, desmopressin, chlorpropamide, clofibrate
Infections
   Central nervous system and pulmonary infections, as above
   Acquired immunodeficiency syndrome
Idiopathetic

Diagnosis

Clinical Findings

Not all patients with SIADH are symptomatic. The likelihood of becoming symptomatic depends on the change in the sodium concentration, more from the rate at which it changes rather from the absolute change of sodium. Symptoms range from mild constitutional symptoms (e.g., fatigue, anorexia, nausea, mild headache), to more serious signs (e.g., seizures, coma, and death). Generally, when the sodium concentration decreases to less than 125 mmol/L, minor symptoms develop. More serious neurologic symptoms, such as coma, seizures, decreased reflexes, and altered mental status, appear as the sodium concentration decreases to 115 mmol/L. When the sodium level is less than 115 mmol/L, sudden death is a risk.

Laboratory Findings

In the evaluation of hyponatremia and SIADH, three key tests are those that measure levels of plasma osmolality, urine osmolality, and urine sodium. These tests will reveal a low plasma osmolality and an elevated urine osmolality. The kidney, as already described, is excreting increased sodium, so the urinary sodium level will be high, exceeding 20 mmol/L. Other laboratory values (e.g., hematocrit, blood urea nitrogen, uric acid) are decreased secondary to dilution. Besides these laboratory values, the diagnosis of SIADH requires that the patient have no other cause for the hyponatremia, such as congestive heart failure, cirrhosis, renal failure, adrenal insufficiency, thyroid disease, or electrolyte imbalance.

Treatment
Therapy for both acute and chronic hyponatremia includes correction of the underlying cause.

Short-Term Therapy
Further treatment depends on the patient's clinical picture. If the patient is mildly symptomatic, one can fluid restrict the patient to up to 1 L/day. If the hyponatremia is severe and the patient is symptomatic, fluid restriction is not adequate to restore the patient's sodium concentration. One must add sodium in excess of water, usually in conjunction with furosemide. This can be done with the addition of a 3% saline solution. Other authors give different rates at which fluids should be infused, but a consensus seems to exist that the change in sodium concentration should not exceed 8 to 12 mmol/L in the first 24 hours. One must keep in mind two main points: the rate should be fast enough to resolve symptoms, but not so rapid as to cause complications such as central pontine myelinolysis. One guideline is to infuse the fluid at a rate of 0.5 to 1 ml/kg/min to increase the sodium concentration by 2 mmol/L, until symptoms resolve or the sodium concentration increases by half of the deficit [72]. Adrogue and Madias [76] have provided the following formula to predict the change in sodium from 1 L of fluid: change in serum sodium 5 (fluid sodium concentration 2 serum sodium concentration)/total body water 1 1.

The infusion can be stopped when symptoms resolve or when the sodium concentration increases to 125 to 130 mmol/L. Sodium concentration and urine output should be monitored closely, every 1 to 2 hours, to ensure that the rate of sodium elevation is appropriate and to detect whether the syndrome resolves, because it can subside abruptly.

Central pontine myelinolysis remains a potential danger of sodium replacement. Certain factors, such as alcoholism, malnourishment, and debilitation, can place patients at increased risk. Additionally, existence of the syndrome for longer than 2 days increases the risk of this complication if the sodium level is corrected too rapidly. Several studies have considered this adverse effect. A multicenter prospective study by Sterns et al. [75] that looked at patients with severe hyponatremia showed that neurologic complications, including central pontine myelinolysis, occurred in patients with chronic hyponatremia whose sodium concentration was corrected faster than 12 mmol/L over a 24-hour period or 18 mmol/L over a 48-hour period.

Long-Term Therapy
One can use two main interventions in long-term management of SIADH. The first is fluid restriction, as already mentioned, at times with the use of loop diuretics; however, many patients are unable to comply with the fluid restriction. Therefore many patients require medication, either demeclocycline or fludrocortisone. Demeclocycline blocks antidiuretic hormone in the kidney. The dose is 600 to 1,200 mg/day, and it may take 1 to 2 weeks to see its effect. A study by Forrest et al. [77] that compared demeclocycline with lithium, which had been used for SIADH, revealed that demeclocycline is superior to lithium in the treatment of SIADH. Fludrocortisone can also be used, at a dose of 0.1 to 0.3 mg twice a day.

Future Therapy
An AVP antagonist is currently under investigation for treatment of SIADH. Saito et al. [78] have shown that administration of an AVP antagonist labeled OPC-31260 increases the serum sodium concentration and treats this syndrome. Further studies have been reported and are still under way.

REFERENCES

Evaluation of the Hypothalamic–Pituitary System

1. (*1C*) **Livesey JH** et al. Effect of time, temperature and freezing on the stability of immunoreactive LH, FSH, TSH, growth hormone, prolactin and insulin in plasma. Clin Biochem 1980;13: 151–155.

   Endogenous LH, FSH, TSH, GH, prolactin, and insulin were measured by RIA in human plasma samples stored at 4°C, 20°C, and 37°C for up to 8 days or repeatedly frozen and thawed. At 4°C, the concentrations of all hormones were stable for at least 8 days; at 20°C, only LH, FSH, and TSH were stable for 8 days; at 37°C, only TSH was stable for 8 days. All tested hormones except insulin were stable during five freeze–thaw cycles

2. (*1C*) **Hindmarsh PC** et al. Comparison between a physiological and pharmacological stimulus of growth hormone secretion: The response to stage IV sleep and insulin-induced hypoglycemia. Lancet 1985;2:1033–1035.

   Peak GH response to insulin-induced hypoglycemia was compared with peak GH concentration during the first cycle of stage IV sleep in 75 children. Sixty-five children had concordant results: in 38, GH concentrations exceeded 15 mU/L, and in 27, they were less. Results were discordant in 10 children. Results of sleep sampling under electroencephalographic control of the assessment of GH secretion are comparable with conventional pharmacologic studies in terms of efficiency, sensitivity, and percentage of false-negative results. Sleep sampling has the advantage of being a physiologic test of secretion.

3. (*1C*) **Nieman LK** et al. A simplified morning ovine corticotropin releasing hormone stimulation test for the differential diagnosis of adrenocorticotropin-dependent Cushing syndrome. J Clin Endocrinol Metab 1993, 77:1308–1312.

   A retrospective review of 118 patients with proven Cushing disease or ectopic ACTH was done to develop criteria for interpretation of a morning ovine CRH test for differential diagnosis of ACTH-dependent Cushing syndrome. A sensitivity of 93% and a specificity of 100% were noted.

Imaging of the Hypothalamic–Pituitary System

4. (*1C+*) **Webb SM** et al. Computerized tomography versus magnetic resonance imaging: a comparative study in hypothalamic-pituitary and parasellar pathology. Clin Endocrinol 1992;36:459–465.

   This study compared hypothalamic–pituitary CTs and MRIs in 40 patients referred for evaluation of pituitary and parasellar lesions by two independent neuroradiologists. More than 40 parameters relating to the bony margins, cavernous sinuses, carotid arteries, optic chiasm, suprasellar cisterns, pituitary, pituitary stalk, and extension of the lesion were evaluated. Both neuroradiologists coincided in their reports in 32 patients. In the eight patients with Cushing disease, MRIs were positive in five, and CTs, in two. The authors concluded that in patients suspected of having Cushing syndrome or hyperprolactinemia (due to microadenomas), MRI is clearly preferable to CT. In macroadenomas, both scans are equally diagnostic, but MRI offered more information on pituitary morphology and neighboring structures.

5. (*1C+*) **Nichols DA** et al. Comparison of MRI and CT in the preoperative evaluation of pituitary adenomas. Neurosurgery 1988;22:380–385.

   Twenty surgically verified pituitary adenomas were imaged in a systematic comparative fashion with MRI and CT before surgery. The study group included 11 microadenomas, four macroadenomas, two recurrent microadenomas, and three recurrent macroadenomas. The MRI and CT examinations were evaluated for presence of a mass lesion, pituitary stalk displacement, cavernous sinus displacement or invasion, hemorrhage, cystic degeneration within the adenoma, bony erosion, detection of suprasellar extension, and displacement of suprasellar structures. MRI was superior to CT for detecting the extrasellar extent of tumor. Within the sella turcica, MRI and CT were equivalent for lesion detection.

6. **Thorner MO** et al. The anterior pituitary. In: Williams' textbook of endocrinology. 9th ed. Philadelphia: WB Saunders, 1988.

   Excellent and comprehensive overview of the normal pituitary gland anatomy and imaging correlation.

Pituitary Tumors

7. (*1C+*) **Freda PU, Wardlaw SL**. Diagnosis and treatment of pituitary tumors. J Clin Endocrinol Metab 1999;84:3859–3866.

   This excellent review summarizes the treatment options and prognosis of all pituitary tumors.

8. (*1C*) **Turner HE** et al. Angiogenesis in pituitary adenomas and the normal pituitary gland. J Clin Endocrinol Metab 2000;85:1159–1162.

   This state-of-the-art study demonstrated the novel finding that pituitary adenomas are less vascular than normal anterior pituitary tissue, and that, depending on tumor type, size is related to vascular density. The authors also discuss the exciting possibility that endogenous inhibitors of angiogenesis are responsible for the tumor behavior and their role in determining angiogenic phenotype.

9. (*1C+*) **Laws ER Jr, Thapar K**. Pituitary surgery. Endocrinol Metab Clin North Am 1999;28: 119–131.

Surgical management of pituitary adenomas is discussed as a safe and effective method for treating patients affected by these lesions. The goals of overall management are discussed in relation to the understanding of pituitary pathophysiology.

10. (*1C+*) **Comtois R** et al. The clinical and endocrine outcome to transsphenoidal microsurgery of nonsecreting pituitary adenomas. Cancer 1991;68:860–866.

This study analyzed the results of 126 patients who underwent transsphenoidal surgery for primary treatment of pituitary adenomas unassociated with clinical or biochemical evidence of hormonal overproduction from 1962 to 1987. Endocrine evaluation revealed the presence of hypogonadism in 75%, adrenal insufficiency in 36%, and hypothyroidism in 18%. Plasma prolactin was increased in 65%. Sella enlargement was documented in all cases, with 33% with invasive adenomas. After surgery, vision was normalized or improved in 75% of the patients, whereas thyroid, adrenal, and gonadal function improved in fewer than 50% and worsened in 15%. Permanent DI occurred in 5%. The recurrence rate in patients with a mean follow-up of 6.4 years was 21%. These data suggest that transsphenoidal microsurgery by a skilled neurosurgeon is an effective and safe initial treatment for patients with nonsecreting pituitary adenoma, and it may reverse hypopituitarism.

11. (*1C+*) **Turner H** et al. Audit of selected patients with non-functioning pituitary adenomas treated without irradiation: A follow-up study. Clin Endocrinol 1999;51:281–284.

The data base for this study was drawn from the progress notes and the imaging of an original cohort of 65 patients from 1994 who had undergone transsphenoidal surgery for nonfunctioning adenomas between July 1979 and 1992. The patients had not received irradiation. Mean follow-up was 76 months. The data demonstrated that pituitary tumor regrowth had occurred in 21 (32%) of 65 patients during a mean follow-up of 76 months. Tumor regrowth was detected at a mean of 5.4 years. Eight patients required a second surgical procedure. Those authors concluded that despite careful selection of patients with nonfunctioning pituitary adenomas, tumor regrowth occurs in a significant proportion, so that continued follow-up is essential. Radiotherapy should be recommended for all patients with nonfunctioning pituitary adenomas, because the regrowth rate approaches 50% at 10 years.

12. (*1C+*) **Brada M** et al. The long-term efficacy of conservative surgery and radiotherapy in the control of pituitary adenomas. Clin Endocrinol 1993;38:571–578.

In this retrospective study, the long-term efficacy and toxicity of surgery and conventional external beam radiotherapy were assessed in 411 patients with pituitary adenomas between 1962 and 1986. The authors concluded that conventional external beam radiotherapy combined with surgery is safe and effective in the control of pituitary adenomas.

13. (*1C+*) **Lillehei KO** et al. Reassessment of the role of radiation therapy in the treatment of endocrine inactive pituitary macroadenomas. Neurosurgery 1998;43:432–439.

This prospective clinical trial evaluated the rate of tumor recurrence in patients with pituitary macroadenomas treated with total surgical resection but not with adjuvant radiotherapy between December 1987 and July 1994. The mean follow-up duration was 5.5 years. Immunocytochemical analysis revealed that 66% of the tumors were weak gonadotroph cell adenomas, 22% were nonfunctional adenomas, 9% were silent prolactinomas, and 3% were silent corticotroph cell adenomas. Thirty-two of 38 patients elected not to receive adjuvant radiotherapy. During that time, recurrence developed in 6% within 24 months of surgery and was successfully treated by using radiation therapy, with one requiring additional surgery. This study demonstrated a 6% 5-year recurrence rate in patients with endocrine-inactive pituitary macroadenomas treated with total surgical resection alone. Those authors concluded that it is reasonable to reserve radiation therapy for patients with recurrence.

14. (*1C+*) **Gittoes N** et al. Radiotherapy for non-functioning tumors. Clin Endocrinol 1998;48:331–337.

Pituitary radiotherapy is often used as adjuvant treatment in the postoperative period for patients with clinically nonfunctioning pituitary tumors. A retrospective review of patient records was performed on 126 patients with nonfunctioning adenomas treated at two institutions in the United Kingdom. One hospital routinely administered radiation therapy within 12 months of initial pituitary surgery, whereas the other rarely used it. The main outcome measure was regrowth of pituitary tumors after surgery. These authors determined the efficacy of radiation therapy in preventing the regrowth of these tumors. The rate of progression-free survival was 93% at both 10 years and at 15 years for the group treated with radiation therapy, and it was 68% and 33%, respectively, for the group not treated with radiation therapy.

15. (*1C*) **Nelson PB** et al. Endocrine function in patients with large pituitary tumors treated with operative decompression and radiation therapy. Neurosurgery 1989;24:398–400.

In this study, 30 patients who underwent operative decompression and radiation therapy for large sellar and suprasellar tumors were investigated prospectively in terms of their endocrine outcome. Ten of these patients had panhypopituitarism before and after treatment. The other 20 patients had partial hormonal deficits before treatment. Ten (50%) of the 20 patients who had partial preoperative deficits eventually had delayed onset of worsening in their endocrine function; nine of 10 experienced panhypopituitarism, and 1 patient had decreased thyroid function. The mean time from surgery until onset of delayed worsening in endocrine function was 26.1 months. None of the 10 patients with delayed onset of pituitary function deterioration had evidence of tumor recurrence by CT. Those authors concluded that delayed-onset radiation effect was the most likely cause of the slow decline in endocrine function.

16. **Sibal L** et al. Pituitary apoplexy: A review of clinical presentation, management and outcomes. Pituitary 2005;7:157–163.

   This retrospective chart review illustrates the high (90%) incidence of hypopituitarism associated with pituitary apoplexy over a period of 20 years, and the need for clinicians to be vigilant in diagnosing and replacing pituitary hormones in individuals who experience this.

17. **Thorner MO** et al. Manifestations of anterior pituitary hormone deficiency. In: Williams' textbook of endocrinology. 9th ed. Philadelphia: WB Saunders, 1998.

   Excellent and comprehensive overview of pituitary gland insufficiency, testing, and replacement.

18. *(1A)* **Salomon F** et al. The effects of treatment with recombinant human growth hormone on body composition and metabolism in adults with growth hormone deficiency. N Engl J Med 1989;321:1979–1803.

   This study was conducted as a double-blind, placebo-controlled trial, investigating the effects of 6 months of GH replacement in 24 adults with GH deficiency. All patients were receiving appropriate thyroid, adrenal, and gonadal hormone replacement. Lean body mass and basal metabolic rate increased significantly, whereas fat mass decreased in the GH-treated group compared with findings in the placebo group after 6 months of GH therapy. Cholesterol levels also were lower with GH treatment. It was concluded that GH has a role in the regulation of body composition in adults, probably through its anabolic and lipolytic actions.

19. *(1C+)* **Borson-Chazot F** et al. Decrease in carotid intima-media thickness after one year growth hormone (GH) treatment in adults with GH deficiency. J Clin Endocrinol Metab 1999;84:1329–1333.

   This was a multicenter open trial involving 22 GH-deficient patients treated with replacement for 2 years. A decrease in carotid artery intima–media thickness was observed in 21 of 22 patients. GH treatment resulted in a moderate decrease in waist circumference and body fat mass. Conventional cardiovascular risk factors were unmodified except for a transient 10% decrease in LDL cholesterol at 6 months. The decrease in intima–media thickness may indicate a reversal in the atherosclerotic process.

20. *(1C+)* **Murray RD** et al. Dose titration and patient selection increases the efficacy of GH replacement in GHD adults. Clin Endocrinol 1999;50:749–757.

   This trial was an open study of GH replacement in 65 severely GH-deficient patients who had GH initiated with a low dose (0.8 U/day) and titrated by 0.4-U increments to normalize the IGF-1. After initiation of GH, serum IGF-1 levels increased significantly, and lipid levels decreased, whereas other metabolic parameters were largely unchanged. Improvement in quality of life in GH-deficient adults was proportional to the degree of impairment before initiating therapy. The authors concluded that the use of low-dose titration and selection of a population with greater morbidity reduces the occurrence of overreplacement and increases the efficacy of treatment.

21. *(1A)* **Whitehead HM** et al. Growth hormone treatment of adults with growth hormone deficiency: Results of a 13 month placebo-controlled cross-over study. Clin Endocrinol 1992;36:45–52.

   This double-blind placebo-controlled crossover study investigated the effect of GH replacement in 14 GH-deficient adults. Patents were treated for 6 months with GH replacement and 6 months with placebo, separated by a 1-month washout period. Body weight, fat, lean body mass, muscle volume, exercise capacity, maximum oxygen consumption, muscle strength, bone mineral content, IGF-1, GH antibodies, and psychological well-being were all assessed. Lean body mass, exercise capacity, and maximum oxygen consumption significantly increased. IGF-1 levels increased, whereas glucose tolerance, fasting lipids, electrolytes, renal and liver function, psychological well-being, and spinal bone mineral density remained unchanged. Those authors concluded that the beneficial effects of GH replacement on body composition and exercise capacity in GH-deficient adults are significant and that this therapy should be considered in appropriate patients.

22. *(1B)* **Drake WM** et al. Optimising growth hormone replacement therapy by dose titration in hypopituitary adults. J Clin Endocrinol Metab 1998;83:3913–3919.

   This important study evaluated two GH-replacement regimens and explored gender differences in GH susceptibility. Fifty adult-onset hypopituitary patients were given GH by using a dose-titration regimen schedule compared with 21 patients previously treated by using conventional weight-based dosing. Titrated patients initiated GH at 0.8 IU/day subcutaneously, with dose adjustments every 4 weeks to achieve an appropriate serum IGF-1 level. Maintenance doses were significantly higher in women than in men, and the time to achieve maintenance dose was significantly shorter in men (4 weeks vs. 9 weeks). The median maintenance dose was lower overall than in a group of 21 patients initially started on GH by using a weight-based dosing schedule, with subsequent adjustment of dose during clinical follow-up. The titration schedule for dosing resulted in rapid achievement of lower maintenance doses than those achieved by using conventional weight-based regimens without loss of efficacy. It was particularly important in female patients who demonstrated decreased overall sensitivity to GH and required higher doses to achieve the same effects as male patients.

Disorders of the Prolactin System

23. **Schlechte JA.** Clinical practice: Prolactinoma review. N Engl J Med 2003;349:2035–2041.

   A comprehensive review of the current clinical practice in the diagnosis and treatment of prolactinoma.

24. (*1C+*) **Greer ME** et al. Prevalence of hyperprolactinemia in anovulatory women. Obstet Gynecol 1980;56:65–69

A 1-year prospective study of 119 patients with at least 3 months of anovulation. They were screened with serum prolactin determinations. In patients with anovulation with or without galactorrhea, a hyperprolactinemia prevalence rate of 15% was established. The range of prevalence was 43% in those with galactorrhea to 9% in those without galactorrhea.

25. (*1C+*) **Montgomery J** et al. Prevalence of hyperprolactinemia in schizophrenia: Association with typical and atypical antipsychotic treatment. J Clin Psychiatry 2004;65:1491–1498.

Patients with a known diagnosis of schizophrenia and other related psychotic disorders were retrospectively analyzed. The total number of patients was 422. Antipsychotics known to elevate prolactin were associated with higher prevalence rates of hyperprolactinemia, and "prolactin-sparing" medications had lower prevalence rates.

26. **Molitch ME.** Medication-induced hyperprolactinemia. Mayo Clin Proc 2005;80:1050–1057.

A review of medical literature of medications that can cause hyperprolactinemia. It included medications such as antipsychotic, antidepressant, and antihypertensive agents, and drugs that increase bowel motility. The hyperprolactinemia in these cases is commonly symptomatic.

27. (*1C+*) **Vallette-Kasik S** et al. Macroprolactinemia revisited: A study on 106 patients. J Clin Endocrinol Metab 2002;87:581–588.

The 1,106 consecutive patients investigated for hyperprolactinemia over a 10-year period were analyzed. Among them, 106 patients had macroprolactinemia, a prevalence of about 10%. These 106 patients were prospectively followed up and compared with 262 hyperprolactinemic patients without macroprolactinemia.

28. **Gibney J** et al. Clinical relevance of macroprolactin. Clin Endocrinol 2005;62:633.

A review article on the nature, methods of measurement, and bioactivity of macroprolactin. It also reviews the epidemiology and natural history of patients with macroprolactinemia.

29. (*1C+*) **Vance ML** et al. Drugs five years later. Bromocriptine. Ann Intern Med 1984;100:78–91.

This article includes a review of 13 studies showing that bromocriptine reduced the serum prolactin concentration to normal in 229 (82%) of 280 women with hyperprolactinemia and, in 12 studies, in 66 (71%) of 92 patients with lactotroph macroadenomas.

30. (*1C*) **Di Sarno A** et al. Resistance to cabergoline as compared with bromocriptine in hyperprolactinemia: Prevalence, clinical definition, and therapeutic strategy. J Clin Endocrinol Metab 2001;86:5256–5261.

In total, 207 patients were studied. Cabergoline was used in 120 patients (56 macroadenomas, 60 microadenomas, and four nontumoral hyperprolactinemias), and bromocriptine was used in 87 patients (28 macroadenomas, 44 microadenomas, and 15 nontumoral hyperprolactinemias). Normalization of serum prolactin and reduction in tumor size was significantly higher in the cabergoline group (82.1% vs. 46.4% among patients with macroprolactinomas, and 90% vs. 56.8% ($p < 0.001$) among those with microprolactinomas).

31. (*1C*) **Sabuncu T** et al. Comparison of the effects of cabergoline and bromocriptine on prolactin levels in hyperprolactinemic patients. Intern Med 2001;40:857–861.

A head-to-head comparison of cabergoline and bromocriptine was made in this study. Cabergoline was found to be much more efficacious and tolerable. After 12 weeks, prolactin reduction was more than 93% in the cabergoline group vs. more than 87.5% in the bromocriptine group ($p < 0.05$).

32. (*1C*) **Jasonni VM** et al. Vaginal bromocriptine in hyperprolactinemic patients and puerperal women. Acta Obstet Gynecol Scand 1991;70:493–495.

Fifteen hyperprolactinemic and seven puerperal women were treated with bromocriptine per vagina because of intolerance to oral treatment. In both groups, hyperprolactinemia was normalized without the typical side effects of bromocriptine.

33. (*1C+*) **Colao A** et al. Withdrawal of long-term cabergoline therapy for tumoral and nontumoral hyperprolactinemia. N Engl J Med 2003;349:2023–2033.

The study population included 200 patients (25 patients with nontumoral hyperprolactinemia, 105 with microprolactinomas, and 70 with macroprolactinomas). Withdrawal of cabergoline was considered if prolactin levels were normal, magnetic resonance imaging (MRI) showed no tumor (or tumor reduction of 50% or more, with the tumor at a distance of more than 5 mm from the optic chiasm, and no invasion of the cavernous sinuses or other critical areas), and if follow-up after withdrawal could be continued for at least 24 months. Recurrence rates 2 to 5 years after the withdrawal of cabergoline were 24% in patients with nontumoral hyperprolactinemia, 31% in patients with microprolactinomas, and 36% in patients with macroprolactinomas. Renewed tumor growth did not occur in any patient.

34. **Molitch ME.** Management of prolactinomas during pregnancy. J Reprod Med 1999;44(12 suppl):1121–1126.

A review article of treatment and follow-up of prolactinomas in pregnancy.

35. (*1C*) **Turkalj I** et al. Surveillance of bromocriptine in pregnancy. JAMA 1982;247:1589–1591.

Information was collected on the outcome of 1,410 pregnancies in 1,335 women to whom bromocriptine had been given, primarily in the early weeks of pregnancy. The incidence rate of spontaneous abortions, extrauterine pregnancies, and minor and major malformations is comparable with that quoted for normal populations.

36. (*2C*) **Ciccarell E** et al. Long-term treatment with cabergoline, a new long lasting ergoline derivative in idiopathic or tumorous hyperprolactinemia and outcome of drug induced pregnancy. J Endocrinol Invest 1997;20:542–547.

   No adverse effect was noted in women who became pregnant while undergoing treatment with cabergoline.

Acromegaly

37. **Melmed S.** Acromegaly. N Engl J Med 1990;322:966–977.

   Comprehensive review article on the topic.

38. **Melmed S** et al. Guidelines for acromegaly management. J Clin Endocrinol Metab 2002;87:4054-4058.

   This consensus statement was developed by neuroendocrinologists and neurosurgeons regarding therapeutic options for acromegaly.

39. **Giustina A** et al. Criteria for cure of acromegaly: A consensus statement. J Clin Endocrinol Metab 2000;85:526–529.

   In February 1999, a workshop was held in Cortina, Italy, to develop a consensus defining the criteria for cure of acromegaly. Invited international participants included endocrinologists, neurosurgeons, and radiotherapists skilled in the management of acromegaly. This statement summarizes the consensus achieved in these discussions.

40. (*1C+*) **Swearingen B** et al. Long-term mortality after transsphenoidal surgery and adjunctive therapy for acromegaly. J Clin Endocrinol Metab 1998;83:3419–3426.

   In this retrospective review of 162 patients, surgical cure was seen in 91% of microadenomas and in 48% of macroadenomas. Adjunctive therapy was required in 40%. Biochemical remission was achieved in 83% at a mean of 7.8 years. Mortality regression analysis of patients cured with surgery approached age- and gender-matched U.S. population samples.

41. (*1C+*) **Kreutzer J** et al. Surgical management of GH-secreting pituitary adenomas: An outcome study using modern remission criteria. J Clin Endocrinol Metab 2001;86:4072–4077.

   This retrospective analysis of 57 patients, at a mean of 37.7 months postoperatively, revealed remission by normal IGF-1 in 70.2%; random GH less than 2.5 mg/L in 66.7%, and glucose-suppressed GH less than 1 mg/L in 61.1%. Tumor size at diagnosis predicted persistence of disease.

42. (*1C+*) **Barker F** et al. Transsphenoidal surgery for pituitary tumors in the United States, 1996-2000: Mortality, morbidity, and the effects of hospital and surgeon volume. J Clin Endocrinol Metab 2003; 88:4709-4719

   This retrospective analysis of 5,497 pituitary operations revealed that higher-volume hospitals and neurosurgeons had better short-term outcomes after transsphenoidal surgery.

43. (*1A*) **Newman C** et al. Octreotide as primary therapy for acromegaly. J Clin Endocrinol Metab 1998;83:3034–3040.

   This multicenter study using daily octreotide compared 26 patients receiving primary octreotide with 81 receiving adjunctive therapy. Responders were defined as having GH levels decreasing to at least 2 standard deviations below baseline mean GH. No significant difference was found in response rates in the primary (70%) and adjunctive (60%) groups. Both groups achieved similar improvement in clinical symptoms during 3 years of follow-up.

44. (*1A*) **Colao A** et al. Long-term effects of depot long-acting somatostatin analog octreotide on hormone levels and tumor mass in acromegaly. J Clin Endocrinol Metab 2001;86:2779–2786.

   Depot octreotide was given to 36 patients, 15 de novo and in 21 who had previously been surgically treated, for up to 24 months. Including both groups, GH below 2.5 mg/L was seen in 69.4%, whereas IGF-1 levels were normal in 61.1% at last observation. Similar percentages were achieved for both groups. Tumor volume decreased in 12 of 15 in the de novo group and five of nine in the operated-on group.

45. **Melmed S** et al. A critical analysis of pituitary tumor shrinkage during primary medical therapy in acromegaly. J Clin Endocrinol Metab 2005;90:4405-4410.

   This systematic literature review highlights the efficacy of somatostatin analogues in decreasing tumor size as primary therapy or before surgery or radiation therapy.

46. (*1C+*) **Abe T, Ludecke DK.** Effects of preoperative octreotide treatment on different subtypes of 90 GH-secreting pituitary adenomas and outcome in one surgical centre. Eur J Endocrinol 2001;145:137–145.

   This retrospective study compared 90 patients who received at least 3 months of preoperative daily octreotide versus 57 who had not received therapy. At a mean follow-up of 51 months, endocrine remission was achieved slightly more frequently in the pretreated group for microadenomas (100% vs. 92.9%), resectable macroadenomas (95.2% vs. 87.5%), and invasive potentially resectable macroadenomas (81.4% vs.73.9%).

47. (*1A*) **Kristof RA** et al. Does octreotide treatment improve the surgical results of macroadenomas in acromegaly? Acta Neurochir 1999;141:399–405.

This prospective controlled study evaluated surgical outcomes in 13 octreotide-treated patients versus 11 controls. Therapy was given for a mean of 16 weeks preoperatively. Postoperative remission rates were not significantly different in the treated (55%) versus untreated controls (69%).

48. **Ben-Shlomo A, Melmed S.** The role of pharmacotherapy in perioperative management of patients with acromegaly. J Clin Endocrinol Metab 2003;88:963–966.

This review discusses somatostatin analogue therapy before resection of somatotroph adenomas or non-pituitary surgery requiring anesthesia in patients with acromegaly. Effects on postoperative IGF-1 and GH control rates and cardiovascular, pulmonary, and glycemic parameters are evaluated.

49. (*1C+*) **Barrande G** et al. Hormonal and metabolic effects of radiotherapy in acromegaly: Long-term results in 128 patients followed in a single center. J Clin Endocrinol Metab 2000;85:3779–3785.

Conventional external beam radiation therapy was delivered to 128 patients in this retrospective single-center study. Basal GH less than 2.5 mg/L was seen in 35% at 5 years, 53% at 10 years, and 66% at 15 years. At 10 years, relative deficiencies were seen in gonadotropins in 80%, TSH in 78%, and ACTH in 82%.

50. **Laws E** et al. Stereotactic radiosurgery for pituitary adenoma: A review of the literature. J NeuroOncol 2004;69:257–272.

Stereotactic radiosurgery can lead to a more rapid normalization of hormone levels with a lessened chance of hypopituitarism, radiation-induced neoplasia, and cerebrovascular injury when compared with fractionated radiation therapy.

51. (*1A*) **Abs R** et al. Cabergoline in the treatment of acromegaly: A study in 64 patients. J Clin Endocrinol Metab 1998;83:374–378.

This prospective open-label study revealed IGF-1 less than 300 mg/L in 39%. If tumors secreted both GH and prolactin, the level of IGF-1 was less than 300 mg/L in 50%. In the subset of patients with initial IGF-1 less than 750 mg/L, 53% achieved an IGF-1 level less than 300 mg/L. Duration of treatment was between 3 and 40 months.

52. (*2A*) **Trainer PJ** et al. Treatment of acromegaly with the growth hormone-receptor antagonist pegvisomant. N Engl J Med 2000;342:1171–1177.

IGF-1 decreased by 50.1% (626.7%) in the 15-mg SC daily group and 62.5% (621.3%) in the 20-mg group in this 12-week randomized double blind study. Normal IGF-1 was achieved in 81% of the 15-mg/day group and 89% of the 20-mg/day group.

53. (*2A*) **Van der Lely AJ** et al. Long-term treatment of acromegaly with pegvisomant, a growth hormone receptor antagonist. Lancet 2001;358:1754–1759.

Pegvisomant was given for 6 to18 months. IGF-1 decreased 50% or more in all groups, with normal IGF-1 levels in 97% of those treated for at least 12 months.

54. **Clemmons D** et al. Optimizing control of acromegaly: Integrating a growth hormone receptor antagonist into the treatment algorithm. J Clin Endocrinol Metab 2003;88:4759-4767.

This review discusses pegvisomant in a new treatment algorithm for acromegaly.

Cushing Disease

55. (*1C+*) **Lindholm J** et al. Incidence and late prognosis of Cushing's syndrome: A population-based study. J Clin Endocrinol Metab 2001;86:117–123.

The aim of the study was to assess the incidence and late outcome of Cushing syndrome, especially that of Cushing disease. Information was collected on patients diagnosed with Cushing syndrome in Denmark over a period of 11 years. The annual incidence was noted to be 1.2 to1.7 per million people for Cushing disease, 0.6 per million for adrenal adenoma, and 0.2 per million for adrenal carcinoma. Of 139 patients with nonmalignant disease, 11.1% died during follow-up. Excessive mortality was observed mainly during the first year. The perceived quality of health was decreased in patients with CD.

56. **Arnaldi G** et al. Diagnosis and complications of Cushing's syndrome: A consensus statement. J Clin Endocrinol Metab 2003;88:5593–5602.

In October 2002, a workshop was held in Ancona, Italy, to reach a consensus on the management of Cushing syndrome. The consensus statement on diagnostic criteria and the diagnosis and treatment of complications of this syndrome reached at the workshop was summarized in the article.

57. **Newell-Price J** et al. The diagnosis and differential diagnosis of Cushing's syndrome and pseudo-Cushing's states. Endocr Rev 1998;19:647–672.

A comprehensive review of the different tests in the diagnosis of Cushing syndrome.

58. (*1C+*) **Dichek HL** et al. A comparison of the standard high dose dexamethasone suppression test and the overnight 8-mg dexamethasone suppression test for the differential diagnosis of adrenocorticotropin-dependent Cushing's syndrome. J Clin Endocrinol Metab 1994;78:418–422.

Forty-one patients who were subsequently proven at surgery to have Cushing syndrome were studied (34 CD and seven EAS). High-dose DST and the 6-day high-dose DST (including a 2-day high-dose DST) were done on these patients. Optimal criteria for the diagnosis of CD were developed for both tests.

59. (1C+) **Newell-Price J** et al. Optimal response criteria for the human CRH test in the differential diagnosis of ACTH-dependent Cushing syndrome. J Clin Endocrinol Metab 2002;87:1640–1645.

One hundred fifteen consecutive patients with proven ACTH-dependent CS were studied, 101 with CD and 14 with EAS. The response to hCRH was also studied in 30 normal volunteers with no clinical evidence of CS, and the results were compared. After basal sampling at ?15 and 0 min, hCRH (100 ?g, i.v.) was administered at 0900 h, and serum cortisol and ACTH were measured at 15-min intervals for 2 h. The results were then analyzed to determine the sensitivity and specificity of the test.

60. (1C) **Hall WA** et al. Pituitary magnetic resonance imaging in normal human volunteers: Occult adenomas in general population. Ann Intern Med 1994;120:817–820.

High-resolution MRI scans of 100 normal volunteers and 57 patients with Cushing disease were evaluated independently by three blinded reviewers to determine the prevalence of focal lesions of the pituitary gland that suggest the presence of pituitary adenoma in people with no symptoms. In patients with Cushing disease, abnormalities in the pituitary MRI were reported in about 56% of cases, but not all these abnormalities correlated with surgical findings. Of normal volunteers, 10% had abnormalities in pituitary MRI.

61. (1C+) **Oldfield EH** et al. Petrosal sinus sampling with and without corticotropin-releasing hormone for the differential diagnosis of Cushing syndrome. N Engl J Med 1991;325:897–905.

A prospective study of 281 patients with Cushing syndrome was done to evaluate the bilateral inferior petrosal sinus sampling. Bilateral sampling was successfully accomplished in 278 patients, with no major morbidity; 262 of these patients underwent sampling before and after administration of ovine CRH. The diagnosis of 246 patients was confirmed surgically. The results were then compared to evaluate the sensitivity and specificity of the test.

62. (1C+) **Ilias I** et al. Jugular venous sampling: an alternative to petrosal sinus sampling for the diagnostic evaluation of adrenocorticotropic hormone-dependent Cushing's syndrome. J Clin Endocrinol Metab 2004;89:3795–3800.

This study included 74 patients with surgically proven CD, 11 with surgically confirmed, and three with occult EAS. Patients underwent JVS and IPSS with administration of CRH on separate days. Ratios of central-to-peripheral ACTH in venous samples were calculated. At 100% specificity, BIPSS correctly identified 61 of 65 patients with Cushing disease (sensitivity, 94%). When patients with abnormal venous drainage were excluded, sensitivity was 98%. JVS had a sensitivity of 83% and 100% specificity. They concluded that centers with limited sampling experience may choose to use the simpler JVS and refer patients for IPSS when the results are negative.

63. (1C+) **Ilias I** et al. Cushing's syndrome due to ectopic corticotropin secretion: Twenty years' experience at the National Institutes of Health. J Clin Endocrinol Metab 2005;90:4955–4962.

A study was performed at a tertiary care clinical research center that reflect their experience with EAS from 1983 to 2004. This includes 90 patients, aged 8 to 72 years, including 48 females, who were included in the study. Imaging localized tumors in 67 of 90 patients. Surgery confirmed an ACTH-secreting tumor in 59 of 66 patients and cured 65%. This article also describes the characteristics of the biochemical testing in EAS and the mortality rate.

64. (1C+) **Swearingen B** et al. Long-term mortality after transsphenoidal surgery for Cushing's disease. Ann Intern Med 1999;130:821–824.

In total, 161 patients (129 women and 32 men; mean age, 38 years) were treated for Cushing disease between 1978 and 1996. All had transsphenoidal adenomectomy with or without adjunctive therapy. The cure rate for microadenoma was 90%. There were no perioperative deaths. Long-term survival rates were similar to those of controls matched for age and gender.

65. (1C+) **Hammer G** et al. Transsphenoidal microsurgery for Cushing's disease: Initial outcome and long-term results. J Clin Endocrinol Metab 2004;89:6348–6357.

A retrospective analysis of patients who had transsphenoidal microsurgery for Cushing disease. A median follow-up was obtained for 11.1 years. They mentioned the initial cure rate and the risk factors associated with low cure. The long-term mortality was higher in patients with persistent disease compared with the general population, whereas it was the same in patients with initial cure.

66. (1C+) **Bachicchio D** et al. Factors influencing the immediate and late outcome of Cushing's disease treated by transsphenoidal surgery: A retrospective study by the European Cushing's Disease Survey Group. J Clin Endocrinol Metab 1995;80:3114–3119.

A retrospective survey of 668 patients treated at 25 European centers. The surgical mortality rate was 1.9%, the major surgical morbidity was 14%, and the initial cure rate was 76%. The long-term cure rate was 67% during 6 to 104 months of follow-up.

67. (Review) **Vance ML.** Pituitary radiotherapy. Endocrinol Metab Clin North Am 2005;34:479–487.

A review of the various methods of pituitary radiotherapy; its efficacy and its complications.

68. **Morris D, Grossman A.** The medical management of Cushing's syndrome. Ann N Y Acad Sci 2002;970:119–133.

A review of the drugs available for treating excessive circulating glucocorticoids.

Diabetes Insipidus

69. **Pivonello R** et al. Central diabetes insipidus and autoimmunity. J Clin Endocinol Metab 2003;88:1629–1636

Central DI is considered idiopathic in approximately 33% of cases. This study evaluated 150 cases of CDI including 64 believed to be idiopathic. Autoantibodies to AVP-secreting cells were present in 33% of the idiopathic cases, with the greatest likelihood of this autoimmunity being present in patients with onset of disease at younger than 30 years, history of other autoimmune conditions, and pituitary stalk thickening on MRI.

70. **Garofeanu C** et al. Causes of reversible nephrogenic diabetes insipidus: A systematic review. Am J Kidney Dis 2005;45:626-637.

This review of 155 studies found that the most common reversible causes of NDI were medications. Lithium, antibiotics, antifungals, antineoplastic agents, and antivirals were leading causes. Hypercalcemia and hypokalemia also were reversible causes. NDI usually resolved with withdrawal of the medication or correction of the metabolic abnormality; however, NDI due to long-term lithium therapy was commonly irreversible.

71. **Robertson G.** Antidiuretic hormone: Normal and disordered function. Endocrinol Metab Clin North Am 2001;30:671–694.

This thorough review describes the physiology of antidiuretic hormone and the disease states that result from abnormal function of this substance.

Syndrome of Inappropriate Antidiuretic Hormone Secretion

72. **Robertson G.** Antidiuretic hormone: Normal and disordered function. Endocrinol Metab Clin North Am 2001;30:671–694.

This thorough review describes the physiology of antidiuretic hormone and the disease states that result from abnormal function of this substance.

73. **Miller M.** Syndromes of excess antidiuretic hormone release. Crit Care Clin 2001;17:11–23.

This article gives an excellent explanation of hyponatremia and the approach to it, particularly among the critically ill.

74. (*1C*) **Comis R** et al. Abnormalities in water homeostasis in small cell anaplastic lung cancer. Cancer 1980;45:2414–2421.

An observational study of 41 patients with small cell lung carcinoma. All patients in the study were given a standard water-load test; as a result, 68% of these patients had an abnormal test result, and 46% had clinical evidence of SIADH.

75. (*1C+*) **Sterns R** et al. Neurologic sequelae after treatment of severe hyponatremia: A multicenter perspective. J Am Soc Nephrol 1994;4:1522–1530.

A multicenter observational study of 56 patients with serum sodium levels less than 105 mM that looked at side effects of therapy that corrected the hyponatremia. This study concluded that chronic hyponatremia and rapid correction within the first 2 days significantly increased the risk of complications.

76. **Adrogue H, Madias N.** Hyponatremia. N Engl J Med 2000;342:1581–1589.

This article provides a detailed explanation of hyponatremia, including its causes, the approach to it, and its management.

77. (*1C+*) **Forrest J** et al. Superiority of demeclocycline over lithium in the treatment of chronic syndrome of inappropriate secretion of antidiuretic hormone. N Engl J Med 1978;298:173–177.

This study compared the efficacy of demeclocycline with lithium in the treatment of 10 patients with chronic SIADH. It showed that demeclocycline is more effective in treatment of this syndrome.

78. (*1C*) **Saito T** et al. Acute aquaresis by the nonpeptide arginine vasopressin (AVP) antagonist OPC-31260 improve hyponatremia in patients with syndrome of inappropriate secretion of antidiuretic hormone (SIADH). J Clin Endocrinol Metab 1997;82:1054–1057.

This was an observational study of 11 patients who were given 0.25 to 0.5 mg/kg of OPC-3160 and then observed for serum sodium levels and urine volume/osmolality. It showed that the AVP antagonist increased urine volume and decreased urine osmolality. This medication at the 0.5-mg/kg dose also increased the serum sodium concentration by 3 mEq/L. The drug's effect lasted 4 hours.

Thyroid Disorders

M. Regina Castro and Hossein Gharib

EVALUATION OF THYROID FUNCTION

Thyrotropin

Thyroid-stimulating hormone (TSH), or thyrotropin, is the single most useful measurement in the evaluation of thyroid function. Produced by the anterior pituitary, TSH stimulates the thyroid gland to produce the thyroid hormones thyroxine (T4) and triiodothyronine (T3), and its secretion is, in turn, closely regulated by the serum concentrations of these hormones. This measurement has been recommended by the American College of Physicians as a screening test in women older than 50 years, in whom the prevalence of unsuspected hypothyroidism appears to be significant [1]. TSH determination every 5 years in women and men older than 35 is a cost-effective measure to detect early thyroid failure; its diagnostic yield increases with advancing age and is higher in women than in men [2]. In hospitalized patients, however, screening with TSH leads to many false-positive results [3].

Limitations of TSH testing include the following:

- Central hypothyroidism. Measurement of TSH alone may be misleading in these patients. Central hypothyroidism is suspected when free T4 (FT4) values are low, and the TSH level is low, normal, or less elevated than would be expected in a patient with hypothyroidism [4]. In these patients, secreted TSH has reduced biologic activity but remains immunoactive in the assay [5].
- Thyrotoxicosis due to inappropriate TSH secretion. Measurement of TSH alone in patients with a TSH-secreting pituitary adenoma may be misleading. High levels of serum FT4 and T3, along with inappropriately normal or elevated serum TSH levels, an elevated α-subunit, and finding of a pituitary adenoma on MRI will confirm the diagnosis.
- Patients treated for hyperthyroidism, in whom serum TSH levels may remain suppressed for 3 months or longer after patient is clinically euthyroid. Because of this delay in recovery of the pituitary thyroid axis, during the first several months of treatment, clinical decisions should be based on measurement of FT4 and T3, until steady-state conditions are met.
- Drugs that affect serum TSH concentrations. Dopamine inhibits TSH and can reduce TSH levels in hypothyroid patients into the normal range. Glucocorti-

coids may slightly reduce TSH into the subnormal range. Short-term amio-
darone use can transiently increase TSH concentration.
- Patients with nonthyroidal illness [6] (see section on euthyroid sick syndrome).

Free Thyroxine

Thyroxine is extensively bound to plasma proteins, and only a very small fraction circulates in the free state. The free hormone fraction, however, determines its biologic
activity, making its measurement diagnostically more relevant than the total serum
level because of the many binding-protein abnormalities that can alter total thyroid
hormone levels, independent of thyroid status. Although many methods of estimation
of serum FT4 concentration are available, none, including equilibrium dialysis and
ultrafiltration, regarded as the standard criterion or reference methods, gives a true
indication of the effects of binding competitors that inhibit binding of T4 to thyroxine-
binding globulin [7].

Total Thyroxine and Triiodothyronine

Serum total T4 and T3 values reflect not only thyroid hormone production but
also serum levels of thyroid hormone–binding proteins. Discrepancy between normal
serum free and high total thyroid hormone concentrations usually reflect elevated
levels of binding proteins, a condition commonly referred to as *euthyroid hyperthyroxinemia*. T3 estimation is most useful when FT4 values are normal and TSH levels
suppressed (T3 toxicosis and subclinical hyperthyroidism) [8]. In euthyroid patients
with acute medical illness, low T3 levels may reflect decreased peripheral conversion
of T4 to T3. A high T3/T4 ratio (>20 ng/μg) suggests Graves disease as the underlying
cause of hyperthyroidism.

Thyroid Autoantibodies

The test for thyroid peroxidase antibodies (TPOAbs) is the most sensitive measurement for autoimmune thyroid disease. When they are measured by a sensitive assay,
more than 95% of patients with Hashimoto's thyroiditis and 85% of patients with
Graves disease have detectable levels of TPOAbs [8].

TSH receptor antibodies (TRAbs) can be found in most patients with Graves disease,
although such determination is seldom necessary to confirm the diagnosis. TRAbs may
be predictive of the risk of relapse of Graves hyperthyroidism after treatment with
antithyroid drugs [9]. TRAbs also are useful in predicting fetal and neonatal thyroid
dysfunction in pregnant women with a history of autoimmune thyroid disease [10].

Thyroglobulin antibody (TgAb) measurement is used primarily as an adjunct test to
serum thyroglobulin (Tg) in the follow-up of patients with differentiated thyroid cancer,
because even very low levels of these antibodies can interfere with Tg determination,
causing falsely low or high values [11]. The sudden increase or appearance of TgAbs in
a previously negative TgAb patient may be the first indication of recurrence [8].

Thyroglobulin

Thyroglobulin is the precursor of thyroid hormone synthesis and is present in the
serum of all unaffected people. Serum Tg concentrations reflect three factors: the mass
of differentiated thyroid tissue; any physical damage or inflammation of the thyroid
gland; and the level of TSH-receptor stimulation, given that most steps in Tg biosynthesis and secretion are TSH dependent [12]. An elevated Tg level is a nonspecific indicator of thyroid dysfunction. Tg is helpful in distinguishing factitious hyperthyroidism,
resulting from exogenous thyroid hormone administration and from endogenous hyperthyroidism, because in the former case, serum Tg levels are usually low, whereas in the
latter, serum Tg concentrations are typically increased. Tg measurement is used primarily as a tumor marker in the follow-up of patients with differentiated thyroid cancer
after thyroidectomy, to detect recurrent or metastatic disease. Serum Tg, measured
during TSH stimulation—endogenous TSH after thyroid hormone withdrawal or recombinant human TSH administration—is more sensitive for detecting differentiated
thyroid cancer than is basal Tg measured during LT4 suppressive therapy [13].

THYROID IMAGING

Ultrasonography

Ultrasonography (US) is the test of choice for evaluation of thyroid size and morphology; it is the most sensitive test in the detection of thyroid nodules, capable of detecting lesions 2 to 3 mm in diameter. It is also useful in guiding fine-needle aspiration (FNA) biopsies of palpable and nonpalpable thyroid nodules. US features predictive of malignancy in thyroid nodules include hypoechogenicity; presence of microcalcifications; a thick, irregular, or absent halo; irregular margins; regional adenopathy; and intranodular vascular spots [14]. US cannot, unequivocally distinguish benign from malignant nodules, and FNA is needed to confirm the diagnosis. US also is used for evaluation of regional lymph nodes, both in the preoperative assessment and in the postoperative surveillance of thyroid cancer. It has been found in some studies to be more sensitive than other surveillance modalities such as Tg measurement and whole-body scanning (WBS) [15]. The major limitations of US are the high degree of observer dependency and its inability to visualize retrotracheal, retroclavicular, or intrathoracic lesions.

Scintigraphy

Scintigraphy (using technetium 99 [^{99m}Tc]) is the standard method for functional imaging of the thyroid. The two isotopes most commonly used are iodine 123 (^{123}I) and ^{99m}Tc-pertechnetate, the latter being preferable because of lower cost and greater availability. ^{99m}Tc scanning provides a measure of the iodine-trapping function in the thyroid or in a nodule within the gland. Thyroid scanning is commonly used to demonstrate that a palpable enlargement represents an entire lobe rather than a nodule; to localize functional thyroid tissue; to identify the cause of hyperthyroidism: homogeneously increased uptake in Graves, irregular uptake in multinodular goiter or thyroid nodules; to identify functioning thyroid nodules: because "hot" or hyperfunctioning nodules are rarely malignant, such finding would obviate the need for FNA biopsy; and to follow the evolution of characteristics of nodular goiter [16].

Computed Tomography

Computed tomography (CT) scans are useful in the evaluation of thyroid cancer recurrence, especially in delineating the extent of retrosternal involvement and defining the presence and extent of lymph node metastases, tracheal invasion, compression or displacement, and vascular invasion. CT also is helpful in assessing tumors not clearly arising from the thyroid, and bulky tumors with possible invasion of local structures. CT is less sensitive than US in detecting intrathyroidal lesions.

Radioiodine Uptake

The main role of radioiodine (RAI) uptake is to evaluate hyperthyroidism, to distinguish subacute or silent thyroiditis from toxic goiter, to provide data to determine whether RAI therapy is feasible and, if so, to aid in the dose calculation. Thyroid uptake reflects a combination of iodine transport into the thyroid follicular cells, its oxidation and organification, and its release from the thyroid. Increased uptake is usually seen in association with hyperthyroidism; Hashimoto thyroiditis; iodine deficiency; subacute, silent, or postpartum thyroiditis in the recovery phase; choriocarcinoma and hydatidiform mole; and during treatment with lithium carbonate. Decreased uptake occurs after use of iodine-containing substances; in the thyrotoxic phase of subacute, silent, or postpartum thyroiditis; in Hashimoto thyroiditis with widespread parenchymal destruction; in thyroid agenesis, or after therapeutic ablation; and with the use of antithyroid drugs [16].

^{131}I Whole-Body Scanning (WBS)

^{131}I WBS is used early in the diagnostic workup of patients with suspected recurrent or metastatic thyroid cancer. Its sensitivity varies widely between studies, averaging 50% to 60%, depending on the dose of the isotope used and site of tumor location, being highest for bone and lung and lowest in lymph node metastases [17]; its overall specificity is high (90%–100%) [18]. When used in combination with Tg measurement after TSH stimulation, its sensitivity increases substantially, detecting up to 93% of cases with disease or tissue limited to the thyroid bed and 100% of cases with metastatic disease [13].

[^{18}F]Fluorodeoxyglucose Positron Emission Tomography

This imaging modality is useful in patients with suspected recurrent or metastatic thyroid cancer, in whom other imaging modalities, such as ^{131}I WBS, have failed to localize the tumor [19]. Its sensitivity in such cases approaches 94%, and its specificity, 95% [20]. It is particularly helpful in patients with Hürthle cell carcinomas, in whom this study was found to be more sensitive than WBS [21].

HYPERTHYROIDISM

Definition

Hyperthyroidism is a syndrome that results from the metabolic effects of sustained excessive circulating concentrations of thyroid hormones, T4, T3, or both. Subclinical hyperthyroidism refers to the combination of undetectable serum TSH concentration and normal serum T3 and T4 concentrations, regardless of the presence or absence of clinical symptoms.

Etiology

Hyperthyroidism may result from endogenous overproduction alone or in combination with secretion of thyroid hormones or may be iatrogenic, as a result of administration of thyroid hormones or other drugs capable of inducing thyroiditis. The most common causes of endogenous hyperthyroidism include Graves disease, toxic multinodular goiter, toxic adenoma, and thyroiditis. Subacute thyroiditis can appear in a painful (granulomatous) form, viral in origin, and a painless form, which may occur sporadically, or more commonly in the postpartum period. In this condition, a high prevalence (50%–80%) of TPOAbs in patients' sera, evidence of lymphocytic infiltration of the gland, and frequently in association with other autoimmune diseases, suggest an autoimmune etiology. Exogenous thyroid hormone, given as suppressive therapy for thyroid cancer or benign thyroid nodules, or because of overreplacement in hypothyroid patients, or surreptitious use in others, may result in overt or subclinical hyperthyroidism.

Epidemiology

Graves disease accounts for between 60% and 80% of patients with hyperthyroidism. It is up to 10 times more common in women, with highest risk of onset between the ages of 40 and 60 years. Its prevalence is similar among Caucasians and Asians and lower among blacks [22]. Autonomous adenomas and toxic multinodular goiter are more common in Europe and other areas of the world where residents are likely to experience iodine deficiency; their prevalence is also higher in women and in patients older than 60 years.

Pathophysiology

Graves disease is an autoimmune disorder in which autoantibodies bind to and stimulate the TSH receptor, resulting in increased intracellular cyclic adenosine monophosphate (cAMP) levels with subsequent thyroid growth, goiter formation, and increased thyroid hormone synthesis and secretion. With the use of more sensitive assays, these antibodies have been found in more than 90% of patients with Graves disease. The pathogenesis of toxic nodular goiter is an area of active investigation. Thyroid autonomy has been postulated as the main pathogenic mechanism in toxic adenomas and is thought to be due to somatic mutations that constitutively activate the cAMP cascade. Such mutations have been clearly described [23], and in some cases of multinodular goiter, several mutations have been documented in the same patient. Other growth factors, iodine intake, and immune mechanisms may also contribute to the pathogenesis of toxic multinodular goiter.

Diagnosis

Clinical manifestations of hyperthyroidism include nervousness, irritability, tremor, fatigue, tachycardia or palpitations, heat intolerance, and weight loss, often despite increased appetite. Atrial fibrillation, cardiac failure, and weakness also are common in older patients. In addition to these symptoms, Graves disease usually appears with a finding of a firm, diffuse goiter in up to 90% of patients, ophthalmopathy in about 50%, and in 1% to 2% with a localized dermopathy over the anterolateral aspects of the shin [22]. In patients with toxic adenoma, a palpable nodule is often found on clinical examination, whereas in toxic multinodular goiter, a firm heterogeneous goiter of variable size is more common. Some patients with multinodular goiters may have retrosternal goiters. Patients with toxic adenomas or multinodular goiters may have few or no clinical symptoms and may be diagnosed only on the basis of laboratory findings. Subacute (granulomatous) thyroiditis may first be seen with an exquisitely tender thyroid gland, often preceded by a viral upper respiratory infection, or in its more common, painless form, seen in the postpartum period, with transient hyperthyroidism, followed by a variable period of hypothyroidism and subsequent spontaneous resolution.

Laboratory findings in hyperthyroidism are summarized in Table 2.1. Suppressed TSH and elevated FT4 and FT3 levels are seen in overt hyperthyroidism, but in subclinical hyperthyroidism, serum FT4 and FT3 concentrations are typically normal. When Graves disease is suspected but the diagnosis remains uncertain, measurement of TRAb may be helpful. Patients with symptoms of hyperthyroidism, elevated FT3 and FT4 levels, and normal or elevated TSH (inappropriate TSH secretion) may have a pituitary TSH-secreting tumor, or selective pituitary resistance to thyroid hormone. Similar findings, in the absence of signs or symptoms of hyperthyroidism, may be seen in syndromes of generalized resistance to thyroid hormone. RAI uptake and scan are useful in determining the etiology of hyperthyroidism. Increased uptake in a homogeneous pattern is seen in Graves disease, whereas in subacute thyroiditis and hyperthyroidism due to exogenous thyroid hormone administration, the uptake is usually low. Patients with toxic adenomas demonstrate a localized area of increased uptake, whereas in multinodular goiter, uptake may be normal, but the pattern, heterogeneous.

Treatment

Antithyroid Drugs

Antithyroid drugs are the treatment of choice for Graves disease in most countries in the world. The most commonly used in the United States are propylthiouracil (PTU) in doses starting at 100 to 150 mg every 8 hours, and methimazole at doses from 10 to 40 mg once daily. When treating hyperthyroidism, the lowest dose needed to achieve and maintain clinical euthyroidism should be used, because higher doses have not been shown to decrease relapse rates but may increase frequency of adverse effects [24]. Methimazole has the advantage of once-daily dosing, resulting in improved compliance, but PTU is preferred during pregnancy because it is less likely to cross the placenta. Their major disadvantage is the high incidence of relapse of hyperthyroidism (≤60%) after discontinuation of therapy. Longer duration of treatment may result in higher remission rates [25], although prolonging treatment beyond 18 months does not seem to provide additional benefit [26]. Long-term treatment appears to be safe [27] and a reasonable option for patients whose hyperthyroidism can be controlled with a low dose of these drugs. Side effects include allergic reactions, hepatitis, arthritis, and agranulolysis.

Antithyroid Drugs Plus Levothyroxine LT4

A study from Japan reported a significant reduction in relapse (from 35% to <2%) with the addition of LT4 after 6 months of treatment with methimazole and continuing this drug for 3 years after methimazole was stopped [28]. A subsequent study failed to confirm these findings [29]. Although controversy exists about the usefulness of antithyroid drugs (ATDs) in Graves disease before definitive therapy with ^{131}I,

Table 2.1. Laboratory Tests for Hyperthyroidism

Etiology	Thyroid-function Tests		Radioiodine Uptake/Scan	Additional Helpful Tests
	TSH	FT4, T3		
Endogenous				
Graves disease	↓↓	↑↑	↑ or N/Homogeneous	TSI (TSAb)
Subacute thyroiditis	→	↑	↓ RAI uptake	ESR
Toxic multinodular goiter	→	N or ↑	N or ↑/Heterogeneous	US or CT
Toxic adenoma	→	N or ↑	Focal increased uptake; rest of gland may have ↓ suppressed uptake	US
Pituitary TSH adenoma	N or ↑	↑	↑/Homogeneous	Pituitary MRI; α-subunit TRH stimulation test
Exogenous				
Iodine induced (including i.v. dye and drugs such as amiodarone)	→	↑	↓↓ RAI uptake	Urinary iodine excretion
Surreptitious thyroid hormone, excessive replacement, or suppressive doses	→	↑	↓ RAI uptake	Serum thyroglobulin

such treatment does not seem to protect against worsening thyrotoxicosis, nor to affect time-to-cure or relapse rates [30].

Radioiodine (RAI)

RAI has been used for treatment of hyperthyroidism for more than six decades. It is the preferred treatment modality in the United States for patients with Graves hyperthyroidism and is commonly used throughout the world. RAI is appropriate treatment for Graves disease, toxic nodules, and toxic multinodular goiters [31]. It is effective and safe and significantly reduces thyroid volume, although patients with large goiters and severe hyperthyroidism may require several doses [32]. Its major disadvantage is development of permanent hypothyroidism in a significant proportion of patients, requiring life-long replacement with thyroid hormone. Some researchers believe that RAI therapy may transiently worsen Graves ophthalmopathy, a problem that can be reduced by administration of prednisone [33].

Surgery

Surgery is the treatment of choice for hyperthyroid patients with large goiters who have symptoms of compression, those with a coexistent suggestive thyroid nodule, for patients who have contraindications to, or refuse medical therapy or RAI, and in pregnant women, whose symptoms cannot be controlled with, or who experience allergic reactions to, antithyroid drugs. It is safe and effective, with an overall success rate of 92% [34]. Complications include hypoparathyroidism, vocal cord paralysis, and hypothyroidism.

β-Blockers

β-Blockers are useful to control the adrenergic symptoms of hyperthyroidism and may be used as initial adjunctive therapy and discontinued after definitive therapy with antithyroid drugs, RAI, or surgery have succeeded in controlling those symptoms. β-Blockers are safe and effective in the preoperative treatment of these patients and result in faster relief of hyperthyroid symptoms when compared with results of conventional preparation with antithyroid drugs [35].

HYPOTHYROIDISM

Definition

Hypothyroidism is a clinical syndrome that results from decreased thyroid hormone production and secretion, most commonly due to a disorder of the thyroid gland (primary hypothyroidism), and it is accompanied by elevated TSH levels. In fewer than 5% of patients, hypothyroidism results from hypothalamic or pituitary disease (secondary hypothyroidism), in which case, low serum thyroid hormone levels are accompanied by inappropriately normal, or even low, serum TSH levels. Subclinical hypothyroidism refers to a state in which increased serum TSH levels are accompanied by normal serum levels of FT3 and FT4, in a patient who is generally asymptomatic.

Etiology

Hashimoto thyroiditis is the leading cause of hypothyroidism. Treatment of thyrotoxicosis with ^{131}I, thyroidectomy, drugs (such as lithium and iodine-containing drugs), or contrast agents can also lead to primary hypothyroidism. Central hypothyroidism results from hypothalamic or pituitary diseases.

Epidemiology and Pathophysiology

Hypothyroidism is one of the most common endocrine disorders. Its prevalence increases with age, and it is much more common in women than in men. Up to 2% of women between 70 and 80 years of age have overt hypothyroidism. The prevalence of subclinical hypothyroidism in women older 50 years is higher, between 5% and 10% [1]. Hashimoto thyroiditis is an autoimmune disorder due to lymphocytic infiltration of the thyroid gland with subsequent atrophy of its follicular cells and fibrosis. Between 50% and 80% of patients with subclinical hypothyroidism test positive for TPOAbs.

Diagnosis

Measurement of serum TSH level is the most sensitive test to diagnose primary hypothyroidism. Patients with "subclinical hypothyroidism" have normal serum FT4 and T3 concentrations and are usually asymptomatic, whereas those with overt disease typically have low serum thyroid hormone levels and nonspecific symptoms, such as cold intolerance, weight gain, constipation, dryness of the skin, fatigue, and periorbital edema. Population screening for subclinical thyroid disease has not been universally accepted because the benefits of subsequent therapy have not been clearly established in prospective clinical trials. In central hypothyroidism, low serum thyroid hormone levels are seen along with inappropriately normal or low serum TSH levels. Pituitary MRI is recommended to exclude the presence of pituitary or hypothalamic disease or tumors.

Treatment

LT4

Levothyroxine (LT4) is the treatment of choice for hypothyroidism. The usual replacement dose is 1.6 to 4.2 mcg/kg/day and should be titrated to maintain serum TSH levels within normal range [36]. Serum TSH levels between 0.5 and 2.0 mIU/L are generally considered the optimal target [8]. Whether subclinical hypothyroidism should be treated remains controversial. Some studies suggest that early treatment may reverse mild symptoms of hypothyroidism [37] and improve serum lipids [38,39], whereas others have shown no effect in total or low-density lipoprotein (LDL) cholesterol levels [37].

LT4 plus Liothyronine (T3)

The use of combination LT4–T3 in the treatment of hypothyroidism has been proposed as an alternative to LT4-only therapy, as a more physiologic form of thyroid hormone replacement [40]. Initial reports of improved mood and neuropsychological function with this combination [40] have not been confirmed by further controlled studies [41–43], despite patients' preference for this combination in some studies [44].

THYROID NODULES

Etiology

Autonomously functioning (toxic) adenomas may occur as the result of mutations in the TSH receptor or in the gene for the α subunit of the G protein, leading to constitutive activation of the cAMP cascade and enhanced response to TSH. These mutations offer a growth and functional advantage to the cells affected, leading to development of an autonomously functioning nodule, inhibition of TSH secretion, and decreased function of the rest of the gland. Toxic multinodular goiter results from gradual multiplication of autonomous follicles with varying degrees of function.

Epidemiology

Thyroid nodules are common in clinical practice. Their prevalence largely depends on the method of screening, and the population evaluated. By palpation, the least sensitive method, their prevalence has been estimated around 4% [45]. With high-resolution US, it has been reported to be as high as 67% [46]. Autopsy data from patients with no history of thyroid disease have indicated a prevalence of 50% [47]. Increasing age, female gender, iodine deficiency, and a history of head and neck radiation seem to increase consistently the risk of developing thyroid nodules. The Framingham study estimated the annual incidence rate, by palpation, at 0.09% [45]. This means that in 2006, approximately 300,000 new nodules will be discovered in the United States.

Diagnosis

Thyroid nodules are usually discovered by palpation of the neck during routine physical examination. Most clinically palpable thyroid nodules are at least 1 cm in diameter. Nodules may be incidentally diagnosed during US of the neck done for unrelated conditions (so-called incidentalomas). TSH is the best test to determine whether a palpable nodule is hyperfunctioning; if so, TSH will be suppressed. Confirmation with scintigraphy is recommended.

FNA biopsy of thyroid nodules is the most important, cost-effective, and useful test in determining whether a nodule is benign or malignant. The mean sensitivity of FNA to detect thyroid cancer is 83% (65%–98%); its specificity, 92% (72%–100%); and overall diagnostic accuracy, 95% [48]. Its two major limitations are the inadequate or insufficient result and the suspicions or indeterminate cytologic findings, which occur in 15% and 20% of cases, respectively. Repeated US-guided biopsy may help overcome the first of these problems, but surgical excision is often needed to obtain a definitive diagnosis. Thyroid incidentalomas are common. The incidence of cancer in such nodules ranges between 6% and 9% [14]. Prevalence of cancer was similar in nodules larger or smaller than 1 cm; irregular margins on US, microcalcifications, and intranodular vascular spots were independent predictors of malignancy, and 87% of cancers presented a solid hypoechoic appearance. FNA of nodules with at least one risk factor identified 87% of cancers [14].

Treatment

Surgery

All thyroid nodules thought to be malignant and most found suspicious by FNA biopsy should be referred for surgical excision. The extent of the surgical procedure required is a matter of debate, with some authors advocating total or near-total thyroidectomy, and others supporting a more limited approach with lobectomy of the affected side. Benign solitary or multiple thyroid nodules do not require surgery, unless they produce symptoms of compression or hyperthyroidism. Surgical excision is a reasonable option for patients with large or hyperfunctioning nodules [49].

Suppressive Therapy with Levothyroxine

Controversial evidence exists regarding the effectiveness of thyroid hormone–suppressive therapy in reducing thyroid nodule size. One meta-analysis suggested an apparent therapeutic benefit of LT4 suppressive therapy in a subset (20%–23%) of patients, with 1.9 to 2.5 times greater probability of achieving at least a 50% reduction in nodule size, when compared with placebo [50]. Another report found no statistically significant effect [51]. Predictors of response have not been identified. Potential adverse effects on the cardiovascular and skeletal systems should be considered before recommending such treatment [52,53]. Suppressive therapy is not indicated for hyperfunctioning nodules. The only controlled trial of suppressive therapy in nontoxic multinodular goiters showed a better than 13% decrease in thyroid volume in 58% of patients treated with LT4 compared with only 5% of those given placebo [54].

Radioiodine Therapy

RAI is effective in reducing thyroid volume by up to 60% in patients with nontoxic multinodular goiter and in improving compressive symptoms in most of them [55]. It is successful in the treatment of nearly 90% of single toxic adenomas, although the relatively high doses usually required result in long-term hypothyroidism in 10% to 20% of cases [49]. It is also 80% to 100% effective in the treatment of toxic multinodular goiter, although often several treatments may be necessary [56].

Percutaneous Ethanol Injection (PEI)

Percutaneous ethanol injection should be reserved for patients who cannot, or will not, undergo standard therapy. Local pain, risk of recurrent laryngeal nerve damage, and the need for repeated treatments make PEI unsuitable for routine treatment of solid thyroid nodules. However, this procedure appears to be safe and effective in the treatment of predominantly cystic nodules, resulting in substantial reduction of nodule volume and amelioration of cosmetic and compressive symptoms in up to 80% of patients [57,58].

Laser Thermal Ablation (LTA)

Ultrasound-guided LTA has emerged as an alternative therapeutic option in the management of patients with benign hypofunctioning thyroid nodules associated with compressive symptoms, who are poor surgical candidates or refuse such intervention. This procedure has resulted in 45% to 60% reduction in nodule volume 6 months after treatment [59,60]. The procedure requires considerable skill of the operator and is currently performed in only a few specialized centers.

THYROID CANCER

Definition and Classification

Thyroid carcinomas are malignant neoplasms of the thyroid epithelium. Papillary and follicular cancers, collectively termed *differentiated thyroid cancer*, arise from the follicular epithelial cells. Other follicular cell–derived thyroid cancers include the oxyphilic, or Hürthle cell variant, and the undifferentiated, anaplastic carcinoma. Medullary thyroid cancer (MTC) originates from the parafollicular, calcitonin-secreting cells (C cells). Papillary thyroid cancer (PTC) is the most common histologic type in the United States, accounting for 80% of thyroid cancers, followed by follicular thyroid carcinoma (FTC) with 10% to 15%, MTC with about 5%, and anaplastic <5%. Of MTC patients, 75% have sporadic disease, and 25% have the hereditary or familial forms [multiple endocrine neoplasia 2A (MEN 2A), MEN 2B, and familial MTC].

Epidemiology

Thyroid cancer usually is first seen as a palpable nodule in the thyroid gland. Although thyroid nodules are very common, thyroid cancer is rare, constituting only 1% to 2% of all malignant neoplasms. It is 3 times more common in women than in men. Its annual incidence is approximately 0.5 to 10 per 100,000 in the world; some 18,000 new cases are diagnosed each year in the United States, resulting in nearly 1,200 annual deaths [61]. Occult thyroid cancer, defined as any unapparent tumor found on a specimen by a pathologist, has been described in 0.5% to 13% of autopsy studies in the United States. Genetic (i.e., family history of thyroid cancer) or environmental factors (i.e., exposure to ionizing radiation) may be associated with the development of thyroid cancer in some populations. Nodule size larger than 4 cm, fixation to adjacent structures, enlarged regional lymph nodes, vocal cord paralysis, rapid growth, and age younger than 15 years or older than 60 years predict a higher risk of malignancy.

Diagnosis

Thyroid Function Tests

All patients with a thyroid nodule should have serum TSH levels measured. If high, TPOAbs should be obtained to exclude coexisting Hashimoto thyroiditis. Patients with low serum TSH and elevated FT4 levels may have a toxic nodule. Because the risk of malignancy in these hyperfunctioning nodules is low, a thyroid scan confirming the hyperfunctioning status may obviate the need for FNA biopsy.

Fine-Needle Aspiration Biopsy (FNA)

Most thyroid cancers appear as a palpable thyroid nodule, often asymptomatic, and are discovered during routine examination of the neck. FNA biopsy remains the single most accurate, reliable, and cost-effective test to diagnose thyroid cancer. In the first case, repeated FNA, under US guidance, may increase the biopsy yield and provide an accurate diagnosis. However, specimens in which repeated aspiration fails to provide an adequate sample should be excised, particularly if nodules are large, solid, or have other features suggestive of malignancy. Suggestive nodules should be excised, given that the rate of malignancy in these nodules may be as high as 30% [48].

Tumor Markers

Thyroglobulin, a glycoprotein produced in the thyroid gland in response to TSH stimulation, can be reliably used as a tumor marker of differentiated thyroid cancer only after total thyroid ablation, such as after thyroidectomy and ablative ^{131}I therapy. In these cases, serum Tg, in the absence of TgAb, is a reliable marker for the local recurrence of thyroid cancer, or for nodal or distant site metastasis. Sensitivity of Tg increases with TSH stimulation, either after T4 withdrawal or recombinant TSH administration, compared to TSH suppression [12,63]. Tg measurement in needle washouts has been used to confirm the presence of metastatic thyroid cancer after FNA biopsy of suggestive cervical lymph nodes in patients with a history of thyroid cancer [64,65]. It has been found to be more sensitive than FNA cytology of lymph nodes and has the advantage of being unaffected by the presence of anti-Tg antibodies in the serum [65].

Calcitonin, a product of the parafollicular C cells, is the most sensitive marker for the diagnosis and monitoring of MTC, because most patients with MTC have elevated basal calcitonin levels, and higher levels can be found even in subclinical disease. Injection of calcitonin secretagogues, such as calcium and pentagastrin (no longer available in the United States), result in increased serum calcitonin levels in patients with MTC, allowing the early detection of C-cell hyperplasia, even before the development of MTC. Provocative testing is now replaced with genetic testing for screening first-degree relatives of patients with MTC in the setting of mutation-positive familial MTC syndromes [66]. In the 5% of families with familial MTC but an undetected genetic mutation, screening for affected members should be done with calcitonin measurement after secretagogue administration. Peak secretogogue-stimulated values greater than known reference ranges. Mild elevations in basal or stimulated calcitonin levels should be interpreted with caution.

Carcinoembryonic antigen (CEA) is a poorer biochemical tumor marker of MTC. When used along with calcitonin, it is useful for monitoring MTC, because persistent increase of these markers after curative surgery suggests residual or metastatic disease. The levels seem to correlate with tumor burden, being higher in patients with clinically evident MTC than in occult disease.

Treatment

Surgery

Surgical excision of all tumor tissue in the neck is the primary therapy for patients with thyroid cancer. The extent of the initial thyroid resection is still a matter of debate. No prospective controlled trials have been performed to settle this controversy. Although some authors argue that unilateral lobectomy is sufficient for most patients with PTC and FTC in the low-risk category, given the low cause-specific mortality and high complication rates with more extensive surgery [67], most clinicians [68–70] advocate total or near-total thyroidectomy, because it decreases local recurrence, nodal metastases, and improves disease-free survival rates [70,71]. Unilateral lobectomy results in higher overall long-term recurrence rates (30% vs. 1% after total thyroidectomy followed by ^{131}I therapy). Papillary carcinomas are often multifocal and bilateral [72].

Near-total thyroidectomy facilitates ablation with ^{131}I and further follow-up with Tg and ^{131}I WBS to detect recurrent or metastatic disease. Lobectomy alone appears to be adequate surgery for unifocal papillary microcarcinomas confined to the thyroid and without vascular invasion [69].

Total thyroidectomy with central neck lymphadenectomy is recommended in all patients with biopsy-proven or suspected MTC, because patients with familial MTC have bilateral multifocal disease, and those presumed to have sporadic disease represent the index case of familial MTC 10% to 20% of the time.

Radioiodine Remnant Ablation

Despite the widespread use of RAI in the postoperative treatment of patients with differentiated thyroid cancer, the indication for initial ablation and subsequent ^{131}I diagnostic and therapeutic interventions remains unclear, because of lack of controlled, prospective studies. Most retrospective studies have shown decreased recurrence and disease-specific mortality with the early use of adjunctive ^{131}I therapy [69,73]. In a review of 1,599 patients followed at the M.D. Anderson Cancer Center, treatment with ^{131}I was the single most powerful prognostic indicator for disease-free interval and increased survival [55]. Advantages of ^{131}I remnant ablation are as follows:

- Elimination of residual uptake in the thyroid bed, facilitating ^{131}I concentration by cervical or pulmonary metastases.
- Facilitation of high TSH levels needed to enhance optimal tumor ^{131}I uptake.
- Allowing use of Tg as reliable tumor marker in the absence of any residual normal thyroid tissue.

[131]I WBS also is used in the follow-up of thyroid cancer patients, to evaluate for the presence of residual or metastatic disease. Although therapeutic doses of ^{131}I have been the standard of care in the treatment of recurrent or metastatic disease detected by diagnostic WBS, the benefit of treating Tg-positive, whole-body scan–negative patients remains unclear. Such therapy may reduce tumor burden, but reduction in morbidity or mortality has not been demonstrated, and potential side effects may negate any benefit.

Thyroid Hormone Suppression of TSH

Decreased recurrence rates have been seen in thyroid cancer patients treated with LT4 as adjuvant therapy compared with findings in patients who did not receive such treatment [69,73,74]. In addition, one study found that constant TSH suppression to 0.05 mU/ml or less resulted in a longer relapse-free survival than when TSH levels were 1 mU/ml or higher and that the degree of TSH suppression was an independent predictor of recurrence [75]. However, no controlled study has yet determined the optimal level of TSH suppression that produces maximal survival benefit while minimizing potential adverse effects of prolonged suppressive therapy.

EUTHYROID SICK SYNDROME

Definition and Etiology

The term *euthyroid sick syndrome* (ESS) refers to abnormalities in thyroid function tests seen in patients with serious systemic nonthyroidal illnesses. There are often the result of variable disturbances in the hypothalamopituitary–thyroid axis, thyroid hormone binding to serum proteins, tissue uptake, or thyroid hormone metabolism [76]. The most common abnormalities include low serum T3 and increased reverse T3 levels, and with more severe and prolonged illness, T4 levels also decrease, portending a worse prognosis. TSH levels are usually normal but may be mildly or frankly suppressed.

Pathophysiology

Although the mechanisms of the abnormalities found in ESS are not clear, several pathogenic factors have been implicated, including decreased peripheral T4 to T3 conversion, abnormalities in serum thyroid-binding proteins, decreased TRH response and TSH release, low tissue uptake, altered metabolism of thyroid hormones, and increased circulating cytokines.

Diagnosis

Exclusion of thyroid disease in acutely ill patients may be challenging. Nonthyroidal illnesses may demonstrate a spectrum of thyroid-function abnormalities, commonly seen in patients with intrinsic thyroid pathology. Low serum T3 levels with normal T4 and TSH levels are the most common finding in ESS. Serum TSH levels are typically normal or mildly reduced in 80% of patients. A previous history of thyroid disease, external irradiation, presence of a goiter, or midline neck scar may point to a true primary thyroid condition. In general, it is best not to rely on any single thyroid-function test in the setting of nonthyroidal illnesses [76] and to wait until after recovery from nonthyroidal illnesses before evaluating thyroid status. TSH testing in hospitalized patients may be fairly inaccurate, resulting in low yield of true-positive and many false-positive results [3]. A study of 1,580 medical inpatients, evaluated with TSH on admission, found that 17% had abnormal levels; after monitoring 63% of those with abnormal results and retesting after resolution of illness, 85% were found to be euthyroid [6]. False-positive results are usually due to acute nonthyroidal illnesses and drug interactions, especially glucocorticoids.

Treatment

Triiodothyronine Replacement

Given the increased mortality seen in patients with severe nonthyroidal illnesses and low T4 values [77], some studies have evaluated the effect of thyroid hormone therapy in such patients. A controlled study showed that T3 administration to patients undergoing coronary bypass procedures improves cardiac hemodynamics as well as decreases postoperative ischemia, inotropic requirements, mortality rate, and length of hospital stay [78]. Another study failed to confirm such benefits [79].

REFERENCES

Evaluation of Thyroid Function

Thyroid-Stimulating Hormone

1. *(1C)* **Helfand M, Redfern CC**. Screening for thyroid disease: An update: Clinical guideline, Part 2. Ann Intern Med 1998;129:144–158.

   This study evaluated the benefits of screening asymptomatic patients for thyroid dysfunction with a sensitive TSH test and evaluated the efficacy of treatment for subclinical thyroid dysfunction in the general adult population. Thirty-three studies of screening and 23 controlled studies on treatment of subclinical thyroid dysfunction were included. Screening can detect symptomatic, unsuspected overt thyroid dysfunction, with highest yield in women older than 50 years. In this group, one in 71 women screened could benefit from relief of symptoms. Evidence of the efficacy of treatment for subclinical thyroid dysfunction is inconclusive.

2. *(2C)* **Danese MD** et al. Screening for mild thyroid failure at the periodic health examination: A decision and cost-effective analysis. JAMA 1996;276:285–292.

   This cost–utility analysis was undertaken to estimate cost-effectiveness of periodic screening for mild thyroid failure by measuring serum TSH levels in hypothetical cohorts of women and men screened every 5 years during the periodic examination, beginning at age 35 years. The cost-effectiveness of screening 35-year-old patients with a serum TSH every 5 years was $9,223 per quality-adjusted life years (QALYs) for women and $22,595 per QALY for men; it improved when age at first screening was increased for both genders and was always more favorable for women. Reduced progression to overt hypothyroidism and relief of symptoms increased QALYs, but they did not reduce direct medical costs. The cost-effectiveness of screening for mild hypothyroidism compares favorably with other accepted preventive medical practices

3. *(2C)* **Attia J** et al. Diagnosis of thyroid disease in hospitalized patients. Arch Intern Med 1999; 159:658–665.

   A systematic review of the literature from 1966 to 1996 was undertaken to estimate the prevalence of undiagnosed thyroid disease, to review the usefulness of clinical signs and symptoms, and to elucidate characteristics of sensitive TSH testing among inpatients. Results indicated that the prevalence of thyroid disease among inpatients is 1% to 2%, similar to that of the outpatient population. Absence of clinical features of thyroid disease reduces the pretest likelihood and makes screening even less useful. Presence of clinical features specific for thyroid disease may increase pretest likelihood and yield of testing. Acute illness reduces the specificity of sensitive TSH tests. The positive likelihood ratio of an abnormal TSH result in ill inpatients is about 10 compared with about 100 in outpatients.

4. **Ross DS**. Serum thyroid stimulating hormone measurement for assessment of thyroid function and disease. Endocrinol Metab Clin North Am 2001;30:245–264.

   This review article, covering advantages, usefulness, and limitations of serum TSH assessment, describes several clinical situations in which measurement of TSH as the single test of thyroid function may not provide an accurate estimation of true thyroid functional status. It also provides an overview of subclinical thyroid disease, its epidemiology, natural history, and clinical significance.

5. **Faglia G** et al. Thyrotropin secretion in patients with central hypothyroidism: Evidence for reduced biological activity of immunoreactive thyrotropin. J Clin Endocrinol Metab 1979;48:989–998.

   This prospective cohort study evaluated the function of the pituitary–thyroid axis and the significance of normal or elevated TSH levels in 89 patients with documented hypothyroidism secondary to diverse hypothalamic–pituitary disorders. Serum TSH levels were measured in all patients before and after i.v. administration of 200 mg of TRH. Basal plasma TSH levels were below 1.0 mIU/ml in 35%, between 1.0 and 3.6 mIU/ml in 40%, and slightly elevated (3.7–9.7 mIU/m) in 25% of the cases. TSH response to TRH was absent in 14%, impaired in 17%, normal in 47%, and exaggerated in 23% of the cases, with delayed or prolonged response in 65% of the cases. Serum T3 response to TRH was absent or low in 40 of 53 patients evaluated. Administration of T3 (100 mg/day for 3 days) or dexamethasone (3 mg/day for 5 days), respectively, suppressed or reduced both basal and TRH-induced plasma TSH levels.

6. **Spencer C** et al. Specificity of sensitive assays of thyrotropin (TSH) used to screen for thyroid disease in hospitalized patients. Clin Chem 1987;33:1391–1396.

This prospective controlled cohort study examined the specificity and clinical usefulness of TSH measurement for evaluating thyroid function in 1,580 hospitalized patients and 109 outpatient control subjects with no history or biochemical evidence of thyroid disease. Seventeen percent of hospitalized patients had abnormal TSH results (mean, ± 3 SD) when compared with the log values of normal controls (0.35–6.7 mIU/L). TSH was undetectable (<0.1 mIU/L) in 3% of patients and high (>20 mIU/L) in 1.6%. On follow-up of 329 patients, of whom 62% had abnormal TSH concentrations, only 24% of those with undetectable TSH levels had thyroid disease: 36% were receiving steroids, and 40% had nonthyroidal illnesses. Although half these patients with TSH that exceeded 20 mIU/L had thyroid disease, in 45% of these, the high TSH level was associated with nonthyroidal illnesses and normalized after recovery. TSH sensitivity was 91% when the mean ± 3 SD limits of reference population were used.

Free T4 and Free T3

7. **Stockigt JR**. Free thyroid hormone measurement: A critical appraisal. Endocrinol Metab Clin North Am 2001;30:265–289.

This article reviews the advantages of free thyroid hormone determination, changes in binding proteins that may result in abnormal total thyroid hormone levels and their underlying causes; describes available assays to determine free thyroid hormone levels, advantages and limitations of each, and circumstances in which FT4 levels may be affected, requiring cautious interpretation.

8. **Demers LM, Spencer CA**. Laboratory medicine practice guidelines: Laboratory support for the diagnosis and monitoring of thyroid disease. Clin Endocrinol 2003;58:138–140.

Excellent detailed review on clinical usefulness, methodology, pitfalls, and recommendations on the use of all available tests of thyroid function for the practicing clinician and bioanalyst.

Thyroid Autoantibodies

9. *(1C)* **Feldt-Rasmussen U** et al. Meta-analysis evaluation of the impact of thyrotropin receptor antibodies on long term remission after medical therapy of Graves disease. J Clin Endocrinol Metab 1994;78:98–102.

This meta-analysis reviewed the evidence of 10 prospective and eight retrospective studies including a total of 1,524 patients. The prospective studies demonstrated a 65% risk reduction (RR) in relapse in TRAb-negative patients compared with those with positive antibodies after antithyroid drug therapy. An even greater RR (92%) was seen in retrospective studies. Overall RR was 78% (all studies).

10. **Matsura N** et al. TSH-receptor antibodies in mothers with Graves' disease and outcome in their offspring. Lancet 1988;1:14–17.

Blood was taken from 56 selected newborn babies whose mothers had Graves disease to assess the relation between their thyroid function and the presence of TSH-binding inhibitor immunoglobulins (TBIIs) and TSAbs in maternal serum. All the mothers of these thyrotoxic babies had both antibodies in their serum. Most of the mothers whose thyroid function had been well controlled in pregnancy gave birth to unaffected babies. Fifteen babies had a transient syndrome of low serum T4 and FT4 with normal TSH levels, which tended to be associated with TSH-receptor antibodies in maternal serum (TBII, nine of 15; TSAb, four of 15). Two infants had transient hyperthyroxinemia without hyperthyroidism, and both their mothers showed strong TSAb activity without TBII activity.

11. **Spencer CA** et al. Serum thyroglobulin autoantibodies: Prevalence, influence on serum thyroglobulin measurement, and prognostic significance in patients with differentiated thyroid carcinoma. J Clin Endocrinol Metab 1998;83:1121–1127.

This case–control study investigated the prevalence of TgAb in a normal and differentiated thyroid cancer patient population and the influence of TgAb on serum Tg measurement in 4,453 healthy control subjects and 213 patients with differentiated thyroid cancer. TgAbs and TPOAbs were measured in all differentiated thyroid cancer patients and controls. Serum Tg and TgAb levels were measured in 15 TgAb-negative sera and in 97 TgAb-positive sera. The prevalence of thyroid autoantibodies was increased threefold in patients with differentiated thyroid cancer compared with the general population (40% vs. 14%). Serum TgAb was present in 25% of differentiated thyroid cancer patients and 10% of controls. Serial postsurgical serum TgAb and Tg patterns correlated with presence or absence of disease. TgAb interference was found in 69% of TgAb-positive sera and was more frequent and severe in sera containing high TgAb levels.

Thyroglobulin

12. **Spencer CA, Wang CC**. Thyroglobulin measurement: Technique, clinical benefits, and pitfalls. Endocrinol Metab Clin North Am 1995;24:841–863.

This article reviews in detail advantages, clinical usefulness, and potential pitfalls of Tg measurement as a serum marker in the management of patients with thyroid cancer.

13. *(1A)* **Haugen BR** et al. A comparison of recombinant human thyrotropin and thyroid hormone withdrawal for the detection of thyroid remnant or cancer. J Clin Endocrinol Metab 1999;84: 3877–3885.

This randomized clinical trial compared the effect of recombinant TSH (rTSH) with thyroid hormone withdrawal on the results of ^{131}I WBS and serum Tg levels in 229 adult patients with differentiated thyroid cancer requiring ^{131}I WBS. Patients received 0.9 mg rTSH every 24 hours for two doses (arm I) or every 72 hours for three doses (arm II). Twenty-four hours after the second or third dose, respectively, 4 mCi ^{131}I was given, and a whole-body scan was obtained 48 hours later. At least 2 weeks after the second or third dose, patients were withdrawn from LT4, and when TSH was over 25 mU/L, 4 mCi ^{131}I was administered and WBS performed 48 hours later. ^{131}I WBS results were concordant between the rTSH-stimulated and LT4-withdrawal phases in 89% of patients. Of the discordant scans, 4% of results were superior after rTSH administration, and 8%, after LT4 withdrawal. Based on a serum Tg level above 2 ng/ml, thyroid tissue or cancer was detected during LT4 therapy in 22%; after rTSH stimulation in 52%; and after LT4 withdrawal in 56% of patients with disease or tissue limited to the thyroid bed, and in 80%, 100%, and 100% of patients, respectively, with metastatic disease. Combination of ^{131}I WBS and serum Tg after rTSH stimulation detected thyroid tissue or cancer in 93% of patients with disease or tissue limited to the thyroid bed and in 100% of those with metastatic disease.

Thyroid Imaging

Ultrasound

14. *(1C)* **Papini E** et al. Risk of malignancy in nonpalpable thyroid nodules: Predictive value of ultrasound and color Doppler features. J Clin Endocrinol Metab 2002;87:1941–1946.

This study evaluated 494 patients with nonpalpable hypofunctioning thyroid nodules, identified by US and color Doppler, in clinically euthyroid subjects, over a 5-year period. All patients had FNA biopsy of the nodules. Patients with suggestive or malignant cytology underwent surgery. Thyroid cancer was found in 9% of solitary nodules and 6% of multinodular goiters, and its prevalence was similar in nodules both larger and smaller than 10 mm (9% vs. 7%). At US, 87% of cancers presented as a solid hypoechoic appearance. Irregular margins (RR, 16.83), intranodular vascular spots (RR, 14.29), and microcalcifications (RR, 4.97) were independent predictors of malignancy. FNA of hypoechoic nodules with at least one risk factor identified 87% of cancers.

15. *(1C)* **Frasoldati A** et al. Diagnosis of neck recurrences in patients with differentiated thyroid carcinoma. Cancer 2003;97:90–96.

In this cohort study, the authors compare the sensitivity of Tg measurement after LT4 withdrawal, ^{131}I WBS, and US in the diagnosis of DTC neck recurrences in 494 DTC patients, after total thyroidectomy and subsequent radioablative ^{131}I treatment. Mean follow-up time was 55.1 ± 37.7 months. Neck DTC recurrences were detected in 51 (10.3%) patients and occurred after 44.6 ± 21.4 months from initial treatment. Serum Tg levels increased (≥2 ng/ml) off LT4 therapy in 29 patients (sensitivity, 56.8%), ^{131}I WBS showed neck uptake in 23 patients (sensitivity 45.1%), coexisting distant metastases were detected in nine of 23 patients, and US identified neck recurrence in 48 patients (sensitivity, 94.1%). Neck US is more sensitive than traditional techniques for surveillance of DTC patients, detecting recurrences even in patients with undetectable serum Tg levels and negative whole-body scan, and is recommended as the first-line test in the follow-up of all DTC patients.

Scintigraphy

16. **Meier DA, Kaplan MM**. Radioiodine uptake and thyroid scintiscanning. Endocrinol Metab Clin North Am 2001;30:291–313.

This article reviews current uses of radioactive iodine uptake testing and radionuclide thyroid scanning in thyroid conditions other than thyroid cancer.

17. **Gallowitsch HJ** et al. Thyroglobulin and low-dose iodine-131 and technetium-99m tetrosfosmin whole-body scintigraphy in differentiated thyroid carcinoma. J Nucl Med 1998;39:870–875.

This study was undertaken to compare low-dose ^{131}I scanning and ^{99m}Tc WBS, by using Tg-off-LT4 as a basis for comparison in 58 patients with differentiated thyroid cancer ablated with thyroidectomy and ^{131}I therapy. ^{131}I revealed 19 of 44 tumor sites and three remnants. Sensitivity showed decreasing values for local recurrences (57%), bone (54%), mediastinal (50%), lung (43%), and lymph node (22%) metastases. Moreover, ^{99m}Tc WBS revealed a total of 39 (89%) of 44 malignant lesions. Sensitivity was superior for lung (100%), mediastinal (100%), and lymph node metastases (90%) and inferior for bone metastases (85%). Local recurrences were detected in 86% of patients, and thyroid remnants in 18%. Tg-off-LT4 detected malignant recurrence or metastases in 95% of patients when a cutoff of 3 ng/ml was used, and in 84% by using a cutoff of 10 ng/ml. Specificity was 72% for a cutoff of 0.5 ng/ml, 90% for cutoff of 3 ng/ml, and 100% if a cutoff of 10 ng/ml was used.

18. **Haugen BR, Lin EC**. Isotope imaging for metastatic thyroid cancer. Endocrinol Metab Clin North Am 2001;30:469–492.

This excellent article provides a review of all different isotope imaging modalities currently available for the evaluation of metastatic thyroid cancer, with indications, advantages, and weaknesses of each modality, and provides a suggested algorithm for imaging patients with suspected thyroid cancer recurrence or metastases.

Positron Emission Tomography with [18F]Fluorodeoxyglucose

19. *(2C)* **Hooft L** et al. Diagnostic accuracy of ^{18}F-fluorodeoxyglucose positron emission tomography in the follow-up of papillary or follicular thyroid cancer. J Clin Endocrinol Metab 2001;86: 3779–3786.

Systematic review to determine the diagnostic accuracy of positron emission tomography with 18-fluorodeoxyglucose–positron emission tomography (FDG-PET) in patients suspected of recurrent differentiated thyroid cancer. Fourteen studies with 10 or more subjects, evaluating the accuracy of FDG-PET in differentiated thyroid cancer, were included. All studies claimed a positive role for PET, but at evidence levels 3 or 4 (lowest), precluding quantitative analysis. Methodologic problems included poor validity of reference tests and lack of blinding of test performance and interpretation. The material was heterogeneous with respect to patient variation and validation methods. The most consistent data were found on the ability of FDG-PET to provide an anatomic substrate in patients with elevated serum Tg and negative ^{131}I scans.

20. *(1C)* **Chung JK, Lee JS.** Value of FDG PET in papillary thyroid carcinoma with negative ^{131}I whole-body scan. J Nucl Med 1999;40:986–992

This prospective study evaluated the utility of FDG-PET in localizing metastatic disease in 54 athyrotic PTC patients (33 with metastatic tumors and 21 patients in remission) with negative diagnostic ^{131}I WBS. FDG-PET revealed metastases in 31 patients (sensitivity, 94%), but Tg levels were elevated only in 18 (sensitivity, 55%). PET results were positive in 14 of 15 metastatic patients with normal Tg levels. PET results were negative in 20 patients with disease in remission (specificity, 95%), whereas Tg levels were normal in 16 patients (specificity, 76%). In patients with normal ^{131}I scans, PET detected metastases in cervical lymph nodes in 88%, lung in 27%, mediastinum in 33%, and bone in 9%. In contrast, among 117 patients with ^{131}I scan–positive functional metastases, ^{131}I scan detected metastases in cervical lymph nodes in 62%, lung in 56%, mediastinum in 22%, and bone in 16%. PET showed increased uptake in cervical or mediastinal lymph nodes in all patients with false-negative Tg results. Metastasis was confirmed in all (11) patients with increased FDG uptake in cervical lymph nodes.

21. *(1C)* **Grunwald F** et al. Fluorine-18 fluorodeoxyglucose positron emission tomography in thyroid cancer: Results of a multicentre study. Eur J Nucl Med 1999;26:1547–1552.

This study evaluates the clinical significance of [18F]FDG-PET in DTC, comparing the results with both ^{131}I WBS and [99mTc]2-methoxyisobutylisonitrile (MIBI). Whole-body PET imaging using FDG was performed in 222 patients: 134 with papillary tumors, 80 with follicular tumors, and eight with mixed-cell type tumors. Finally, clinical evaluation was done including histology, cytology, Tg level, US, CT, and subsequent clinical course, to allow comparison with functional imaging results. Sensitivity of FDG-PET was 75% and 85% for the whole patient group and for the group with negative ^{131}I whole-body scans, respectively. Specificity was 90% in the whole patient group. Sensitivity and specificity of WBS were 50% and 99%, respectively. When results of FDG-PET and WBS were considered in combination, tumor tissue was missed in only 7%.

Hyperthyroidism

22. **Weetman AP.** Graves' disease. N Engl J Med 2000;343:1236–1248.

This excellent review covers the pathogenesis of Graves disease, predisposing genetic and environmental factors, epidemiology, clinical manifestations, diagnosis, natural history, therapeutic options, management during pregnancy, and treatment of ophthalmopathy.

23. **Russo D** et al. Genetic alterations in thyroid hyperfunctioning adenomas. J Clin Endocrinol Metab 1995;80:1347–1351.

Thirty-seven thyroid autonomously hyperfunctioning adenomas were screened for mutations in the TSH receptor (TSHR), G alpha s (gsp), and ras genes. Polymerase chain reaction–amplified fragments of the TSHR C-terminal part (exon 10), gsp (exons 8 and 9), and the three ras genes were obtained from the genomic DNA extracted from 37 tumors and their adjacent normal tissues and were studied by direct nucleotide sequencing and hybridization with synthetic probes. A point mutation in the third intracellular loop (codon 623) of the TSHR was found in three (10%) of 37 adenomas studied. This mutation codes for a change in the TSHR structure and is somatic and heterozygotic. Constitutive activation of the TSHR was demonstrated by an increase in basal cAMP levels after transfection of CHO cells with a mutated Ser 623-TSHR complementary DNA. Nine gsp- and one ras-activating mutations also were detected. No simultaneous alteration of the studied genes was present.

Antithyroid Drugs

24. *(1A)* **Reinwein D** et al. A prospective randomized trial of antithyroid drug dose in Graves' disease therapy. J Clin Endocrinol Metab 1993;76:1516–1521.

This prospective, randomized, multicenter trial evaluated whether higher doses of methimazole result in higher long-term remission rates of hyperthyroidism in Graves disease in 309 patients with Graves disease from 18 thyroid clinics in Europe. Patients were given methimazole, 10 or 40 mg, with LT4 for 1 year with 1 year of follow-up. Both doses were equally effective in achieving remission, although euthyroidism was achieved by 3 weeks at higher dosages. No difference was found in relapse rates between the two groups (36% vs. 37%) or in length of time between stopping treatment and relapse, but the rate of adverse reactions was significantly higher in the 40-mg group (26% vs. 15%).

25. *(1A)* **Allannic H** et al. Antithyroid drugs and Graves' disease: A prospective randomized evaluation of the efficacy of treatment duration. J Clin Endocrinol Metab 1990;70:675–679.

This prospective randomized clinical trial compared the efficacy of 18 months versus 6 months of antithyroid drug therapy on remission rates of Graves hyperthyroidism in 94 patients with Graves disease. Carbimazole was given in doses needed to maintain clinical euthyroidism for 6 months (group 1) or 18 months (group 2). Treatment for 18 months resulted in higher remission rates 2 years after discontinuation of treatment (62% vs. 42%; $p < 0.05$).

26. *(1A)* **Maugendre D** et al. Antithyroid drugs and Graves' disease-prospective randomized assessment of long-term treatment. Clin Endocrinol 1999;50:127–132.

This prospective, randomized trial was undertaken to determine benefits of a 42-month compared with an 18-month treatment with carbimazole. The population comprised 142 patients with Graves disease who were given carbimazole at doses needed to achieve euthyroidism for 18 months (group 1) or 42 months (group 2). No difference in relapse rate was found between the two groups (36% vs. 29%, NS), or in percentage of TPOAb-positive patients (53% vs. 46%; p = NS); The percentage of patients with TSAb was lower in group 2 (18% vs. 42%; p = 0.004) at treatment discontinuation.

27. *(1A)* **Azizi F** et al. Effect of long-term continuous methimazole treatment of hyperthyroidism: Comparison with radioiodine. Eur J Endocrinol, 2005;152:695–701.

In this prospective, randomized study, the authors investigated the long-term effects of continuous methimazole (MMI) therapy in 104 patients whose hyperthyroidism recurred within 1 year after discontinuing 18 months of MMI treatment. They were randomized into two groups for continuous ATD and RAI treatment. Numbers of occurrences of thyroid dysfunction and total costs of management were assessed during 10 years of follow-up. At the end of the study, 26 patients were still receiving continuous MMI (group 1), and of 41 ^{131}I-treated patients (group 2), 16 were euthyroid, and 25 became hypothyroid. No significant difference in age, sex, duration of symptoms, and thyroid function was found between the two groups. No serious complications occurred in any of the patients. The cost of treatment was lower in group 1. At the end of 10 years, goiter rate was greater and TPOAb concentration was higher (RR, 1.8) in group 1 than in group 2. Serum total and LDL-cholesterol concentrations were higher (RR, 1.6) in group 2. The authors conclude that long-term treatment of hyperthyroidism with MMI is safe and that complications and expense of the treatment do not exceed those of ^{131}I therapy.

Antithyroid Drugs Plus LT4

28. *(2B)* **Hashizume K** et al. Administration of thyroxine in treated Graves' disease: Effects on the level of antibodies to thyroid-stimulating hormone receptors and on the risk of recurrence of hyperthyroidism. N Engl J Med 1991;324:947–953.

This prospective randomized, placebo-controlled study evaluated the effectiveness of LT4 in decreasing TSAb levels and rate of recurrence of Graves hyperthyroidism after normalizing thyroid hormone secretion with methimazole (MMI) in 109 patients with untreated Graves hyperthyroidism. All patients received MMI and were euthyroid by 6 months. Patients were randomly assigned to receive 100 μg of LT4 and 10 mg of methimazole, or to placebo and 10 mg of MMI. After 1 year, MMI was discontinued; LT4 or placebo was continued for 3 more years. TSAb levels decreased after 1 month of treatment with LT4 and MMI but did not change in patients receiving placebo and MMI ($p < 0.01$). After withdrawal of MMI, TSAb levels decreased further in patients receiving LT4 but increased in those receiving placebo ($p < 0.01$). Within 3 years of discontinuing MMI, hyperthyroidism recurred in 2% of patients receiving LT4 and in 35% of those receiving placebo ($p < 0.001$).

29. (2B) **McIver B** et al. Lack of effect of thyroxine in patients with Graves' hyperthyroidism who are treated with an antithyroid drug. N Engl J Med 1996;334:220–224.

This prospective, randomized controlled trial evaluated whether addition of LT4 to antithyroid drug therapy in Graves disease reduces relapse rates of hyperthyroidism in 111 patients with Graves hyperthyroidism. All patients received 40 mg of carbimazole (CBZ) daily for 1 month. Next, one group received CBZ for 17 months, and the other group received CBZ plus LT4 for 17 months, followed by LT4 alone for 18 months. In the CBZ group, this dosage was adjusted to maintain normal serum TSH levels. In the CBZ–LT4 group, the dose of CBZ was not changed, but 100 mg of LT4 was added and the dosage adjusted to maintain serum TSH levels to less than 0.04 mIU/ml. At the time of analysis, 53 patients had completed at least 3 months of follow-up (median, 12 months) after withdrawal of CBZ. Hyperthyroidism recurred in eight patients in each group with no difference in relapse rates between the groups.

30. **Andrade VA** et al. The effect of methimazole pretreatment on the efficacy of radioactive iodine therapy in Graves' hyperthyroidism: One year follow up of a prospective randomized study. J Clin Endocrinol Metab 2001;86:3488–3493.

This study evaluated the effect of MMI pretreatment on the efficacy of ^{131}I therapy in 61 untreated patients with Graves hyperthyroidism. Exclusion criteria included previous treatment with ^{131}I or thyroidectomy, signs of moderate or severe ophthalmopathy, severe heart disease, debilitating conditions, and large, compressive goiters. [131]I alone (n = 32) or ^{131}I plus pretreatment with methimazole

(30 mg/day; n = 29). [131]I was administered 4 days after drug discontinuation. The calculated ^{131}I dose was 200 μCi/g thyroid tissue as estimated by US, corrected by 24-hour ^{131}I uptake. Serum TSH, T4, and FT4 levels were measured 4 days before ^{131}I therapy, on the day of treatment, and then monthly for 1 year. About 80% of patients from both groups were cured (euthyroid or hypothyroid) 3 months after ^{131}I treatment. After 1 year, the groups were similar in terms of persistent hyperthyroidism (16% vs. 14%), euthyroidism (28% vs. 31%), or hypothyroidism (56% vs. 55%). Relapsed patients had larger thyroid volume (p = 0.002) and higher 24-hour ^{131}I uptake (p = 0.022) and T3 levels (p = 0.002). Multiple logistic regression analysis identified T3 values as an independent predictor of therapy failure.

Radioiodine

31. **Kaplan MM** et al. Treatment of hyperthyroidism with radioactive iodine. Endocrinol Metab Clin North Am 1998;27:205–223.

    This article reviews advantages of ^{131}I for treatment of hyperthyroidism, selection of patients for this therapy, overview of treatment modalities, recommendations regarding pretreatment with antithyroid drugs, selection of dosage in different hyperthyroid conditions, radiation safety concerns, side effects, and follow-up of patients after treatment with radioactive iodine.

32. *(1C)* **Peters H** et al. Reduction in thyroid volume after radioiodine therapy of Graves' hyperthyroidism: Results of a prospective, randomized, multicentre study. Eur J Clin Invest 1996;26: 59–63.

    Ninety-two patients with Graves disease treated with ^{131}I were evaluated by US to assess reduction in thyroid volume. Patients received either a standard ^{131}I activity (555 MBq), or an activity calculated to deliver 100 Gy. Within 1 year of treatment, a median 71% volume reduction was observed, most of which occurred during the first 6 months. The standard group achieved a higher median dose and a more pronounced volume reduction (60% vs. 46% at 6 months, and 74% vs. 66% at 12 months, respectively) than the calculated group. The RR in thyroid size was just as marked in patients with large thyroids as in those with smaller glands, and the goiter prevalence was reduced from 73% to 16%, at 1 year after ^{131}I treatment.

33. *(1A)* **Bartalena L** et al. Relation between therapy for hyperthyroidism and the course of Graves' ophthalmopathy. N Engl J Med 1998;338:73–78.

    This randomized, controlled trial evaluated the effects of MMI, ^{131}I, and ^{131}I plus prednisone in 443 patients with Graves disease and mild (or no) ophthalmopathy. All patients received methimazole for 3 to 4 months and were then allocated to ^{131}I, ^{131}I and prednisone, or MMI. Progression or new ophthalmopathy occurred in 15% of patients treated with ^{131}I and in 3% of those receiving methimazole (p < 0.001); no patients receiving ^{131}I and prednisone developed or had progression of ophthalmopathy (p < 0.001 vs. [131]I). When ophthalmopathy was initially present, 67% of patients receiving ^{131}I plus prednisone improved compared with 4% who received methimazole (p < 0.001), and none receiving ^{131}I alone. In 65% of patients receiving only ^{131}I, transient or worsening ophthalmopathy occurred, and in 5% of patients, persistent diplopia developed.

Thyroidectomy

34. (1C+) **Palit TK** et al. The efficacy of thyroidectomy for Graves' disease: A meta-analysis. J Surg Res 2000;90:161–165.

    Meta-analysis of 35 studies including 7,241 patients who underwent either total thyroidectomy (TT) (n = 538) or subtotal thyroidectomy (ST) (n = 6,703) for Graves disease. Hyperthyroidism persisted or recurred in 7% of patients. All patients who had TT became hypothyroid. Of the patients who underwent ST, 60% became euthyroid, 25% became hypothyroid, and 8% remained hyperthyroid. Permanent recurrent laryngeal nerve injury occurred in 1% of TT patients and 0.7% of ST patients and permanent hypoparathyroidism in 1.6% and 1%, respectively. A 9% decrease in hypothyroidism and 7% increase in euthyroidism was seen for each gram of thyroid remnant (p < 0.0001). Thyroidectomy successfully treated hyperthyroidism in 92% of patients.

β-Blockers

35. *(1A)* **Jansson S** et al. Oxygen consumption in patients with hyperthyroidism before and after treatment with beta-blockade versus thyrostatic treatment: A prospective randomized study. Ann Surg 2001;233:60–64.

    This prospective, randomized controlled trial was undertaken to evaluate the effect of thyrostatic treatment (tiamazole) compared with selective (metoprolol) and nonselective (propranolol) β-blockade on whole-body metabolism in 28 hyperthyroid women undergoing surgery as treatment of their hyperthyroidism. Six euthyroid women, with benign thyroid adenomas, served as controls. Whole-body O_2 consumption and CO_2 production were measured. Tiamazole normalized O_2 consumption and induced signs of anabolism. Propranolol (not metoprolol) reduced elevated O_2 consumption by 54%. Body weight was stable after specific and nonspecific β-blockade, which led to relief of symptoms in 90% of patients.

Hypothyroidism

Levothyroxine

36. *(1C)* **Fish LH** et al. Replacement dose, metabolism and bioavailability of levothyroxine in the treatment of hypothyroidism: Role of triiodothyronine in pituitary feedback in humans. N Engl J Med 1987;316:764–770.

This prospective controlled cohort study was undertaken to determine adequate replacement dose of LT4 in 19 patients with hypothyroidism of different etiologies; 66 healthy volunteers served as controls. Results showed that the mean replacement dose was 112 ± 19 µg/day. TSH levels of patients taking LT4 replacement returned to normal when T3 concentrations were similar to those of controls but when serum T4 levels were higher than those of controls (11.3 vs. 8.7 mg/dL; $p < 0.001$)

Subclinical Hypothyroidism

37. *(2B)* **Cooper DS** et al. L-Thyroxine therapy in sub-clinical hypothyroidism: A double-blind, placebo-controlled trial. Ann Intern Med 1984;101:18–24.

Thirty-three patients with subclinical hypothyroidism were randomly assigned to receive placebo or LT4 therapy (double-blind) and observed during follow-up for 1 year with thyroid function tests, serum lipids, basal metabolic rate, and a questionnaire on hypothyroid symptoms. The placebo group showed no changes in thyroid function or indices of thyroid hormone action. In the LT4-treated group, serum lipids did not change. Symptoms improved in 57% of patients taking LT4 and in 25% patients receiving placebo ($p < 0.05$).

38. *(2B)* **Danese MD** et al. Effect of thyroxine therapy on serum lipoproteins in patients with mild thyroid failure: A quantitative review of the literature. J Clin Endocrinol Metab 2000;85:2993–3001.

Systematic review of the literature (1966–1999) assessing changes in serum lipid levels after treatment with LT4; 13 studies with 247 patients were included. The mean reduction in total cholesterol was 20.20 mmol/L (95% CI, 0.20 mmol/L; 20.09–20.34), and it was directly proportional to its baseline concentration. Studies enrolling hypothyroid undertreated subjects showed larger reductions in total cholesterol after TSH normalization than did studies of untreated patients with subclinical hypothyroidism (20.44 mmol/L vs. 20.14 mmol/L; $p = 0.05$). LDL cholesterol levels decreased 20.26 mmol/L (95% CI, 20.12–20.41). High-density lipoprotein (HDL) and triglyceride levels did not change.

39. *(2A)* **Meier C** et al. TSH-controlled L-thyroxine therapy reduces cholesterol levels and clinical symptoms in subclinical hypothyroidism: A double-blind, placebo-controlled trial. J Clin Endocrinol Metab 2001;86:4860–4866

This randomized, double-blind, placebo-controlled study evaluated the effect of physiologic, TSH-guided, LT4 treatment on serum lipids and clinical symptoms in 66 women with subclinical hypothyroidism. Treatment included LT4 with dosage guided by blinded TSH monitoring, resulting in euthyroid TSH levels (3.1 6 0.3 mIU/L) for 48 weeks. Results indicated that in the LT4 group, total and LDL cholesterol were reduced by 4% ($p = 0.015$) and 8% ($p = 0.004$), respectively. LDL-cholesterol reduction was larger in patients with TSH levels higher than 12 mIU/L or high LDL cholesterol at baseline. HDL cholesterol, triglycerides, apo-AI, and Lp(a) levels remained unchanged. Clinical scores of symptoms and signs of hypothyroidism improved ($p = 0.02$)

LT4 plus T3

40. *(2B)* **Bunevicius R** et al. Effects of thyroxine as compared with thyroxine plus triiodothyronine in patients with hypothyroidism. N Engl J Med 1999;340:424–429.

Randomized, double-blind, crossover study designed to compare the effects of LT4 alone with those of LT4 plus T3 on thyroid hormone actions in the brain, pituitary gland, and other organs in patients with hypothyroidism. Thirty-three patients receiving replacement doses of LT4 for chronic autoimmune thyroiditis ($n = 16$) or suppressive doses of LT4 after near-total thyroidectomy for thyroid cancer ($n = 17$) were randomized to receive LT4 alone for 5 weeks, then LT4 + T3 for 5 weeks, or vice versa, and then to the alternative treatment. LT4 was given as 50-µg tablets at each patient's usual total dose, but 50 µg of the dose was replaced by a capsule containing either 50 µg of LT4 or 12.5 mg of T3. On the last day of each treatment period, all patients had measurements of TSH, thyroid hormones, cholesterol, triglycerides, and SHBG, and assessments of cognitive function and psychological state. Among 17 scores on tests of cognitive performance and assessments of mood, six were better or closer to normal after treatment with LT4 + T3. Similarly, among 15 visual-analogue scales used to indicate mood and physical status, results for 10 were better after treatment with LT4 + T3.

41. *(1B)* **Sawka AM** et al. Does a combination regimen of thyroxine (T4) and 3,5,3′ triiodothyronine improve depressive symptoms better than T4 alone in patients with hypothyroidism? Results of a double-blind, randomized, controlled trial. J Clin Endocrinol Metab 2003;88:4551–4555.

This prospective, randomized, double-blind, placebo-controlled study evaluated whether combination of LT4 + T3 improves depressive symptoms better than LT4 alone in patients with hypothyroidism. Forty hypothyroid individuals with depressive symptoms taking a stable dose of LT4 were randomized to receive LT4 plus placebo or combination of LT4 plus T3 for 15 weeks. Patients receiving combination therapy had their dose of LT4 reduced by 50%, and 12.5 μg of T3 was started twice daily, and doses were adjusted to keep normal TSH levels. Compared with the group taking LT4 alone, the group taking both LT4 plus T3 did not report any improvement in self-rated mood and well-being scores that included all subscales of the Symptom Check List-90, the Comprehensive Epidemiological Screen for Depression, and the Multiple Outcome Study ($p > 0.05$ for all indexes).

42. *(1B)* **Clyde PW** et al. Combined levothyroxine plus liothyronine compared with levothyroxine alone in primary hypothyroidism: A randomized controlled trial. JAMA 2003;290:2952–2958.

    Randomized, parallel-group study design. Forty-six hypothyroid patients (most with autoimmune thyroiditis) were randomized to continue their current dose of LT4 ($n = 23$) or to receive 50 μg less than their usual LT4 dose, with the difference being replaced by T3 at a dose of 6.5 μg twice daily for 4 months ($n = 23$). LT4 doses were adjusted in both groups to maintain normal TSH levels. The HRQL questionnaire scores improved significantly in both the control group (23%; $p < 0.001$) and the combination therapy group (12%; $p = 0.02$), but these changes were statistically similar ($p = 0.54$). In 12 of 13 neuropsychological tests, outcomes between groups were not significantly different; the remaining test (Grooved Peg Board) showed better performance in the control group.

43. *(1B)* **Walsh JP** et al. Combined thyroxine/liothyronine treatment does not improve well-being, quality of life, or cognitive function compared to thyroxine alone: A randomized controlled trial in patients with primary hypothyroidism. J Clin Endocrinol Metab 2003;88:4543–4550.

    Double-blind, controlled trial with a crossover design in which 110 hypothyroid patients were randomized to receive their usual LT4 dose or substituting 10 μg of T3 for 50 μg of the patients' usual T(4) dose. No significant ($p > 0.05$) difference between LT4 and combined LT4/T3 treatment was demonstrated on cognitive function, QOL scores, Thyroid Symptom Questionnaire scores, subjective satisfaction with treatment, or eight of 10 visual analogue scales assessing symptoms. For the General Health Questionnaire-28 and visual analogue scales assessing anxiety and nausea, scores were significantly ($p < 0.05$) worse for combined treatment than for LT4 alone. Serum TSH was lower during LT4 treatment than during combined LT4/T3 treatment, a potentially confounding factor; however, subgroup analysis of subjects with comparable serum TSH concentrations during each treatment showed no benefit from combined treatment compared with LT4 alone.

44. *(1B)* **Escobar-Morreale HF** et al. Thyroid hormone replacement therapy in primary hypothyroidism: A randomized trial comparing L-thyroxine plus liothyronine with L-thyroxine alone. Ann Intern Med 2005;142:412–424.

    Twenty eight women with overt primary hypothyroidism were randomized to receive LT4 100 μg/d (standard treatment), or combination LT4 75 μg/d + T3 5 μg/d, for 8-week periods in a double-blind, crossover design. All patients also received LT4, 87.5 μg/d + T3, 7.5 μg/d (add-on combination treatment), for a final 8-week period. Primary outcomes included serum thyroid hormone levels, results of QOL and psychometric tests, and patients' preference. Combination treatment led to lower FT4 levels, slightly higher TSH levels, and unchanged FT3 levels. No improvement was observed in the other primary end points after combination treatment, with the exception of the Digit Span Test, in which the mean backward score and the mean total score increased slightly. The add-on combination treatment resulted in over-replacement. Levels of TSH decreased by 0.85 mU/L, and serum FT3 levels increased by 0.8 pmol/L compared with standard treatment; 10 patients had levels of TSH that were below the normal range. Twelve patients preferred combination treatment, six patients preferred the add-on combination treatment, two patients preferred standard treatment, and six patients had no preference ($p = 0.015$).

Thyroid Nodules

Epidemiology

45. **Vander JB** et al. The significance of nontoxic thyroid nodules: Final report of a 15 year study of the incidence of thyroid malignancy. Ann Intern Med 1968;69:537–540.

    A sample of 4,469 people from the city of Framingham, Massachusetts, randomly selected from the total population of 10,000 (in 1948), and 740 volunteers were studied with physical examination and laboratory tests every 2 years and observed for up to 15 years. Of the 5,127 participants, 4% had nontoxic thyroid nodules, none of which showed evidence of malignancy after 15 years of follow-up. The 15-year incidence rate of new thyroid nodules was 1.4%.

46. **Ezzat S** et al. Thyroid incidentalomas: Prevalence by palpation and ultrasonography. Arch Intern Med 1994;154:1838–1840.

    This prospective cohort study assessed the prevalence of thyroid nodules in the community and compared findings by palpation and HRUS in 100 asymptomatic North American subjects without known thyroid disease. Of these participants, 21% had palpable nodules (9% solitary nodules, 12% multiple nodules). By US measurement, 22% of patients had solitary nodules, and 45% had multiple nodules. The prevalence of nodules was greater in women (72% vs. 41%; $p < 0.02$). The concordance rate between US and palpation was 49%.

47. **Mortensen JD** et al. Gross and microscopic findings in clinically normal thyroid glands. J Clin Endocrinol Metab 1955;15:1270–1280.

    Thyroid glands from 1,000 subjects without previous evidence of thyroid disease were removed during routine autopsy and examined for macroscopic lesions. Sixty-six subjects were excluded because of clinical evidence that their thyroid may not have been normal and 113 others because of inadequate recording of clinical examination of the thyroid. In the remaining 821 glands, 12% contained a single nodule, and 38% had multiple nodules. The size of these nodules varied from 2 mm to 7.5 cm in diameter, and 36% of nodular glands contained one or more nodules larger than 2 cm. Benign and malignant nodules occurred with about the same frequency, but malignant nodules were more common in women, after the age of 40 years and in patients living in so-called goiter belts. Primary occult carcinoma was found in 17 patients (4% of the nodular thyroid glands).

48. *(1C+)* **Gharib H, Goellner JR**. Fine needle aspiration of the thyroid: An appraisal. Ann Intern Med 1993;118:282–289.

This article is a comprehensive review of the literature and the authors' experience with more than 11,000 biopsies on the usefulness, advantages, limitations, and diagnostic accuracy of FNA biopsy in the diagnosis and management of thyroid nodules and thyroid cancer.

49. **Hermus AR, Huysmans DA**. Treatment of benign nodular thyroid disease. N Engl J Med 1998; 338:1438–1447.

Excellent review of available treatment modalities for toxic and nontoxic uninodular and multinodular thyroid disease, including advantages and disadvantages of each modality.

LT4 Suppressive Therapy

50. *(2B)* **Csako G** et al. Assessing the effects of thyroid suppression on benign solitary thyroid nodules: A model for using quantitative research synthesis. Medicine 2000;79:9–26.

Systematic review of 30 published reports on the efficacy of LT4-suppressive therapy in solitary thyroid nodules. The study's authors also report results of a survey on the opinion of all endocrinologists working at the National Institutes of Health and perform a meta-analysis of five randomized controlled trials that met the following criteria: documentation of TSH suppression, US measurement of thyroid nodules, and assessment of clinically significant (0.50%) reduction in nodule size. The percentage of patients with nodule size reduction exceeding 50% was higher in the treatment groups than in the controls (19% vs. 10%). LT4 suppressive therapy was associated with a 2.11 (CI, 0.90–4.94; p = 0.086) to 2.49 (CI, 1.41–4.40; p = 0.008) times greater probability of achieving at least a 50% reduction in nodule size by using a random and fixed effects models, respectively; effect sizes were heterogeneous.

51. *(2B)* **Castro MR** et al. Effectiveness of levothyroxine suppressive therapy in benign solitary thyroid nodules: A meta-analysis. J Clin Endocrinol Metab 2002;87:4154–4159.

This is a systematic review of the literature and meta-analysis of a randomized controlled trial, fulfilling the following inclusion criteria: solitary thyroid nodules, benign by FNA, treatment and follow-up of at least 6 months, documented suppression of TSH, measurement of thyroid nodule volume by US, and response to therapy defined as an at least 50% reduction 50% in volume from findings at baseline. Six randomized controlled trials (1987–1999) with 346 patients were included in this meta-analysis. The overall effect size showed a relative risk of 1.9 (95% CI, 0.95–3.81) favoring a treatment effect. Results were highly sensitive to changes in statistical analysis, especially if the method used ignored heterogeneity among the effect sizes.

52. **Uzzan B** et al. Effects of bone mass of long-term treatment with thyroid hormones: A meta-analysis. J Clin Endocrinol Metab 1996;81:4278–4289.

This meta-analysis evaluated the effect of long-term LT4 therapy on bone mineral density. It includes 41 controlled, cross-sectional studies, which included about 1,250 patients. Studies with women receiving estrogen therapy were a priori excluded. Suppressive LT4 therapy was associated with significant bone loss in postmenopausal, but not in premenopausal women. Conversely, replacement therapy was associated with bone loss in premenopausal, but not in postmenopausal women. The adverse effect of LT4 was more marked on cortical than on trabecular bone.

53. *(1C)* **Sawin CT** et al. Low serum thyrotropin concentrations as a risk factor for atrial fibrillation in older persons. N Engl J Med 1994;331:1249–1252.

This was a 10-year cohort study of participants in the original Framingham Heart Study. Its purpose was to determine whether a low serum TSH level in adults 60 years of age or older is a risk factor for development of atrial fibrillation. The population consisted of 2,007 adults aged 60 years or older at baseline assessment. About 3% of participants had low (≤0.1 mU/L) TSH levels, 9% had slightly low (0.1–0.4 mU/L) levels, 79% had normal (.0.4–5.0 mU/L) levels, and 9% had high (5.0 mU/L) levels. During follow-up, atrial fibrillation developed in 192 participants. The cumulative incidence of atrial fibrillation in 10 years was 28% in the low-level group, 16% in the slightly low-level group, 11% in the normal-level group, and 15% in the high-level group. When adjusted for age, gender, and all risk factors, the relative risk for new atrial fibrillation in the low-level group compared with that in the normal-level group was 3.1 (95% CI, 1.7–5.5; p < 0.001); for the slightly low-level group, relative risk was 1.6 (CI, 1.0– to 2.5; p = 0.05). Results were similar when subjects taking thyroid hormones were excluded.

54. *(2A)* **Berghout A** et al. Comparison of placebo with L-thyroxine alone or with carbimazole for treatment of sporadic non-toxic goitre. Lancet 1990;336:193–197.

The efficacy of suppressive doses of LT4 (2.5 mg/kg/day) alone or combined with CBZ (40 mg daily) was studied in 78 patients with sporadic nontoxic goiter in a prospective, placebo-controlled, double-blind, randomized controlled trial. Treatment was given for 9 months, with 9 months of follow-up. A response to treatment as measured by US was found in 58% of the LT4 group, 35% of the LT4/CBZ group, and 5% of the placebo group. The mean reduction of thyroid volume in those who responded was 25%. After discontinuing treatment, thyroid volume increased in the responders and had returned to baseline values after 9 months of follow-up. In the placebo group, mean thyroid volume had increased by 20% at 9 months and 27% at 18 months.

Radioiodine

55. *(1C+)* **Nygaard B** et al. Radioiodine treatment of multinodular non-toxic goitre. BMJ 1993;307:828–832.

   This observational study investigated the long-term effect of ^{131}I on thyroid size and function in 69 patients with nontoxic multinodular goiter, causing compressive symptoms or cosmetic concerns, who had contraindication to, or had refused surgery. Fifty-six patients received a single dose of ^{131}I, 12 received two doses, and one received four doses. In nine of 45 patients who received one dose and remained euthyroid, median thyroid volume was reduced by 60% ($p < 0.0001$) by 24 months; half of this amelioration occurred during the first 3 months. Patients treated with two doses, and those in whom hypothyroidism developed, also had a significant reduction in thyroid volume. Cumulative 5-year risk of development of hypothyroidism was 22% (CI, 5%–38%).

56. *(1B)* **Huysmans DAKC** et al. Long-term results of two schedules of radioiodine treatment for toxic multinodular goiter. Eur J Nucl Med 1993;20:1056–1062.

   This prospective study evaluated the long-term effectiveness of low-dose [131]I (150 MBq; group A) and of calculated dose adjusted for thyroid weight (1.85–3.7 MBq/g; group B) in 103 patients with toxic multinodular goiter. Mean follow-up was 4 to 5 years. Hyperthyroidism was successfully reversed in 73% of group A and 88% of group B, with development of hypothyroidism in 7% in each group. Patients treated with calculated doses required significantly fewer treatments (1.3 ± 0.1 vs. 2.2 ± 0.2), and the percentage of patients adequately treated with a single dose was more that twice as high in group B (66% vs. 27%). Euthyroidism was achieved sooner with calculated doses (0.6 years in group B vs. 1.5 years in group A).

Percutaneous Ethanol Injection

57. *(1C)* **Valcavi R, Frasoldati A**. Ultrasound-guided percutaneous ethanol injection therapy in thyroid cystic nodules. Endocr Practice 2004;10:269–275.

   Controlled randomized study involving 281 patients with benign thyroid cystic nodules. Inclusion criteria were local discomfort or cosmetic damage, cystic volume more than 2 ml, 50% or more fluid component, benignity confirmed by US-guided FNA biopsy, and euthyroidism. Exclusion criteria were inadequate, suggestive, or positive FNAB cytology, high serum calcitonin, and contralateral laryngeal cord palsy. By random assignment, 138 patients underwent simple cyst evacuation, and 143 underwent cyst evacuation plus PEI. The amount of ethanol injected was 50% to 70% of the cystic fluid extracted. Before treatment, the mean nodule volume was similar in both groups (21.0 ml PEI vs. 20.0 ± 13.4 ml in simple evacuation group). After 1 year, volumes were 5.5 ± 11.7 ml vs. 16.4 ± 13.7 ml ($p < 0.001$), with a median 85.6% versus 7.3% reduction, respectively ($p < 0.001$), of the initial volume. Compressive and cosmetic symptoms disappeared in 74.8% and 80.0% of patients treated with PEI versus 24.4% and 37.4% of patients treated with simple evacuation, respectively ($p < 0.001$). Side effects were minor.

58. *(1A)* **Bennedbaek FN, Hegedus L**. Treatment of recurrent thyroid cysts with ethanol: A randomized double-blind controlled trial. J Clin Endocrinol Metab 2003;88:5773–5777.

   Sixty-six consecutive patients with recurrent and benign thyroid cysts (≥2 ml) were randomly assigned to either subtotal cyst aspiration, flushing with 99% ethanol, and subsequent complete fluid aspiration ($n = 33$), or to subtotal cyst aspiration, flushing with isotonic saline, and subsequent complete fluid aspiration ($n = 33$). In case of recurrence (defined as cyst volume >1 ml) at the monthly evaluations, the treatment was repeated but limited to a maximum of three treatments. Procedures were US-guided, and patients were followed up for 6 months. Cure (defined as a cyst volume ≤1 ml at the end of follow-up) was obtained in 82% of patients treated with ethanol and in 48% of patients treated with saline ($p = 0.006$). In the ethanol group, 64% of patients were cured after one session only, compared with 18% in the saline group ($p = 0.002$). The chance of success decreased with the number of previous aspirations and with increasing cyst volume. Seven patients (21%) treated with ethanol had moderate to severe pain (median duration, 5 min), and one had transient dysphonia. Indirect laryngoscopy was performed before and after the last session and was normal in all patients. Flushing with ethanol may be a reasonable nonsurgical alternative for thyroid cysts that recur despite repeated aspirations.

Laser Thermal Ablation

59. *(2C)* **Dossing H** et al. Effect of ultrasound-guided interstitial laser photocoagulation on benign solitary solid cold thyroid nodules: A randomized study. Eur J Endocrinol 2005;152:341–345.

   Thirty euthyroid outpatients with a benign cold solitary solid thyroid nodule causing local discomfort were prospectively randomized to one session of LTA ($n = 15$) or observation ($n = 15$) and followed up for 6 months. Thyroid nodule volume and total thyroid volume were assessed by US and thyroid function was determined by routine assays before and during follow-up. Pressure and cosmetic complaints before and at 6 months were evaluated on a visual analogue scale. LTA was performed under US guidance. Nodule volume decreased significantly in the LTA group (median reduction was 44%) after 6 months ($p = 0.001$), and this reduction correlated with a substantial decrease in pressure symptoms and cosmetic complaints with no major side effects. In the control group, a nonsignificant increase in median nodule volume of 7% was noted after 6 months.

60. *(2C)* **Papini E** et al. Ultrasound-guided laser thermal ablation for treatment of benign thyroid nodules. Endocr Practice 2004;10:276–283.

Prospective observational cohort study. Twenty patients fulfilling the following entry criteria were enrolled in the study: (a) presence of a hypofunctioning thyroid nodule with a volume exceeding 8 ml, (b) benign cytologic findings, (c) local compression symptoms or patient concern, and (d) refusal of or ineligibility for surgical treatment. Under US monitoring, LTA was performed. Nodule volume was assessed by US at 1 and 6 months after LTA. Mean nodule volume reduction in comparison with baseline was 43.8% ± 8.1% at 1 month and 63.8% ± 8.9% at 6 months. LTA induced burning cervical pain, which rapidly decreased after the laser energy was turned off. Three patients (15%) required treatment with betamethasone for 48 hours. No patient had local bruising, cutaneous burning, or dysphonia.

Thyroid Cancer

61. **Mazzaferri EL, Kloos R.** Current approaches to primary therapy for papillary and follicular thyroid cancer. J Clin Endocrinol Metab 2001;86:1447–1463.

This is an excellent review, covering risk stratification, staging systems, approaches to initial surgical management, ^{131}I remnant ablation, diagnostic WBS, ^{131}I therapy for residual disease, and thyroid hormone–suppressive therapy in the management of papillary and follicular thyroid cancer.

Diagnosis

62. **Belfiore A, La Rosa GL**. Fine-needle aspiration biopsy of the thyroid. Endocrinol Metab Clin North Am 2001;30:361–400.

This article covers indications, technique, complications, cytologic diagnosis, diagnostic accuracy, and pitfalls of thyroid FNA biopsy and provides guidelines on how to use the information obtained by this procedure in the clinical management of thyroid nodules.

63. **Torrens JI, Burch HB.** Serum thyroglobulin measurement: Utility in clinical practice. Endocrinol Metab Clin North Am 2001;30:429–467.

This article provides information to allow a meaningful interpretation of Tg levels in the diagnosis and management of several thyroid disorders, with emphasis on differentiated thyroid cancer. Immunologic characteristics of Tg and TgAb and of several Tg assays and their potential pitfalls are discussed. Practical guidelines are provided for use of serum Tg in clinical practice

64. *(1C)* **Frasoldati A** et al. Role of thyroglobulin measurement in fine-needle aspiration biopsies of cervical lymph nodes in patients with differentiated thyroid cancer. Thyroid 1999;9:105–111.

In this prospective cohort, the authors measured Tg in the needle washout FNA biopsy of enlarged neck lymph nodes (LNs) in 23 patients awaiting surgery for DTC ($n = 33$ LN), 47 patients previously thyroidectomized for thyroid tumor ($n = 89$ LNs), and 60 patients without thyroid disease ($n = 94$ LNs). Immediately after aspiration biopsy, the needle was rinsed with 1 ml of normal saline solution, and Tg levels were measured on the needle washout (FNAB-Tg). FNAB-Tg levels were markedly elevated in metastatic LN both in patients awaiting thyroidectomy (metastatic vs. negative LN, mean ± SEM, 16,593 ± 7,050 ng/ml vs. 4.91 ± 1.61 ng/ml; $p < 0.001$) and in thyroidectomized patients (11,541 ± 7,283 ng/ml vs. 0.45 ± 0.07 ng/ml; $p < 0.001$). FNAB-Tg sensitivity, evaluated through histologic examination in 69 LNs, was 84.0%. The combination of cytology plus FNAB-Tg increased FNAB sensitivity from 76% to 92.0%.

65. *(1C)* **Baskin HJ.** Detection of recurrent papillary thyroid carcinoma by thyroglobulin assessment in the needle washout after fine-needle aspiration of suspicious lymph nodes. Thyroid 2004;14:959–963.

US was performed on 74 postoperative patients followed up for stage I and II PTC. All patients were clinically free of cancer 1 to 43 years after a total thyroidectomy and were screened with US and Tg measurement while taking thyroid hormone suppression. US revealed findings suggestive of recurrent disease in the LNs of the neck in 21 patients. Material for cytology and Tg analysis was obtained by US-guided FNA on these 21 patients, seven of whom tested positive for Tg in their needle washout. Only three of the seven had detectable serum Tg, and only five of the seven had positive cytology. Presence of Tg in the needle washout proved to be more sensitive than cytology in diagnosing cancer in the LN and was not affected by positive TgAb in the serum.

66. **Ledger GA** et al. Genetic testing in the diagnosis and management of multiple endocrine neoplasia type II. Ann Intern Med 1995;122:118–124.

This review covers advances in the early diagnosis and treatment of MTC in patients with MEN 2 syndromes, clinical features, biochemical screening, and the usefulness and limitations of genetic testing, especially DNA and linkage analysis, as a means of early detection of individuals affected with the familial forms of MTC. It also reviews the correlation between results of genetic and biochemical testing and current screening recommendations in this disorder.

Surgery

67. **Shaha AR** et al. Prognostic factors and risk group analysis in follicular carcinoma of the thyroid. Surgery 1995;118:1131–1136.

Review of 228 previously untreated patients with FTC during a 55-year period. Fifty-nine (26%) patients had Hürthle cell histology. Sixty-two patients were in the low-risk group, 84 in the intermediate-risk group, and 82 in the high-risk groups, with 10-year survival rates of 98%, 88%, and 56%, respectively, and 20-year survival rates of 97%, 87%, and 49%, respectively. Adverse prognostic factors included age older than 45 years ($p < 0.001$), Hürthle cell variety ($p = 0.05$), extrathyroidal extension, tumor size that exceeds 4 cm, and presence of distant metastasis ($p < 0.001$). Gender, focus, and lymph node metastasis did not affect prognosis.

68. **Samaan NA** et al. The results of various modalities of treatment of well-differentiated thyroid carcinomas: A retrospective review of 1599 patients. J Clin Endocrinol Metab 1992;75:714–720.

This study of 1,599 patients with differentiated thyroid cancer analyzed impact of age, gender, histologic diagnosis, extent of disease at diagnosis, and surgical intervention on the cancer, and impact of surgical treatment, ^{131}I, and radiotherapy on outcomes. Patients were predominantly female (2.3:1), with papillary (81%) and intrathyroidal carcinomas (42%) at the time of diagnosis. Median follow-up was 11 years. Of these patients, 66% had total thyroidectomy, 7% received external radiation, and 46% had ^{131}I as part of treatment of the original disease; overall recurrence rate was 23%, and the death rate, 11%. Treatment with ^{131}I was the single most powerful prognostic indicator for increased disease-free intervals and overall survival ($p < 0.001$). Other predictors of better outcome included younger age, female gender, localized intrathyroidal papillary disease, and near-total or total thyroidectomy.

69. **Mazzaferri EL, Jhiang SM**. Long-term impact of initial surgical and medical therapy on papillary and follicular thyroid cancer. Am J Med 1994;97:418–428.

Patients with PTC and FTC ($n = 1,355$) treated at the U.S. Air Force hospital or Ohio State University hospital over the course of 40 years were evaluated to determine treatment outcomes. After 30 years, survival rate was 76%, recurrence rate 30%, and cancer death rate 8%. Recurrences were most frequent at the extremes of age (<20 and >59 years). Cancer mortality rates were lowest in patients younger than 40 years and thereafter increased with each decade of life. Thirty-year cancer mortality rates were highest in FTC patients. When patients with distant metastases at diagnosis were excluded, FTC and PTC mortality rates were similar (10% vs. 6%, respectively). The likelihood of cancer death was (a) increased by age older than 40 years, tumor size 1.5 cm or larger, local tumor invasion, regional lymph node metastases, and delay in therapy of more than 12 months; (b) reduced by female gender, surgery more extensive than lobectomy, and ^{131}I plus thyroid hormone therapy; and (c) unaffected by tumor histologic type. Remnant ablation with ^{131}I reduced the recurrence rate to less than one third the rate after thyroid hormone therapy alone ($p < 0.001$). Low ^{131}I doses (e.g., 29–50 mCi) were as effective as high doses (51–200 mCi) in controlling tumor recurrence. After ^{131}I therapy, recurrence and likelihood of cancer death were reduced by at least half.

70. **Hay ID** et al. Unilateral total lobectomy: Is it sufficient surgical treatment for patients with AMES low-risk papillary thyroid carcinoma? Surgery 1998;124:958–964.

This retrospective study evaluated the outcome in 1,685 patients with PTC considered low risk by AMES criteria, initially treated during 1940 through 1991 and followed up for 54 postoperative years or less (mean, 18 years). In the study, 1,656 (98%) patients had complete primary tumor resection; 634 (38%) had involvement of regional nodes. Additionally, 195 (12%) patients had undergone unilateral lobectomy; bilateral lobar resection accounted for 1,468 (near-total, 60%; total thyroidectomy, 18%). Thirty-year rates for cancer-specific mortality and distant metastasis were 2% and 3%, respectively. The 20-year rates for local recurrence and nodal metastasis were 4% and 8%, respectively. Although the cancer-specific mortality or distant metastasis rates did not differ significantly between unilateral lobectomy and bilateral lobar resection, the 20-year rates for local recurrence and nodal metastasis were 14% and 19%, significantly higher ($p = 0.0001$) in unilateral lobectomy than the 2% and 6% rates seen after bilateral lobar resection.

71. *(2C)* **Miccoli P** et al. Completion total thyroidectomy in children with thyroid cancer secondary to the Chernobyl accident. Arch Surg 1998;133:89–93.

After the nuclear disaster in Chernobyl, 47 children with differentiated thyroid cancer from Belarus were evaluated in Italy. About half had had previous hemithyroidectomy, and 19 underwent completion thyroidectomy. Serum Tg was measured before and after reoperation, and a withdrawal ^{131}I WBS was performed. Result on histologic examination was positive for PTC in six (29%) patients, three with residual cancer in the remaining lobe and three with nodal metastases. A post-therapy WBS demonstrated lung and nodal metastases in 28% and 33% of patients, respectively. Hypoparathyroidism developed in four of 19 patients who underwent a completion thyroidectomy; unilateral laryngeal nerve palsy developed in one patient. Among 22 children with previous total thyroidectomy, a diagnostic whole-body scan showed lung metastases in 45% and lymph node metastases in 14% ($p =$ NS compared with those who underwent completion thyroidectomy). Completion thyroidectomy allowed the diagnosis and treatment of recurrent thyroid cancer and lung or nodal metastases in 61% of patients in whom residual differentiated thyroid cancer had not been previously recognized.

72. **Katoh R** et al. Multiple thyroid involvement (intraglandular metastasis) in papillary thyroid carcinoma: A clinicopathologic study of 105 consecutive patients. Cancer 1992;70:1585–1590.

Whole thyroids resected from 105 nonselected, consecutive patients were sectioned at 2- to 3-mm intervals and histologically reviewed. Intraglandular cancer foci, other than the tumor regarded as the primary focus, were demonstrated in 78% of patients. These small foci were distributed around the primary lesion and were also found frequently (61%) in the opposite lobe as bilateral disease. In the opposite lobe, a similar incidence (approximately 30%) of disease was seen.

Radioidine Remnant Ablation

73. *(1C+)* **Mazzaferri EL**. Thyroid remnant ^{131}I ablation for papillary and follicular thyroid carcinoma. Thyroid 1997;7:265–271.

This study compared outcomes in 1,004 patients with differentiated thyroid cancer and no apparent residual tumor after initial thyroidectomy who underwent remnant ablation with [131]I (n = 151) with outcomes in those who were either treated with thyroid hormone alone (n = 755) or given no postoperative medical therapy (n = 98). Tumor recurrence and cancer deaths were lower (p < 0.001), and fewer patients had distant metastases (p < 0.002) after remnant ablation than after other forms of treatment, an effect observed only in patients with primary tumors of 1.5 cm or larger. Cancer recurrence was influenced by absence of cervical lymph node metastases [hazard ratio (HR), 0.8], tumor stage (HR, 1.8), and treatment of the thyroid remnant (HR, 0.9); cancer-specific death rates were independently affected by age (HR, 13.3), recurrence of cancer (HR, 16.6), time-to-treatment (HR, 3.5), thyroid remnant ablation (HR, 0.5), and tumor stage (HR, 2.3).

LT4 Suppressive Therapy

74. *(1C+)* **Cooper DS** et al. Thyrotropin suppression and disease progression in patients with differentiated thyroid cancer: Results from the National Thyroid Cancer Treatment Cooperative Registry. Thyroid 1998;8:737–744.

A cohort of 683 patients (617 with PTC and 66 with FTC) were observed during annual follow-up for a median of 4.5 years. Cancer status was defined as no residual disease; progressive disease at any follow-up time; or death of thyroid cancer. A mean TSH score was calculated for each patient by averaging all available TSH values, where 1 is undetectable, 2 is subnormal, 3 is normal, and 4 is elevated TSH. The degree of TSH suppression did not differ between PTC and FTC patients but was higher in PTC patients who were initially classified as being at higher risk for recurrence. For all stages of PTC, disease stage, patient age, and ^{131}I therapy predicted disease progression, but TSH score category did not. TSH score category independently predicted disease progression in high-risk patients, but was no longer significant when ^{131}I therapy was included in the model.

75. *(1C)* **Pujol P** et al. Degree of thyrotropin suppression as a prognostic determinant in differentiated thyroid cancer. J Clin Endocrinol Metab 1996;81:4318–4323.

One hundred forty-one patients who underwent LT4 therapy after thyroidectomy were observed on a follow-up basis from 1970 to 1993. Patients received LT4 (mean dose, 2.6 μg/kg/day). TSH suppression was evaluated by TRH stimulation test until 1986, and thereafter by a sensitive TSH assay. Relapse-free survival (RFS) was longer in the group with constantly suppressed TSH (all TSH values, <0.05 mU/L) than in the group with nonsuppressed TSH (all TSH values, >1 mU/L; p < 0.01). The level of TSH suppression was analyzed by studying the percentage of undetectable TSH values (<0.05 mU/L) during follow-up. Patients with greater TSH suppression (>90% of undetectable TSH values) had a trend toward a longer RFS (p = 0.14), whereas patients with less TSH suppression (<10% of undetectable TSH values) had a shorter RFS (p < 0.01). In multivariate analysis, the degree of TSH suppression independently predicted RFS (p = 0.02).

Euthyroid Sick Syndrome

76. **Chopra IJ**. Euthyroid sick syndrome: Is it a misnomer? J Clin Endocrinol Metab 1997;82:329–334.

This article covers the concept and laboratory abnormalities of the euthyroid sick syndrome, its pathogenesis, clinical significance, and difficulties surrounding the diagnosis of thyroid disease in patients affected by systemic nonthyroidal illness. It also reviews the evidence for and against thyroid hormone replacement in this condition.

77. **Slag MF** et al. Hypothyroxinemia in critically ill patients as a predictor of high mortality. JAMA 1981;245:43–45.

This prospective cohort study evaluated 86 critically ill patients admitted to an intensive care unit. Exclusion criteria included expected poor outcome (concurrent malignancy or so-called DNR status), chronic renal failure, transfusion of blood products in the previous 48 hours, simple arrhythmias, drug overdose, and known thyroid disease or current treatment with thyroid hormone. Patients had blood specimens obtained within the first 24 hours of admission to the intensive care unit and assays of thyroid-function tests were performed (T4, T3, TBG, TSH, T3 resin uptake, rT3 and FT4 index calculated). Thirty-five clinically euthyroid subjects from an outpatient clinic were used as controls (33 men and two women; age range, 21–74 years). Of these patients, 22% had a low T4 level (8%, <3 mg/dl, and 14%, 3–5 mg/dl), and of these, 30% also had a low FT4 index. The overall mortality rate was 25%. Low T4 values were highly correlated with mortality. An initial T4 level less than 3 mg/dl correlated with 84% mortality (p < 0.01), and the mortality rate decreased as T4 levels increased. Of patients with a low T3 level, 44% died during the hospital admission. Neither T3 nor rT3 levels correlated with or predicted mortality.

Thyroid Hormone Supplementation

78. *(2B)* **Mullis-Jansson SL** et al. A randomized double-blind study of the effect of triiodothyronine on cardiac function and morbidity after coronary bypass surgery. J Thorac Cardiovasc Surg 1999;117:1128–1134.

This double-blind, randomized, placebo-controlled study was undertaken to define the effect of T3 on hemodynamics and outcome after coronary artery bypass grafting in 170 patients undergoing elective coronary artery bypass grafting. Intravenous T3 (0.4-mg/kg bolus plus 0.1-mg/kg infusion over a 6-hour period) or placebo was administered. Patients receiving T3 had higher cardiac index, lower inotropic requirements, and incidence of postoperative myocardial ischemia (4% vs. 18%; $p = 0.007$) and pacemaker dependence (14% vs. 25%; $p = 0.013$). Seven patients in the placebo required postoperative mechanical assistance compared with none in the T3 group ($p = 0.01$).

79. *(2B)* **Bennet-Guerrero E** et al. Cardiovascular effects of intravenous triiodothyronine in patients undergoing coronary artery bypass graft surgery: A randomized, double-blind, placebo-controlled trial: Duke T3 Study Group. JAMA 1996;275:687–692.

This randomized, double-blind, placebo-controlled trial evaluated whether T3 administration improves hemodynamic variables and decreases inotropic drug requirements in 211 patients undergoing coronary artery surgery at high risk for requiring inotropic drug support. Treatment consisted of T3 infusion (0.8 mg/kg i.v. followed by 0.12 mg/kg/h for 6 h), dopamine (positive control, 5 μg/kg/min for 6 h), or placebo. FT3 serum levels decreased significantly during cardiopulmonary bypass in all groups and increased to twice normal range ($p < 0.001$) after initiation of T3. T3 therapy increased heart rate ($p < 0.001$) but did not change hemodynamic variables or inotropic drug requirements.

Adrenal Disorders

Dana Erickson, Shailesh Pitale, and Steven A. DeJong

EVALUATION OF ADRENAL FUNCTION
Dana Erickson

Evaluation of Glucocorticoid Function

Cortisol

Normal production of cortisol by adrenal glands has diurnal variation. This fact, along with variations of "normal values" in multiple commercially available laboratory cortisol assays, explains the difficulties with diagnosis of adrenal pathology based on a single cortisol value. In general, a morning plasma cortisol less than 3 µg/dl is associated with high probability of adrenal insufficiency [1]. A midnight cortisol value of more than 7.5 µg/dl is useful for diagnosis of Cushing syndrome [2]. Additional limiting factors in interpretation of cortisol assays are caused by conditions that change the concentration of cortisol-binding protein: estrogen use, critical illness. In these instances, measurements of plasma free cortisol might be more appropriate [3].

Salivary cortisol reflects serum free cortisol. Various laboratory assays and collection methods reflect the need for each particular laboratory validation. This test performed late at night appears to be particularly useful as a screening test for Cushing syndrome [4].

Twenty-four–hour urinary cortisol collection assay is the best single test for the diagnosis of Cushing syndrome (values 2 to 3 times normal are typically seen in CD). Normal values are laboratory dependent; generally the use of immunoassays or newest high-performance liquid chromatography, or tandem mass spectrometry assays is recommended. The sensitivity and specificity depend on the cut-off value used for CS diagnosis (56%–100% sensitivity) [5]. The limitations of 24-hour collection include incomplete collection, medications that interfere with assay interpretation, periodic hypercortisolism, and pseudo-Cushing states. This test is not very helpful in the diagnosis of adrenal insufficiency.

Adrenocorticotropic Hormone

Measurement of ACTH in plasma is important in the diagnosis of both adrenal insufficiency and CS. Two-site immunoradiometric assays should be obtained (along with serum cortisol values), and samples must be handled rapidly and precisely because of the instability of ACTH at room temperature. In general, levels of ACTH are elevated in primary adrenal insufficiency and low or low normal in secondary adrenal insufficiency. In ACTH-dependent CD, ACTH is typically more than 20 pg/ml; in ACTH-independent CS, typically it is below the low-normal limit of assay. Values in between need repeated testing or further dynamic evaluation.

Dynamic Adrenal Tests
Stimulatory and suppressive laboratory tests are of major value in diagnosis and further workup of glucocorticoid disorders. Specific tests are described under each pathologic condition (see later).

Evaluation of Mineralocorticoid Function
Resistant or multidrug hypertension as well as spontaneous hypokalemia in a patient should raise the suspicion for primary hyperaldosteronism. Screening with simultaneous random plasma aldosterone concentration (PAC) to plasma renin activity (PRA) ratio showing a value above 20 indicates positive screening test for primary hyperaldosteronism. Recent meta-analysis, however, raised uncertainty about the screening test characteristics and described lack of standardization [6]. Confirmatory test with sodium loading (NaCl tbl or 3 days high-salt diet) and 24-hour urinary collection for aldosterone should follow (urinary aldosterone >14 µg/24 h has sensitivity of 96% and specificity of 93% for diagnosis of hyperaldosteronism) [7]. Mineralocorticoid deficiency is suspected when hyperkalemia and hyponatremia are present in appropriate clinical situations. No dynamic evaluation is recommended for mineralocorticoid deficiency.

Evaluation of Adrenal Medulla
Measurements of catecholamines and their metabolites are essential in the diagnostic evaluation of pheochromocytoma. For physiology and metabolism details, see the pheochromocytoma subchapter.

The utility of various available biochemical tests has been evaluated in various studies. The results of these tests depend on the type of assay used, proficiency, and lack of analytic interference of the particular laboratory. Plasma free metanephrines have the highest sensitivity (97%–99%) but a lower specificity (85%–89%) [8]. Severe stress and various medications could cause false-positive values. Total urinary metanephrines combined with fractionated free urinary catecholamines have also been reported to have a relatively high sensitivity and excellent specificity for catecholamine tumors diagnosis [9]. Urinary fractionated metanephrine use is limited by lack of specificity (69%), whereas urinary vanillylmandelic acid assays lack sensitivity (65%) [8]. Plasma catecholamine use is limited by multiple compounding factors.

Evaluation of Adrenal Androgen Production and Congenital Adrenal Hyperplasia
An elevated level of serum dehydroepiandrosterone and dehydroepiandrosterone sulfate (DHEA-S) indicates adrenal androgen overproduction. In cases of suspected congenital adrenal hyperplasia (CAH), intermediate products of steroid biosynthesis are elevated [10]. The 17-hydroxyprogesterone (basal or post-ACTH) is elevated in 21-hydroxylase deficiency; 11-deoxycortisol is elevated in 11-hydroxylase deficiency; 17-hydroxypregnenolone, in 3β-hydroxysteroid dehydrogenase deficiency; and progesterone and pregnanolone, in 17-hydroxylase deficiency. The cut-offs for partial or complete deficiency of enzymes vary, and genotyping of patients has somewhat changed the traditional interpretation of results [11]. The clinical presentation of CAH and degree of biochemical abnormalities depend on the type and degree of enzymatic defect.

ADRENAL IMAGING
Steven A. DeJong

Imaging studies of the adrenal gland have undergone significant advancement over the past several years. Computed tomography (CT) scanning of the adrenal gland has often been the only imaging study needed in the evaluation of a patient with adrenal gland pathology. The abundant perinephric fat, as often seen in patients with CS, allows excellent visualization of the gland. Adrenal magnetic resonance imaging (MRI) and scintigraphy can now provide significant additional information in the evaluation of patients with functional and incidentally discovered adrenal tumors. Although clinical patient information and biochemical testing are the foundation of adrenal evaluation, imaging studies can confirm, visualize, and characterize adrenal pathology to direct medical or surgical intervention [12,13]. In addition, the widespread use of cross-sectional imaging increased the detection of incidental adrenal masses, and accurate characterization of these lesions is of significant clinical importance.

Computed Tomography Scanning

Despite their small size, the adrenal glands are visualized in nearly 100% of patients with CT scanning. The V-shaped right adrenal gland is usually seen directly posterior to the inferior vena cava and measures approximately $1 \times 2 \times 0.5$ cm. This gland is nearly the same width as the diaphragmatic stripe. The left adrenal gland, which has a similar size and shape, is located anterior to the upper portion of the kidney and directly adjacent to the aorta. Adrenal CT scanning remains an excellent initial study in the patient with adrenal disease, and 1-cm contiguous scans are routinely used to demonstrate the location, size, and tissue characteristics of most adrenal masses. This technique can also identify lymphadenopathy, obvious malignancy, and local invasion or distant metastasis associated with adrenal tumors [14]. Thinner scans using 3- to 5-mm slices are often necessary to detect and evaluate smaller functional tumors such as aldosteronomas. Most pheochromocytomas or adrenal adenomas causing Cushing syndrome are 2 to 5 cm in diameter, whereas most aldosteronomas are 8 mm to 2 cm in size. The main limitation of CT scanning is its periodic inability to separate benign from malignant, and functional from nonfunctional tumors of the adrenal. Cysts and myelolipomas are the only benign conditions readily identified with CT scanning. An adrenal lesion with a large amount of macroscopic fat is suggestive of a myelolipoma. Benign adrenal adenomas often demonstrate loss of enhancement on delayed imaging after standard contrast-enhanced CT imaging of the adrenal gland. Benign adrenal adenomas have an attenuation value of less than 30 to 40 HU on a contrast-enhanced CT scan and demonstrate more than 60% washout 15 minutes after initial enhancement [15]. Although contrast enhancement may increase accuracy, patients with suspected pheochromocytoma should undergo α-adrenergic blockade before contrast administration to eliminate the small risk of contrast agents precipitating a hypertensive crisis. Primary adrenal malignancy should be considered in large adrenal masses with calcification, necrosis, or hemorrhage. CT of the adrenal gland has reported sensitivity, specificity, and accuracy rates of 84%, 98%, and 90%, respectively [3,5]. Percutaneous biopsy of the adrenal gland, when indicated, can be safely performed by using CT guidance techniques. The left adrenal gland is usually more difficult to access for biopsy with this technique because of its posterior location [16].

Magnetic Resonance Imaging

MRI is gaining widespread acceptance as the initial study in the evaluation of adrenal masses because of its superb soft-tissue contrast, natural enhancement of certain pathologic adrenal masses, and the lack of ionizing radiation. MRI characterizes adrenal tumors by their signal characteristics on different pulse sequences and by their enhancement characteristics. It also allows multiplanar imaging to depict the relation between the adrenal mass and the kidney [17]. MRI accurately identifies benign adrenal adenomas, myelolipomas, adrenal cysts, malignant or metastatic adrenal tumors, and pheochromocytomas and commonly augments information obtained with CT [18]. MRI reliably distinguishes between adenoma and metastasis in most cases and allows accurate oncologic staging, limited adrenal biopsies, and initiation of appropriate treatment regimens in the affected patient population. Chemical-shift techniques using breath-hold T_1-weighted GRE images can rapidly and reliably identify benign adrenal adenomas through the accurate detection of their characteristic high intracellular lipid content [17,19]. Normal adrenal glands and adrenal tumors larger than 1 cm in diameter can be visualized in more than 90% of patients with these images, but MRI is not able to distinguish functional from nonfunctional cortical adenomas of the adrenal. T_2-weighted images, however, can demonstrate unique signal intensities. Hyperintense T_2-weighted images suggest the presence of pheochromocytoma, and MRI can also be useful in locating extra-adrenal pheochromocytomas. The MRI signal intensity of adrenal cortical carcinomas is variable, and they generally are heterogeneous on T_1- and T_2-weighted images. These tumors often appear as large, necrotic, poorly marginated retroperitoneal masses of uncertain origin where MRI fails to identify a normal ipsilateral adrenal gland [20]. These aggressive neoplasms often invade into the renal vein or inferior vena cava, and this venous extension can also be demonstrated on MRI. MRI is also an attractive imaging modality for children and pregnant patients with adrenal disease because of its lack of ionizing radiation.

Adrenal Cortical Scintigraphy

Hormone production in the adrenal cortex begins with cholesterol. Several radiolabeled cholesterol analogues have been developed to allow localization and functional information regarding adrenal cortical tumors. The only one currently approved for use in the United States is [131I]-6β-iodomethylnorcholesterol (NP-59). Adrenal scintigraphy is usually performed after the diagnosis of a functional adrenal cortical tumor is well established. Information obtained with scintigraphy is usually correlated with conventional images using CT scanning or MRI. Adrenal scintigraphy is often useful in differentiating unilateral adrenal adenomas from bilateral adrenal hyperplasia in patients with Cushing syndrome or primary hyperaldosteronism. Unfortunately, NP-59 can be difficult to obtain, and studies using this material are usually expensive, time consuming, and involve significant radiation exposure to the patient. The material, however, is safe to administer, and the accuracy rate of NP-59 to identify and distinguish correctly a Cushing adrenal adenoma or an aldosteronoma from bilateral adrenal hyperplasia approaches 90% [21]. Detection of aldosteronomas with NP-59 requires discontinuation of diuretic and antihypertensive medication, and accuracy rates are increased if the patients are pretreated with dexamethasone.

Adrenal Medullary Scintigraphy

Metaiodobenzylguanidine (MIBG), a radiolabeled derivative of guanethidine with no pharmacologic effect, was developed in 1980. It is the most frequently used substance to image the adrenal medulla and other sympathetic tissues. It is incorporated into sympathetic nerve cells as a catecholamine precursor. [131I]MIBG is the most commonly used isotope, but recent studies suggest that ^{123}I is more accurate with less radiation exposure to the patient. Single-photon emission computed tomography (SPECT) technology may also improve the sensitivity and accuracy of this imaging tool. MIBG scanning is diagnostic for neoplasms producing excess catecholamine and has successfully detected pheochromocytomas, neuroblastomas, and other neuroendocrine tumors such as paragangliomas, carcinoid tumors, and medullary carcinomas of the thyroid. The most common role for MIBG is in patients with a biochemical diagnosis of pheochromocytoma and normal conventional adrenal imaging studies. MIBG can identify paragangliomas and metastatic pheochromocytomas to guide further imaging. The sensitivity and specificity of MIBG scanning for pheochromocytoma and neuroblastoma are between 80% and 100%. An alternative to MIBG is radiolabeled octreotide [111I(indium)]-DTPA (diethylenetriaminepenta-acetate) octreotide, which can detect paragangliomas and neuroendocrine tumors containing cell-surface receptors for somatostatin [22].

Positron Emission Tomography

Several different radiopharmaceuticals can detect increased cellular activity in hyperfunctional adrenal states more specifically than does conventional imaging. These agents can also target specific adrenal enzymes that are expressed in adrenal tumor cells. As an example, [18F]fluorodopamine PET scanning allows tumor visualization within minutes of injection of the imaging agent, and spatial resolution is excellent.

[18F]FDG scanning is also effective in differentiating benign from malignant adrenal lesions with high accuracy [24]. PET scanning also correctly localizes adrenal and extra-adrenal pheochromocytomas that lack the ability to concentrate MIBG [23,25].

Adrenal Vein Sampling

Adrenal vein sampling is useful in patients with functional tumors of the adrenal glands such as in patients with Cushing syndrome or primary hyperaldosteronism. These patients have normal or equivocal findings on CT, MRI, or adrenal scintigraphy imaging studies that cannot distinguish between a unilateral aldosteronoma requiring adrenalectomy and bilateral adrenal hyperplasia treated medically [26]. Although the left adrenal vein is accessible in nearly all patients, the right adrenal vein can be more difficult to cannulate. Patients with primary hyperaldosteronism receive an infusion of cosyntropin, and blood from both adrenal veins and the distal inferior vena cava (IVC) is measured for both aldosterone and cortisol. Adrenal vein cortisol should be 5 times greater than IVC cortisol to verify the position of the venous catheter in the adrenal vein. The ratios of aldosterone to cortisol for both adrenal veins are compared, and a ratio of 4:1 or greater reliably identifies a small unilateral aldosteronomas, whereas a ratio of less than 3:1 usually indicates bilateral adrenal hyperplasia [27]. Selective venous sampling in patients with Cushing syndrome is performed in a similar manner without the infusion of cosyntropin. Cortisol levels from both adrenal veins and the IVC are compared to distinguish between bilateral adrenal hyperplasia and adrenal adenoma in patients with Cushing syndrome.

PRIMARY HYPERALDOSTERONISM
Steven A. DeJong

Definition and Etiology

Primary hyperaldosteronism is the excessive autonomous adrenal secretion of aldosterone, resulting in suppression of plasma renin activity (PRA). The exact cause is unknown. This syndrome results in a rare form of surgically correctable hypertension, polyuria, weakness, hypokalemia, sodium retention, and mild metabolic alkalosis. A small, benign, unilateral, aldosterone-producing adrenal tumor, first described by Jerome Conn in 1955, is the most common cause of primary hyperaldosteronism in 70% to 80% of patients. Idiopathic bilateral macronodular or micronodular hyperplasia of the adrenal cortex causes primary hyperaldosteronism in 20% to 30% of patients [28]. Other less common causes of primary hyperaldosteronism include glucocorticoid-suppressible hyperaldosteronism, a rare familial form of hypertension that affects 1% to 3% of patients with primary hyperaldosteronism [29], and aldosterone-producing adrenal carcinoma [30].

Epidemiology

The prevalence of primary hyperaldosteronism in unselected patients with hypertension is 1% to 2%. About 1% of all adrenal masses discovered incidentally are found to be aldosterone-producing adrenal adenomas. Aldosteronomas occur more commonly in female patients, by a 2:1 ratio, and are rare in children. Bilateral idiopathic adrenal hyperplasia causing primary hyperaldosteronism is more common in men and usually appears in patients at an older age than does aldosteronoma. High blood pressure is present, but this sign is a common medical problem and is not sufficiently specific to identify this endocrinopathy. Although hypertension in these patients is often of moderate severity, multiple medical regimens to control blood pressure are usually unsuccessful, causing the diagnosis of primary hyperaldosteronism to be considered [29].

Pathophysiology

Aldosterone is the final product in the biosynthesis of mineralocorticoids produced from the zona glomerulosa of the adrenal cortex. Factors stimulating the synthesis and release of aldosterone include angiotensin II, potassium, ACTH, and decreased renal perfusion or circulating blood volume. The clinical manifestations of primary hyperaldosteronism arise from the autonomous production of aldosterone, causing altered sodium and potassium homeostasis. Aldosterone normally enhances the reabsorption of sodium from the distal renal tubules in exchange for potassium and hydrogen excretion. Excessive aldosterone secretion leads to sodium and water retention and increased potassium and hydrogen excretion. The result is volume expansion and hypertension, suppressed PRA, hypokalemia, and metabolic alkalosis [28]. Serum sodium levels remain normal because of a parallel increase in the water content of the blood. Hypokalemia is responsible for most of the clinical symptoms of primary hyperaldosteronism, such as proximal muscle weakness and cramps, polyuria, polydipsia, nocturia, headache, and fatigue.

Diagnosis

Unlike most endocrine disorders, primary hyperaldosteronism does not have characteristic symptoms or signs, but this disorder should be considered in all patients with hypertension, unprovoked hypokalemia, and metabolic alkalosis. The use of antihypertensive medications that specifically block aldosterone secretion, such as spironolactone and other similar diuretics, must be stopped for 4 to 6 weeks before testing. Screening studies such as PRA, measurement of aldosterone and potassium levels, and 24-hour urine collection for aldosterone, potassium, and sodium should begin the evaluation. Nearly all patients with primary hyperaldosteronism have a serum potassium level less than 4.0 mEq/L; most range from 2.5 to 3.5 mEq/L [28,29]. Despite hypokalemia and a total body deficit of potassium, the 24-hour urine collection for potassium demonstrates inappropriate kaliuresis. Diuretic-induced hypokalemia that does not respond to potassium replacement also suggests the presence of primary hyperaldosteronism.

Plasma aldosterone levels are usually elevated, and PRA is suppressed. Low PRA excludes the presence of secondary hyperaldosteronism, characterized by increased renin and aldosterone levels, resulting from renal artery stenosis, cirrhosis, intravascular volume loss, congestive heart failure, and other disorders that decrease renal perfusion. Plasma aldosterone levels usually exceed 30 ng/L, and PRA is usually less than 1 ng/L. A ratio of plasma aldosterone to PRA that exceeds 30 to 50 is highly suggestive of excess endogenous aldosterone production [28,29]. Oral or intravenous sodium chloride administration may be necessary in some hypertensive patients in whom the distinction between primary and secondary hyperaldosteronism is less clear. A persistently elevated urinary aldosterone level during sodium loading confirms the diagnosis of autonomous aldosterone secretion. In addition, the inability to reduce plasma aldosterone levels and increase PRA after the administration of captopril, an angiotensin-converting enzyme (ACE) inhibitor, also suggests primary hyperaldosteronism [29].

After the diagnosis of primary hyperaldosteronism is confirmed, the main cause of this syndrome, either unilateral adrenal adenoma or idiopathic bilateral adrenal hyperplasia, must be determined because of significant treatment implications [31]. Postural testing can be used in this distinction because aldosterone-producing adrenal adenomas are unresponsive to the effects of angiotensin II. Plasma levels of aldosterone are measured in patients assuming a supine position and then again after 4 hours of standing. Angiotensin II and PRA increase in the standing position, but patients with aldosterone-producing adrenal adenomas have no increase in their aldosterone levels during this test. Conversely, aldosterone levels in patients with idiopathic bilateral adrenal hyperplasia usually increase. Postural testing can correctly differentiate between unilateral and bilateral adrenal disease in 75% to 85% of patients with primary hyperaldosteronism [28,31]. CT scanning of the adrenal glands has largely replaced postural testing in many centers as the initial study of choice to identify the aldosteronoma, but postural testing is helpful in equivocal cases or when a nonfunctional adrenal adenoma is suspected. Measurement of 18-hydrocorticosterone (18-OH-β) also can distinguish adrenal adenoma from bilateral adrenal hyperplasia. Plasma levels of 18-OH-β greater than 100 ng/dl are indicative of unilateral adrenal adenoma, with a sensitivity rate of 50% to 80%. Postural testing and serum 18-OH-β levels alone, however, fail to localize the aldosteronoma [32].

Imaging of the adrenal glands, after diagnostic confirmation of primary hyperaldosteronism, is best performed with high-resolution CT scanning of both adrenal glands, which has an 80% to 90% sensitivity rate in detecting aldosteronomas. These tumors are usually 0.8 to 2 cm in diameter and require thinner scans than the conventional 1-cm CT sections. It is important to visualize the contralateral adrenal gland adequately because enlargement of both glands may suggest idiopathic bilateral adrenal hyperplasia. The sensitivity of MRI is equal to that of CT scanning for these patients [29].

Patients with biochemically confirmed primary hyperaldosteronism and either no adrenal mass, bilateral adrenal masses, or equivocal findings on CT or MRI should undergo adrenal vein sampling for aldosterone and cortisol levels to determine the origin of the primary hyperaldosteronism. Adrenal vein sampling for aldosterone has a diagnostic sensitivity of 96% but does require significant technical expertise, as the short right adrenal vein can be challenging to cannulate. ACTH is administered, and aldosterone and cortisol levels are measured from both adrenal veins and the IVC. An adrenal vein/IVC cortisol ratio of 3:1 ensures proper placement of the catheter into the respective adrenal vein. A unilateral aldosterone-producing adenoma produces a ratio of aldosterone to cortisol that is 4 to 5 times greater than that of the opposite side [32]. Bilateral adrenal disease reveals bilateral elevation of this ratio and no appreciable gradient. One study compared CT and adrenal vein sampling in 24 patients with primary hyperaldosteronism [33]. CT led to diagnosis of unilateral adenoma in 19 patients and hyperplasia in seven. After adrenal venous sampling, unilateral adenoma was diagnosed in 22 patients. Of the seven patients with bilateral nodules, adrenal venous sampling correctly identified the unilateral adenoma in six.

Iodocholesterol scanning with [6β-^{131}I]iodomethyl-19-norcholesterol (NP-59) after dexamethasone suppression is a less-used imaging study to differentiate adenoma from hyperplasia. This study has a reported sensitivity of 88% and can identify unilateral uptake in larger adrenal aldosteronomas and bilateral uptake in adrenal hyperplasia [28,29]. In a study of 41 patients who were examined by using CT and iodocholesterol scanning with NP-59 after dexamethasone suppression, scintigraphy correctly identified bilateral and unilateral lesions in 92% of cases compared with 58% by CT [34]. Aldosterone-producing adrenal carcinoma often demonstrates no uptake on adrenal scintigraphy [30]. Unfortunately, this study depends heavily on the size of the adenoma, and its declining use is limited by the availability of the radioisotope.

Treatment

The hypertension and hypokalemia associated with idiopathic bilateral adrenal hyperplasia is best treated medically with potassium-sparing diuretic agents such as spironolactone, amiloride, and other antihypertensive agents. These medications can be associated with adverse side effects like gynecomastia and impotence [29]. The hypertension responds poorly to bilateral adrenalectomy in these patients, and adrenal insufficiency often develops. Unilateral aldosteronomas are treated with laparoscopic or open adrenalectomy [35]. Adrenal resection is performed after a 1- to 2-week course of spironolactone at 25 to 400 mg/day in divided doses to correct the associated volume and metabolic derangements. The laparoscopic approach is the method of choice because of fewer wound complications, less patient discomfort, shorter hospitalizations, and a more rapid return to work and normal activity. Most patients with an aldosteronoma become normotensive and normokalemic shortly after surgery. Resolution of preoperative hypokalemia usually occurs within 5 to 7 days of adrenalectomy in 95% of patients, and cure of hypertension over several months is expected in 70% to 80% of patients with normal renal function [35,36]. The remaining 20% to 30% of patients usually experience improvement in blood pressure control, and they often require fewer antihypertensive medications after adrenalectomy. Aldosterone-producing adrenal carcinomas occur in 1% of patients with primary hyperaldosteronism and have an overall

5-year survival rate of 35%. These tumors are often large with aggressive invasive features and require open adrenalectomy for complete resection or debulking [30].

CUSHING SYNDROME
Dana Erickson

The constellation of clinical features that result from persistent, inappropriate elevation of glucocorticoids is described as Cushing syndrome (CS).

Etiology and Pathogenesis
Exogenous administration of glucocorticoids (iatrogenic or factitious) is the most common cause of CS. Approximately 80% of patients with endogenous CS have ACTH-dependent disease, most frequently caused by pituitary microadenomas (i.e., Cushing disease; see Chapter 1) [37]. Overproduction of ACTH in ACTH-dependent Cushing may also be due to ectopic overproduction of ACTH or corticotropin-releasing hormone (CRH), caused by certain malignancies (Table 3.1). The excessive ACTH or CRH production leads to overproduction of cortisol by adrenal glands. In ACTH-independent CS (15%–20% of endogenous causes), autonomous increase in cortisol production by adrenal glands is found, resulting in suppression of ACTH. The etiology of this autonomous cortisol overproduction is represented by: adrenal adenomas, adrenal carcinomas, bilateral or unilateral macronodular adrenal hyperplasia, and micronodular adrenal hyperplasia. The expression of certain ectopic promiscuous receptors (gastric inhibitory polypeptide, vasopressin, β-adrenergic receptors, serotonin, and luteinizing hormone receptors) in adrenocortical cells explains some of the causes of macronodular adrenal hyperplasia [38]. Certain conditions such as affective disorders, stress, and obesity can lead to mild elevations in plasma or urinary cortisol levels, the so-called pseudo-Cushing state. The entity of subclinical CS is described in the section on adrenal incidentalomas.

Clinical Features
The clinical manifestations of hypercortisolism are common to all forms of CS and include hypertension; central obesity; diabetes mellitus [39], acne; androgenic hirsutism; signs of protein catabolism such as myopathy, osteopenia, or osteoporosis; cutaneous lesions (i.e., wide violaceous striae, tinea versicolor, verrucous vulgaris,

Table 3.1.   Causes of Cushing Syndrome

Exogenous: oral, injectable, inhalational, topical
Endogenous
   ACTH dependent
      Pituitary ACTH production: Cushing disease
      Ectopic ACTH production: Small cell lung carcinoma
                      Carcinoid
                      Pancreatic cancer
                      Pheochromocytoma
                      Medullary thyroid carcinoma
      Ectopic CRH production
   ACTH independent (adrenal glucocorticoid overproduction)
      Adrenal adenoma
      Adrenal carcinoma
      Bilateral micronodular hyperplasia
      Bilateral macronodular hyperplasia

ACTH, adrenocorticotropic hormone; CRH, corticotropin-releasing hormone.

ecchymosis); hyperpigmentation; and psychiatric manifestations (depression, cognition, and vegetative function). These classic features may not be present in ectopic ACTH production from malignancies, because of shorter duration of hypercortisolemia.

Evaluation

Diagnostic Tests

Measurement of 24-hour urinary free cortisol is the most reliable screening test for CS. The sensitivity is reported to be between 56% and 100%, and the specificity varies depending on study population, assays, and laboratory cutoffs for elevation [40]. A value that is more than 3 times the upper limit of normal is typically considered to be indicative of CS.

Loss of circadian rhythm with high plasma cortisol level (7.5 mg/dl) between 10 p.m. and midnight is an early indicator of CS [2]. Late-night salivary cortisol requires further refinement but appears very promising. Diagnostic accuracy of this test once again depends on laboratory assay, particular statistical analysis and study population (reported sensitivity of 92% to 100% and specificity of 84.9% to 100%) [4].

The overnight dexamethasone suppression test (dexamethasone, 1 mg PO administered at 11 p.m., followed by 8 a.m. plasma cortisol) is used as a screening test for CS [41]. Various criteria for normal suppression (traditionally <5 μg/dl or recently <1.8 μg/dl) applied to various study populations and frequently lack of matching controls influence sensitivity and specificity of the test [42]. Data regarding salivary post–1-mg dexamethasone cortisol test are very limited.

In the 2-day low-dose dexamethasone test, dexamethasone, 0.5-mg tablet, is taken every 6 hours for 2 days, followed by plasma cortisol determination at 8:00 a.m. Normal response includes plasma cortisol level suppression to less than 5 μg/dl (or more stringent cut-off of <1.8 μg/dl) and urinary free cortisol suppression below the lower limit of normal [31–43]. Dexamethasone—0.5 mg every 6 hours for 2 days followed 2 hours later by intravenous ovine CRH, 1 μg/kg—yields plasma cortisol of less than 1.4 mg/dl at 15 minutes in patients with pseudo-Cushing [44].

Localization Tests

Baseline ACTH Level

An inappropriately normal or elevated baseline plasma ACTH level (i.e., >20 pg/ml) indicates ACTH-dependent CS. Cushing disease usually appears with ACTH levels less than 200 pg/ml, whereas ACTH levels in ectopic ACTH syndromes range from 200 to 1,000 pg/ml. A low ACTH level (typically <5 pg/ml) represents ACTH-independent CS.

High-Dose Dexamethasone Suppression

The high-dose dexamethasone suppression (HDDS) test is done to differentiate between pituitary ACTH overproduction and ectopic ACTH production and occasionally in ACTH-independent CS. Dexamethasone, 2 mg orally every 6 hours for 2 days, is followed by plasma cortisol estimation at 8 a.m. Plasma cortisol below 50% of basal values, 24-hour urinary free cortisol less than 90% of basal values, or 24-hour 17-hydroxysteroid excretion less than 69% indicates Cushing disease [45]. Absence of response to HDDS indicates ectopic ACTH or adrenal CS. In the overnight HDDS test, a single dose of 8-mg dexamethasone is given at 11 p.m., and 8 a.m. plasma cortisol is measured the next day. The test is interpreted the same way as is standard HDDS testing. In a limited series, the sensitivity and specificity of the overnight HDDS test are similar to those of the standard HDDS test; however, a higher plasma cortisol suppression (>68%) cut-off was used for the latter [46]. Effectiveness analysis of both tests points toward the limitations of these tests by using standard criteria in interpretation [47]. Note that the pretest probability of pituitary Cushing disease is high, which limits the usefulness of these tests.

Invasive testing including inferior petrosal or cavernous sinus sampling (highest sensitivity and specificity), as well as CRH stimulation tests, is discussed in the section on Cushing disease in Chapter 1.

Radiologic Imaging

Thin-section CT (3-mm cuts) or MRI of the adrenal glands to look for the cause of adrenal autonomy is the next step in evaluation of patients with ACTH-independent CS. Imaging of ACTH-dependent CS is discussed in Chapter 1.

Treatment

The goal of therapy is to eradicate the cause of CS. Treatment of pituitary Cushing disease is described in Chapter 1. Optimal therapy in cases of ACTH-independent CS includes surgical removal of adrenal adenoma or carcinoma. In cases of ACTH-independent bilateral hyperplasia (micronodular or macronodular), as well as in certain cases of persistent or recurrent ACTH-dependent disease, bilateral adrenalectomy is the treatment of choice. The laparoscopic approach to surgery has reduced the surgical morbidity of adrenalectomy. The hospital stay is shorter, and complications are much less frequently encountered compared with results associated with open surgery. Mortality is reported at 0.2% [48].

Medical treatment can be used when surgery is contraindicated, if the tumor is metastatic or occult, or if surgery and radiation therapy (for pituitary disease) have failed. Medical therapy may also be used to attempt to stabilize patients preoperatively.

Medications used to reduce cortisol production are divided into several groups: those inhibiting adrenal steroidogenesis (mitotane, ketoconazole, aminoglutethamide, etomidate, and metyrapone), those acting at pituitary level (cyproheptadine, bromocriptine, somatostatin, valproic acid, possible thiazolidines—all of them very limited use and efficacy), and last, glucocorticoid-receptor antagonist (mifepristone; not commercially available). Ketoconazole is initiated at a dose of 200 mg 3 times daily and then increased to 400 mg 3 times daily with effective plasma cortisol reduction [49]. Liver-function test abnormalities can occur. The therapeutic effect is frequently transient. As with all of adrenal steroidogenesis inhibitors, acute adrenal insufficiency can occur; therefore physiologic glucocorticoid replacement might be necessary. Mitotane is implemented at a dose of 0.5 to 1 g/day and increased by 0.5 to 1 g over a period of a few weeks, maximum 10 g/day; severe gastrointestinal and neurologic side effects occur [50]. Monitoring of mitotane levels and dose adjustment is frequently advocated. The starting dose of aminoglutethamide is 500 mg/day in four divided doses, with increments every few days to a maximum of 2 g/day; it is useful as an adjunctive agent [51].

Last, targeted medical therapy (propranolol, leuprolide) has been reported to decrease cortisol production in selected cases of documented ectopic hormone-receptor expression in bilateral macronodular hyperplasia.

ADRENAL INCIDENTALOMA

Dana Erickson

Definition

An adrenal incidentaloma is a tumor larger than 1 cm in diameter that is discovered serendipitously during routine diagnostic imaging in the absence of symptoms or clinical findings suggestive of adrenal disease. The advent of specialized imaging techniques and the more widespread application of abdominal ultrasound, CT, and MRI has made this entity a more frequently encountered phenomenon in clinical practice. In a large series of 61,054 abdominal CT scans published by the Mayo Clinic, incidental adrenal tumors were visualized in 0.4% [52]. At autopsy, an adrenal mass is found in at least 3% of persons older than 50 years [53].

Etiology

Adrenal masses visualized on imaging studies are of various etiologies (Table 3.2). The mass has to be characterized with respect to functional hormonal status and imaging characteristics. Although most incidentally discovered adrenal masses are nonfunctional, up to 15% may be hormonally active. In a study retrospectively analyzing 1,096 cases of incidentally diagnosed adrenal tumors, 9.2% were found to be cortisol

Table 3.2. Differential Diagnosis of Adrenal Masses

Nonfunctioning mass	Hormonally active mass
Benign adrenal adenoma	Pheochromocytoma
Cyst	Primary aldosteronoma
Myelolipoma	Cushing syndrome
Neurofibroma	Masculinizing or feminizing tumors
Adenolipoma	Micro- or macronodular hyperplasia
Ganglioneuroma	Adrenocortical carcinoma
Hamartoma	Pseudo-adrenal mass
Teratoma	Renal, pancreatic, vascular, neurologic
Infections	origin
Metastatic carcinoma	
Adrenocortical carcinoma	

secreting, 4.2% were pheochromocytomas, and 1.6%, aldosteronomas [54]. Adrenal carcinomas are very rare in this setting, and more than 98% are larger than 4 cm.

Diagnosis

A detailed clinical history and physical examination represent the initial step in evaluation of all patients [53]. Evaluation for possible hormonal hyperfunction should follow. Screening for pheochromocytoma includes measurement of 24-hour total or fractionated urinary metanephrines combined with 24-hour urinary catecholamines or measurement of plasma catecholamines [55,56]. The choice of a particular test could be determined by certain imaging characteristics of tumor and by the clinical context. Screening for primary hyperaldosteronism includes measurements of the plasma aldosterone/renin ratio. The optimal biochemical definition of subclinical CS (SCS) is debatable, and various studies included patients with abnormal overnight 1-mg dexamethasone (>5 µg/dl; recommendation of NIH consensus in 2003) or 3-mg suppression test, abnormal 2-day low-dose dexamethasone suppression test (cutoffs for abnormal plasma and urinary cortisol vary), lack of diurnal variation of cortisol levels, elevated baseline urinary cortisol levels, low baseline ACTH level, or abnormal CRH stimulation test [57]. Over the last several years, several studies have shown that patients with SCS have metabolic abnormalities (impaired glucose tolerance, increased blood pressure, and reduced insulin sensitivity), increased cardiovascular risk factors, higher triglycerides, increased total and LDL cholesterol and fibrinogen levels [58], and possibly reduced bone mass. Last, testing for androgen overproduction should be performed in cases of severe hirsutism.

Certain imaging characteristics are very useful for differentiating malignant and nonmalignant tumors, as described in Table 3.3. Fine-needle aspiration (FNA) can distinguish adrenal tumors from extra-adrenal neoplasms; however, it cannot reliably differentiate a benign adenoma from an adrenal carcinoma. Thus FNA should not be routinely undertaken in the evaluation of an adrenal incidentaloma, unless the index of suspicion for a malignancy outside the adrenal gland is high, and the presence of pheochromocytoma must be excluded before the procedure. Adrenal scintigraphy with iodinated cholesterol derivative (i.e., NP-59) can identify patients with functioning adrenocortical tissue; however, it has very limited availability.

Treatment

Generally, adrenal tumors larger than 4 to 6 cm should be surgically excised if no evidence of metastases from a distant source is found [52,53]. Cutoff at 4 cm had the highest sensitivity (93%) in differentiating between benign and malignant tumors in a large national survey of more than 1,000 patients [54]. Nonfunctioning adenomas are virtually all cured by surgery. Hormonally active tumors as pheochromocytoma,

Table 3.3.   Characteristics of Malignant and Nonmalignant Adrenal Masses

Characteristic	Malignant	Benign
Size	Typically ≥4 cm	<4 cm
CT scan appearance	Heterogeneous Calcified, hemorrhagic	Homogeneous (low density compared with liver)
Margins	Irregular	Round, smooth
Contrast media Enhancement on CT	Marked	Low
CT imaging (Hounsfield units)	>10 HU without contrast and >40 HU 30 min after contrast	<10 HU without contrast and <37 HU after contrast
MRI appearance	Hyperintense	Isointense

aldosteronoma, and even nonfunctioning tumor of less than 4 cm with suggestive imaging characteristics should be surgically removed. Currently, insufficient evidence exists regarding surgical intervention in patients with subclinical CS in the setting of adrenal incidentaloma. Very limited retrospective case analysis showed amelioration of the cardiovascular risk profile after surgical removal of an adrenal mass [58]. If a conservative approach is used, complications should be aggressively addressed by lifestyle modifications and pharmacotherapy. No randomized trials have compared open adrenalectomy with the laparoscopic procedure for benign disease; however, results of recent meta-analysis of published studies illustrate the advantages of the latter [59]. In cases of adrenal cancer, the type of surgical approach as well as use of adjuvant systemic therapy remains controversial [60].

Follow-Up
Patients with nonfunctional tumors smaller than 4 cm in diameter should be followed up with serial CT scans at 3 months and 1 year [53], with a decrease in frequency thereafter (example at 2 years and 4 years; incomplete evidence precludes very specific recommendations). Tumors that enlarge by more than 1 cm (5% of all tumors) during the follow-up period should be surgically removed. Periodical hormonal evaluation is supported by the fact that in approximately 4% of patients, new hormonal abnormalities may develop.

ADRENAL INSUFFICIENCY
Dana Erickson

Definition
Adrenal insufficiency is characterized by deficiency of adrenal hormones. The etiology and the rate of onset of this condition determine the clinical presentation and laboratory findings. Primary adrenal insufficiency, also known as Addison disease, is due to dysfunction at the level of the adrenal glands and is typically associated with a low plasma cortisol level and an elevated plasma ACTH. Secondary adrenal insufficiency is characterized by dysfunction at the level of the hypothalamus or pituitary gland that results in decreased ACTH production and the resulting decline in or lack of cortisol secretion [61].

Etiology and Epidemiology
The most common cause of adrenocortical failure is ACTH deficiency due to prolonged administration of exogenous glucocorticoid therapy (iatrogenic adrenal insufficiency). Various causes of primary and secondary adrenal insufficiency are listed in Table 3.4.

Table 3.4. Etiologic Factors for Adrenal Insufficiency

Primary adrenal insufficiency
  Autoimmune disease (common)
    Isolated
    Polyglandular autoimmune syndromes type I and II
  Infectious etiologies
    Disseminated tuberculosis (common)
    Disseminated fungal infections
    HIV infection
    Other systemic bacterial infections
  Inherited disorders
    Adrenal leukodystrophy (rare)
    Triple A syndrome
    Kearns–Sayre syndrome
  Hemorrhagic infarction
    Sepsis (meningococcemia/*Pseudomonas aeruginosa*)
    Anticoagulant therapy
    Antiphospholipid antibody syndrome
  Metastatic disease
  Iatrogenic
    Drugs: ketoconazole, aminoglutethamide, metyrapone, suramin, and etomidate
  Infiltrative disorders
  Congenital adrenal hyperplasia
  Congenital adrenal hypoplasia (DAX-1–related forms)
  Resistance to ACTH
Secondary and tertiary adrenal insufficiency
  Prolonged administration of exogenous corticosteroids (iatrogenic)
  Isolated ACTH or CRH deficiency (rare)
  Organic hypothalamic or pituitary gland disorders
    Primary or metastatic tumors (including macroadenomas and craniopharyngiomas)
    Infections
    Hypophysitis
    Granulomatous-type disorders
    Sheehan syndrome
  Parasellar lesions (meningiomas)
  Prior radiation or neurosurgery
  Peripheral resistance to glucocorticoids

Autoimmune adrenalitis accounts for most cases of primary adrenal insufficiency in industrialized nations. Antibodies against various steroidogenic enzymes, most frequently CYP21A2 (21-hydroxylase), are present in 65% to 85% of cases of primary autoimmune adrenal insufficiency [62]. Disseminated tuberculosis remains a significant cause of this condition in developing countries worldwide.

The term *relative adrenal insufficiency* has been extensively used in critical care literature. It includes "inadequate" production of corticosteroids during critical care illness, particularly sepsis. The endocrine criteria for definition of the condition vary and are unclear (nonstimulated cortisol during sepsis <20 μg/dl or an increment during cosyntropin stimulation <9 μg/dl). With these various criteria and based on results of recent meta-analysis, which showed improvement in patients' mortality, the use of glucocorticoids and/or mineralocorticoids is recommended in certain situations in critical care literature [63,64]. Note that some of the studies included in the meta-analysis used steroids even in the absence of documented relative adrenal insufficiency; therefore some of the beneficial effect might be explained by "overcoming glucocorticoid resistance at the glucocorticoid receptor level."

Pathophysiology

Secretion of cortisol is controlled primarily through the hypothalamus and pituitary gland, whereas aldosterone is predominantly regulated by the renin–angiotensin system. Primary adrenal insufficiency is characterized by decreased production of both cortisol and aldosterone, with a compensatory increase in ACTH production, whereas secondary adrenal insufficiency is associated with decreased levels of cortisol and ACTH, with preserved mineralocorticoid activity. In autoimmune adrenal insufficiency, the first evidence of a decline in adrenocortical function is an increase in PRA with a low or normal serum aldosterone concentration. This is followed by decreasing plasma cortisol response to ACTH stimulation, increased basal ACTH levels, and finally diminished basal plasma cortisol concentrations and symptoms.

Diagnosis

Clinical Symptoms

Clinical manifestations of adrenal insufficiency depend mainly on the acuteness and the degree of glucocorticoid and mineralocorticoid deficiency. Acute adrenal insufficiency typically leads to shock, usually precipitated by a significant stress (surgery, infection). Decreased production of glucocorticoids and mineralocorticoids results in hypotension (diminished cardiac and peripheral vascular resistance), hypovolemia, hyponatremia, hyperkalemia, and metabolic acidosis. Weakness, fatigue, anorexia, nausea, abdominal pain, weight loss, and orthostatic hypotension are common presenting features of a chronic form of this disease. Other manifestations include diarrhea, muscle aches, dizziness, and hypoglycemia. Hyperpigmentation can be seen in primary adrenal insufficiency, and it is caused by increase in pro-opiomelanocorticotrophic hormone, which leads to increase in melanin levels in skin.

Laboratory Diagnosis

Adrenocortical provocative tests are critical in the diagnosis of adrenal insufficiency (see later).

Plasma cortisol levels are usually at their peak in the early morning (between 4:00 and 8:00 a.m.) and further increase with stress; thus a low plasma cortisol level (<3 μg/dl) provides presumptive evidence of adrenal insufficiency. Conversely, a high morning plasma cortisol concentration (>17 μg/dl) is highly predictive of a normal plasma cortisol response to insulin-induced hypoglycemia or ACTH administration [65]. However, patients with partial adrenal deficiency may demonstrate relatively normal morning levels, whereas low values can be seen in eucortisolemic patients (timing of sampling in regard to diurnal rhythm) and in patients with low cortisol-binding globulin. Likewise, although basal urinary free cortisol and 17-hydroxycorticosteroid (17-OHCS) excretion are usually low in patients with severe adrenal insufficiency, patients with partial deficiencies may have low-normal values. Measurement of the midnight-to-morning urinary cortisol has been proposed as a potential diagnostic approach, but this requires further validation [66].

ACTH (Cosyntropin) Stimulation Test

A normal response to high-dose ACTH (250-mg i.v. or i.m. bolus) stimulation test is an increase in plasma cortisol concentration after 30 to 60 minutes to a peak of at least 18 to 20 μg/dl (500–550 nmol/L). A normal response to high-dose ACTH stimulation excludes primary adrenal insufficiency [67] but not secondary disease. Prolonged secondary adrenal insufficiency leads to adrenal atrophy, which will be seen as sluggish or inappropriate response to ACTH stimulation. However, in patients with mild or recent onset of secondary adrenal insufficiency, ACTH stimulation test results will be normal, and the only reliable tests are the insulin–hypoglycemia test or metyrapone test. The low-dose cosyntropin stimulation test (1 μg i.v. bolus) with measurements of plasma cortisol at 15 and 30 minutes has been proposed to have slightly higher sensitivity than the standard stimulation tests in setting of secondary adrenal insufficiency. Depending on the cutoff used in various studies (peak cortisol of 18–22 μg/dl), the sensitivity of the test varies between 65% and 100%, with specificity of 87% to 96% [68]. The need for meticulous dilution of the currently available cosyntropin vial makes the interpretation and reliability of the test more difficult. Note that recent meta-analysis of available studies showed both types of provocative tests to have similar sensitivities when specificities were set at 95% [69].

A subnormal response confirms the diagnosis of adrenal insufficiency, but further testing is needed to determine the cause of the condition. It is generally helpful to measure a baseline plasma ACTH before administration of cosyntropin.

Metyrapone Test
Refer to the section on evaluation of pituitary function.

Insulin Hypoglycemia Test
Refer to the section on evaluation of pituitary function.

Measurement of Adrenocorticotropic Hormone
Simultaneous measurement of ACTH and cortisol will differentiate primary from secondary causes of hypoadrenalism (plasma ACTH is elevated in primary adrenal insufficiency and low or low normal in secondary and tertiary disease).

Plasma Renin Activity and Aldosterone
The PRA and PRA-to-plasma or -urinary aldosterone ratio was elevated in 100% of the patients with primary adrenal insufficiency [67].

Corticotropin-Releasing Hormone Test
Secondary (pituitary) and tertiary (hypothalamus) adrenal insufficiency could be differentiated through the administration of CRH. ACTH and cortisol responses are minimal or absent with pituitary-related deficiency, whereas an exaggerated response is seen with hypothalamic disease. This is not now clinically useful.

Imaging Studies
In patients with primary adrenal insufficiency, CT of the abdomen with 3-mm cuts of adrenals is the preferred imaging study; when secondary adrenal insufficiency is identified, MRI or CT of the sella turcica and hypothalamus with contrast is performed.

Treatment
The initial goals of therapy in a patient with acute adrenal insufficiency are volume resuscitation and correction of electrolyte abnormalities. Large amounts of 0.9% saline should be rapidly administered at about 2 to 3 L/h until the hypotension is corrected. Once the patient is fluid repleted, saline can be switched to 5% dextrose with 0.45% normal saline. Glucocorticoid deficiency should be addressed expeditiously by intravenous hydrocortisone (100-mg bolus) or dexamethasone (4-mg bolus). The latter can be used if further testing is required because it does not interfere with the measurement of cortisol. The first day, hydrocortisone, 100 mg every 6 to 8 hours, is continued and slowly tapered the next 3 to 4 days, depending on the level of stress. Maintenance dosing usually consists of 15 to 25 mg of hydrocortisone per day orally in two to three divided dosages, with the last dose not later than 5 to 6 p.m., or prednisone, 5 mg, in the morning. The requirement of two or three dosages of hydrocortisone is debatable, a recent study showing a more physiologic cortisol profile with 3 times daily dosing (10 mg–5 mg–5 mg), but a better health-related quality of life with a 20 mg–0 mg–10 mg regimen [70]. Over-replacement with glucocorticoids is a

frequently seen problem and should be avoided. Patients with primary adrenal insufficiency will require treatment with mineralocorticoid agents. Fludrocortisone is typically administered at a dose of 0.1 mg/day, but higher or lower dosage may be required, with adjustments based on symptoms, blood pressure, fluid retention, and serum sodium concentration. Transient glucocorticoid dose increases will be needed for stress or surgery.

Replacement of adrenal androgens is not yet a part of routine clinical practice. The results of several studies (performed only in women) show improvement in fatigue, well-being and sexuality [71], or insulin sensitivity [72] in some studies but not in others [73]. Dosages of 25 to 200 mg of DHES daily have been used, and hirsutism appears to be a major side effect. Treatment is further hampered by lack of pharmaceutically controlled preparations.

PHEOCHROMOCYTOMA
Steven A. DeJong

Definition and Etiology
Pheochromocytomas are catecholamine-producing neuroendocrine tumors that originate from chromaffin cells in the adrenal medulla or extra-adrenal paraganglia. Chromaffin cells develop from neuroectodermal tissue and are associated with the sympathetic ganglia. Although most such cells degenerate after birth, a large collection persists in the adrenal medulla. As a result, 90% of all pheochromocytomas are located in the adrenal medulla, and 98% are located below the diaphragm in the posterior, central middle, or lower abdomen [74]. Extra-adrenal pheochromocytomas, also known as paragangliomas, are usually located along the sympathetic chain from the base of the skull to the bladder, and are more frequently malignant. Paragangliomas derived from parasympathetic tissue often lack the ability to produce catecholamines. The most common extra-adrenal site for a pheochromocytoma is the organ of Zuckerkandl, a collection of paraganglion cells found near the origin of the inferior mesenteric artery and the bifurcation of the aorta [75]. Paragangliomas have been found adjacent to the thoracic or abdominal aorta, in the dome or trigone of the bladder, in the carotid body, and inside the heart. These extra-adrenal tumors are further characterized by an aberrant, unusually large blood supply. Pheochromocytomas are traditionally referred to as "the tumor of 10s," because 10% of these tumors are extra-adrenal, malignant, found in children, and bilateral, multiple, or familial. Recent data, however, suggest that 80% to 85% of pheochromocytomas arise from the adrenal medulla, 15% to 20% are of extra-adrenal origin, and nearly 25% may be hereditary [76]. The cause is unknown, although chromosomal deletions and mutations have been identified in both sporadic and familial pheochromocytomas associated with the multiple endocrine neoplasia type 2 syndromes or von Hippel–Lindau disease [74,75,77].

Epidemiology
A pheochromocytoma can occur at any age and has been described in both newborn and elderly patients. The peak incidence of these tumors occurs during the fourth and fifth decades of life, and they are uncommon after the age of 60 years. Both adrenal glands are affected equally, and no sexual predilection exists, aside from a slight increased female incidence in children. As one of the few rare curable causes of hypertension, pheochromocytomas are identified in only 0.1% to 0.6% of all hypertensive patients [78]. Autopsy studies show a relatively high prevalence of 0.3% to 0.95%, suggesting that a number of these tumors are missed and can result in premature mortality [79]. Biochemical screening results in a prevalence of 1.9%. Approximately one to two per 100,000 people harbor pheochromocytomas, and patients with unrecognized pheochromocytoma risk significant morbidity and mortality [72,75,76]. Approximately 5% of incidentalomas are pheochromocytomas, and 25% of pheochromocytomas are discovered incidentally during unrelated imaging studies [78]. Complications manifested by

hypertensive crisis alone or with shock leading to death may result from pharmacotherapy, anesthesia, childbirth, or surgery performed for other conditions.

Hereditary or familial pheochromocytomas are often bilateral and are frequent components of the inherited syndromes. Pheochromocytomas occur in 25% to 70% of patients with multiple endocrine neoplasia type 2 syndrome, in 25% of patients with von Hippel–Lindau disease, and in fewer than 1% of patients with neurofibromatosis type 1 and von Recklinghausen disease [79]. Specific genetic testing identifying changes in the genetic mutations of the RET proto-oncogene have facilitated prompt accurate identification of patients with the multiple endocrine neoplasia type 2 syndrome and timely treatment of associated pheochromocytoma and other endocrinopathies [82].

Pathophysiology

Catecholamine synthesis begins in the cytoplasm of the chromaffin cells of the adrenal medulla. Phenylalanine and tyrosine undergo a series of hydroxylations and decarboxylations to form norepinephrine, which can be stored in and released from intracellular granules. Conversion from norepinephrine to epinephrine requires the enzyme phenylethanolamine-N-methyl transferase (PNMT), which is found almost exclusively in the adrenal medulla and organ of Zuckerkandl. Epinephrine displays alpha (α) activity, manifested by vasoconstriction, and beta (μ) activity that causes a lesser degree of vasodilation and tachycardia. Norepinephrine acts primarily by α-receptor stimulation, which results in profound vasoconstriction and reflex bradycardia. Epinephrine is 4 to 6 times more potent than norepinephrine and constitutes 85% of adrenal medullary catecholamine production. An epinephrine-producing pheochromocytoma is almost invariably localized to the adrenal medulla [75]. Conversely, extra-adrenal pheochromocytomas often lack the ability to produce epinephrine and thus secrete more norepinephrine. Significant variability is found in the amounts and types of catecholamines released by most pheochromocytomas, which explains the common pattern of paroxysmal symptoms. Pheochromocytomas also have the ability to produce and release other peptides such as calcitonin, vasoactive intestinal peptide, dopamine, neuropeptide Y, parathyroid-related hormone, and ACTH [74,77].

Most tumors that cause hypertension are 3 to 5 cm in diameter, but they can range in size from microscopic adrenal medullary hyperplasia to 30 cm in diameter. They can weigh between 1 g and 4 kg, with an average weight of 100 g [83]. Gross examination reveals a highly vascular gray to pinkish-tan tumor, and areas of hemorrhage, calcification, necrosis, and cystic degeneration are commonly seen. Microscopically, the tumors resemble the cell structure and appearance of the adrenal medulla. The histologic appearance of these tumors, even with capsular or vascular invasion, cannot reliably distinguish benign from malignant lesions. Malignancy is defined by tumor invasion outside the primary site of origin or the demonstration of metastatic disease to lymph nodes, liver, bone, lung, and, rarely, the central nervous system. Malignant pheochromocytomas tend to be larger with more necrosis and are slightly more common in female patients. Malignancy is less common in pheochromocytomas associated with familial syndromes. DNA ploidy studies have been useful in the proper characterization of malignant tumors and may predict prognosis [84].

Diagnosis

The clinical presentation of pheochromocytoma is attributed to the physiology of excess circulating catecholamines; often a significant delay occurs between initial symptoms and final diagnosis [79]. The predominant sign is paroxysmal or sustained hypertension, although as many as 5% of patients with pheochromocytoma are normotensive. Patients with pheochromocytoma discovered incidentally are often normotensive. Other associated symptoms include palpitations, tachycardia, headache, diaphoresis, nausea, abdominal/chest pain, fever, flushing, vomiting, and anxiety or panic attacks [74,77]. Metabolic effects include hyperglycemia, lactic acidosis, and weight loss [85]. Biochemical screening should be performed in hypertensive children, pregnant patients, patients who are resistant to antihypertensive medication, young patients with new-onset hypertension, patients with hypertension associated with new or worsening diabetes, or patients with a hypertensive crisis after anesthesia, surgery, or medication administration. Family members of multiple endocrine neoplasia type 2 syndrome patients should also be screened for pheochromocytoma, and most patients with pheochromocytoma should undergo genetic testing [81,82].

Measurement of plasma catecholamine and 24-hour urinary fractionated catecholamine, metanephrine, normetanephrine, and vanillylmandelic acid (VMA) production remain the cornerstone of the diagnosis of pheochromocytoma. Extra-adrenal paragangliomas are common in patients with predominant elevation of urinary norepinephrine. Plasma free catecholamine (metanephrine and normetanephrine) levels have played an increasingly significant role in detecting pheochromocytoma [86]. In one of the largest studies on biochemical diagnosis of pheochromocytoma, the sensitivity of plasma-free metanephrines was found to be 99%, and specificity was 89%, compared with urinary catecholamines of 86% and 88%, respectively. Plasma catecholamine sensitivity was 84%, with a specificity of 81% [87]. False-positive results often exceed true-positive results, as many physiologic stimuli, drugs, dietary interferences, or any clinical condition that increases circulating catecholamines can produce false-positive testing. Discontinuation or substitution of medications such as tricyclic antidepressants can improve the accuracy of urinary and plasma testing for pheochromocytoma [88]. Provocative testing, by using glucagon, histamine, and other agents, is now unnecessary and is associated with considerable morbidity and mortality. Suppression testing by using clonidine is rarely needed and may cause unexpected hypotension in patients with pheochromocytoma medicated with α-adrenergic and β-blocking agents [89].

Treatment

Medical blockade of excess catecholamine production should be started as soon as the diagnosis of pheochromocytoma is confirmed. Phenoxybenzamine, a long-acting noncompetitive presynaptic and postsynaptic α-adrenergic antagonist, is started 1 to 3 weeks before surgical resection at 10 mg/day and gradually increased until the patient experiences mild postural hypotension. The daily dose can be as high as 1 mg/kg, with the goal of blood pressure control, symptom relief, and volume replacement before surgical intervention. Other agents useful for refractory patients include prazosin, doxazosin, terazosin, labetalol, phentolamine, metyrosine, and calcium channel blockers [88]. Isolated β-blocker therapy, usually in the form of propranolol in doses of 10 to 40 mg every 6 to 8 hours, may be required for patients with tachycardia or cardiac arrhythmias [77,83]. Hypertensive crisis, cardiac arrhythmias, acute cardiac failure/ischemia, pulmonary edema, and cerebral vascular accident can occur if β-blockers are started before complete α-blockade and volume restoration is achieved. Metyrosine can also decrease serum catecholamine levels through inhibition of tyrosine kinase, the rate-limiting enzyme involved in catecholamine synthesis.

Surgical resection after adequate localization and medical preparation remains the definitive treatment for all patients with sporadic or familial pheochromocytoma or paraganglioma. Given that 98% of all pheochromocytomas are found in the abdomen, preoperative tumor localization is safely and successfully accomplished with MRI scanning of the adrenal glands, abdomen, and pelvis [90]. CT scanning of the adrenal glands and entire abdomen with and without contrast is another suitable imaging option for patients whose excess catecholamine production has been medically controlled. It is important to visualize a normal contralateral adrenal gland because 10% to 20% of pheochromocytomas are bilateral; familial disease is commonly bilateral although clinically asynchronous. Occasionally, ^{131}I or preferably [^{123}I]MIBG is needed to identify extra-adrenal tumors in patients with negative CT or MRI imaging or in patients with malignant pheochromocytoma to detect distant sites of tumor metastasis. [^{111}In]Octeotide may also be useful in patients with negative localization studies [91]. Evidence suggests that PET scans, although not advisable as the initial localization study, may be more sensitive than MIBG for visualization of pheochromocytoma. Twenty-nine patients with pheochromocytoma were evaluated with MIBG and PET scans using 2-fluoro-2-deoxy-D-glucose (FDG) [92]. Four patients were found to have positive PET scans and negative levels of MIBG. Of those patients with positive PET and MIBG scans, the PET scans were superior to MIBG in 56% and determined to be as good as or better than in 88% of cases.

The principles of safe extirpation include careful and complete intraoperative monitoring, stress-free anesthesia, complete tumor resection, minimal tumor manipulation, avoidance of tumor seeding, meticulous hemostasis, and early control of the vascular supply and venous drainage of the tumor. Many such tumors can be removed by using a laparoscopic approach in experienced centers to reduce postoperative morbidity and pain, to shorten hospital stay, and to decrease expense compared with traditional laparotomy. The complication rate is less than 8%, operative mortality is 1% to 2%, and the open conversion rate is 5% [93]. Tumors larger than 7 cm in diameter may be malignant and often should be removed with an anterior or thoracoabdominal approach. Laparoscopic bilateral adrenal resection can also be performed if indicated as a single or staged procedure with or without adrenocortical-sparing techniques. Postoperative hypotension and hypoglycemia may develop and may require transient intravenous inotropic and glucose administration, and the overall rate of recurrence is 17% [94].

Malignant pheochromocytomas are often treated with radical surgical removal to improve symptoms and survival, with variable results. Medical control of symptoms is achieved with α-adrenergic blockers, and treatment with chemotherapeutic agents has resulted in disappointing results [88]. Radioactive ablation with high dose [^{131}I]MIBG has been moderately successful to prolong survival and provide effective palliation in some patients, but further studies are needed to confirm benefit [95].

REFERENCES

Evaluation of Adrenocortical Function

1. *(1C)* **Smidt I** et al. Diagnosis of adrenal insufficiency: Evaluation of the corticotropin-releasing hormone tests and basal serum cortisol in comparison to the insulin tolerance test in patients with hypothalamic-pituitary-adrenal disease. J Clin Endocrinol Metab 2003;88:4193–4198.

   The aim of this prospective study was to evaluate diagnostic value of the human CRH test and the basal morning cortisol for diagnosis of adrenal insufficiency in 54 patients and 20 volunteers. In 41 patients, morning basal cortisols were assessed in comparison with ITT. The lower cut point for basal cortisol, providing adrenal insufficiency, was determined as 98 nmol/L (3.6 μg/dl); 100% specificity and 50% sensitivity. The upper cut point for cortisol to confirm adrenal sufficiency was 285 nmol/L (10 μg/dl; 100% sensitivity and 68% specificity).

2. *(1C)* **Papanicolaou D** et al. A single midnight serum cortisol measurement distinguishes Cushing's syndrome from pseudo-Cushing states. J Clin Endocrinol Metab 1998;83:1163–1167.

   Authors report on a cohort of 240 patients with Cushing syndrome and 23 patients with pseudo-Cushing state. Midnight serum cortisol values of more than 7.5 μg/dl had a sensitivity of 96% and specificity of 100% for diagnosis of CS. No obese control study population was included.

3. *(1C)* **Hamrahian A** et al. Measurements of serum free cortisol in critically ill patients. N Engl J Med 2004;350:1629–1638.

   Authors prospectively studied 66 critically ill patients (36 had hypoproteinemia, 30 with near-normal albumin concentration) and 33 healthy volunteers. Baseline and cosyntropin-stimulated serum total cortisol concentrations were lower in hypoproteinemic patients. However, the mean baseline serum free cortical were similar in both groups and several times higher than in normal volunteers. In all patients, cosyntropin-stimulated free cortisol levels were high normal or elevated (including 14 with abnormal cosyntropin tests using measurements of total cortisol).

4. *(1C+)* **Papanicolaou D** et al. Nighttime salivary cortisol: A useful test for the diagnosis of Cushing's syndrome. J Clin Endocrinol Metab 2002;87:4515–4530.

   A large cohort of patients (143 with possible Cushing syndrome and 57 controls) was studied. A midnight salivary cortisol greater than 15.2 nmol/L (550 ng/dl) showed a sensitivity of 93% and excluded all individuals without the disorder by using fluorescence polarization immunoassay.

5. *(1C+)* **Putignano P** et al. Midnight salivary cortisol versus urinary free and midnight serum cortisol as screening tests for Cushing's syndrome. J Clin Endocrinol Metab 2003;88:4153–4157.

   Authors compare diagnostic performance of urinary free cortisol with that of midnight serum cortisol and midnight salivary cortisol in differentiating 41 patients with Cushing syndrome from 33 with pseudo-Cushing syndrome, 199 with simple obesity, and 27 healthy normal weight volunteers. Overall diagnostic accuracy for urinary free cortisol was 95.3%, sensitivity of 90.2%, and specificity of 96% (using a cut-off of 120 μg/24 h or more) and similar to the two other screening tests.

6. *(1C)* **Montori V** et al. Use of plasma aldosterone concentration-to-plasma renin activity ratio as a screening test for primary aldosteronism: A systematic review of literature. Endocrinol Metab Clin North Am 2002;31:619–632.

   Systematic review of literature (16 studies) to establish characteristics of aldosterone–renin ratio used in screening for primary hyperaldosteronism in subjects with presumed essential hypertension. Only 16% of studies had both the ratio and confirmatory tests performed. None of the studies provided valid estimates of the aldosterone–renin ratio test characteristics.

7. *(1C+)* **Bravo E.** The changing clinical spectrum of primary aldosteronism. Am J Med 1983;74: 641–651.

   Prospective study of 80 patients with primary hyperaldosteronism. Authors demonstrated excessive aldosterone excretion after 3 days of salt loading (>14 µg/24 h) with 96% sensitivity and 93% specificity.

8. *(1C)* **Lenders J** et al. Biochemical diagnosis of pheochromocytoma: Which is the best test? JAMA 2002;287:1427–1434.

   Multicenter cohort study of 214 patients with pheochromocytoma (large proportion with hereditary disease) and 644 patients without pheochromocytoma. Sensitivities and specificities of various tests were as follows: 99% and 89% for plasma free metanephrines, 97% and 69% for urinary fractionated metanephrines, 84% and 81% for plasma catecholamines, 77% and 93% for urinary total metanephrines, and 64% and 95% for urinary vanillylmandelic acid, respectively.

9. *(1C)* **Sawka AM** et al. A comparison of biochemical tests for pheochromocytoma: Measurement of fractionated plasma metanephrines compared with the combination of 24-hour urinary metanephrines and catecholamines. J Clin Endocrinol Metab 2003;88:553–558.

   Retrospective analysis of 31 patients with catecholamine-secreting tumors and 261 patients without pheochromocytoma. The sensitivity of fractionated plasma metanephrines and 24-hour urinary total metanephrines and catecholamines (either test positive) were 97% and 90% respectively; however, the specificity for them was 85% versus 98%, respectively. The authors' recommendation is that plasma metanephrine collection is the test of choice in high-risk patients (adrenal vascular mass, familial syndromes).

10. **Speiser P.** Congenital adrenal hyperplasia. N Engl J Med 2003;349:776–778.

    In-depth review of the topic includes details about pathophysiology, various clinical manifestations and biochemical evaluation of enzyme deficiencies. Diagnosis, molecular genetic analysis, and treatment (including prenatal) are described.

11. *(2C)* **Lutfallah C** et al. Newly proposed hormonal criteria via genotypic proof for type II 3beta-hydroxysteroid dehydrogenase deficiency. J Clin Endocrinol Metab 2002;87:2611–2622.

    Cohort of 55 patients with clinical and/or hormonal presentation suggesting compromised 3β-hydroxysteroid dehydrogenase activity underwent genotyping. The hormonal findings for genotype proven (extensive sequencing performed) were provided from infancy to adulthood. For detailed values, please see the article.

Adrenal Imaging

12. *(1A)* **Korobkin M, Francis IR.** Imaging of adrenal masses. Urol Clin North Am 1997;24: 603–622.

    This review article provides an excellent summary of the radiologic options available to image the adrenal gland.

13. *(1C+)* **Francis IR** et al. Integrated imaging of adrenal disease. Radiology 1992;184:1–13.

    This article describes the different radiographic characteristics of adrenal tumors.

14. *(1C)* **Boland GWL** et al. Characterization of adrenal masses using unenhanced CT: An analysis of the CT literature. AJR Am J Roentgenol 1998;171:201–204.

    This article reviews and describes the usefulness and limitations of CT scanning of the adrenal gland. Ten CT reports were analyzed, from which individual adrenal lesion-density measurements were obtained for 495 adrenal lesions (272 benign lesions and 223 malignant lesions). Threshold analysis generated a range of sensitivities and specificities for lesion characterization at different density thresholds. Sensitivity for characterizing a lesion as benign ranged from 47% at a threshold of 2 HU to 88% at a threshold of 20 HU. Similarly, specificity varied from 100% at a threshold of 2 HU to 84% at a threshold of 20 HU. The attempt to be absolutely certain that an adrenal lesion is benign may lead to an unacceptably low sensitivity for lesion characterization. The threshold chosen will depend on the patient population and the cost–benefit approach to patient care.

15. *(1C)* **Caoili EM** et al. Adrenal masses: Characterization with combined unenhanced and delayed enhanced CT. Radiology 2002;222:629–633.

    This is a comprehensive review of the advantages and disadvantages of CT scanning in the detection and characterization of benign, malignant, and metastatic adrenal masses.

16. *(1C)* **Latronico AC, Chrousos GP.** Extensive personal experience: Adrenocortical tumors. J Clin Endocrinol Metab 1997;82:1317–1324.

    The various aspects of benign and malignant adrenal disease from clinical and radiologic perspectives are described.

17. *(1C+)* **Israel GM, Krinsky GA**. MR imaging of renal and adrenal masses. Radiol Clin North Am 2003ˣ:145–159.

This reference is an excellent review of the basic principles and characteristics of MRI for adrenal tumors.

18. *(1C)* **Tsushima Y** et al. Adrenal masses: Differentiation with chemical shift, fast low-angle shot MR imaging. Radiology 1993;186:705–709.

This reference describes the role of MRI techniques in distinguishing benign and malignant adrenal tumors on the basis of MRI appearance.

19. *(1C)* **Varghese JC** et al. MR differentiation of phaeochromocytoma from other adrenal lesions based on qualitative analysis of T2 relaxation times. Clin Radiol 1997;52:603–606.

This article reviews the imaging of pheochromocytoma and describes specific techniques using MRI to distinguish pheochromocytomas from other functional and nonfunctional adrenal tumors.

20. *(1C)* **Siegelman ES**. MR imaging of the adrenal neoplasms. Magn Reson Imaging Clin North Am 2000;4:769–786.

This is a comprehensive review of the advantages of using MRI for evaluation of adrenal masses. The unique characteristics seen on MRI of all of the recognized adrenal lesions are demonstrated, and the reference includes many illustrations.

21. *(1C)* **Reschini E, Catania A**. Clinical experience with the adrenal scanning agents iodine 131-19-iodocholesterol and selenium 75-6-selenomethylcholesterol. Eur J Nucl Med 1991;18:817–823.

This article describes the use of adrenal scintigraphy in the characterization of adrenal tumors. The results of adrenocortical scintigraphy with iodine 131-19-iodocholesterol or selenium 75-6-selenomethyl-cholesterol performed in 94 patients with proven or suspected adrenal disease provided a direct validation of uptake measurements in vivo. The data, collected over a 17-year period, demonstrate that despite the advent of new imaging techniques, adrenal scintigraphy that gives both functional and morphologic information still has an important role in the diagnosis of adrenal disease.

22. *(1C)* **Freitas JE**. Adrenal cortical and medullary imaging. Semin Nucl Med 1995;25:235–230.

This review article provides detailed information about adrenal medullary scintigraphy and its role in the diagnosis of adrenal, extra-adrenal, and metastatic pheochromocytomas.

23. *(1C)* **Shulkin BL** et al. Pheochromocytomas that do not accumulate metaiodobenzylguanidine: Localization with PET and administration of FDG. Radiology 1993;186:711–715.

This study describes the role of PET scanning in the imaging of pheochromocytomas that are unable to concentrate MIBG.

24. *(1C+)* **Yun M** et al. ^{18}F-FDG PET in characterizing adrenal lesions detected on CT or MRI. J Nucl Med 2001;42:1795–1799.

This study details the benefits of using PET scanning in the characterization of incidentally discovered adrenal masses. A useful comparison is made with the us of CT scanning, and specific advantages of PET scanning are identified.

25. *(1C)* **Pacak K** et al. 6-[^{18}F]Fluorodopamine positron emission tomographic (PET) scanning for diagnostic localization of pheochromocytoma. Hypertension 2001;38:6–8.

This reference describes the efficacy of using PET scanning to detect adrenal and extra-adrenal pheochromocytomas.

26. *(1C+)* **Doppman JL, Gill JR Jr**. Hyperaldosteronism: Sampling the adrenal veins. Radiology 1996;198:309–312.

This article provides a review of the use and technique of adrenal vein sampling in the detection and localization of functional adrenal tumors.

27. *(1C)* **Young WF** et al. Role for adrenal venous sampling in primary aldosteronism. Surgery 2004;136:1227–1235.

This article describes the technique and advantages of adrenal vein sampling in a large cohort of patients with primary hyperaldosteronism.

Primary Hyperaldosteronism

28. *(1A)* **Ganguly A**. Primary hyperaldosteronism. N Engl J Med 1998;339:1828–1834.

This extensive review provides detailed information on all aspects of the disease.

29. *(1C+)* **Young WF Jr** et al. Primary hyperaldosteronism: Diagnosis and treatment. Mayo Clin Proc 1990;65:96–110.

This reference is a practical guide to the clinical presentation and treatment of this disorder.

30. *(2C)* **Li JT** et al. Aldosterone-secreting adrenal cortical adenocarcinoma in an 11-year-old child and collective review of the literature. Eur J Pediatr 1994;153:715–717.

This case report describes the aspects of primary hyperaldosteronism seen in patients with adrenocortical carcinoma and review of the current literature on this subject.

31. *(1C)* **Weinberger MH, Fineberg NS**. The diagnosis of primary hyperaldosteronism and separation of two major subtypes. Arch Intern Med 1993;153:2125–2129.

    This publication describes techniques helpful in determining the etiology of hyperaldosteronism. It concludes that the use of the plasma aldosterone/PRA ratio appears to be useful in the screening, diagnosis, and differentiation of unilateral and bilateral forms of primary hyperaldosteronism. These observations may also be applicable to patients receiving some antihypertensive medications.

32. *(1C+)* **Young WF** et al. Role for adrenal venous sampling in primary aldosteronomas. Surgery 2004;136:1227–1235.

    This study provides detailed information on a large patient population undergoing adrenal vein sampling for primary hyperaldosteronism. Many technical aspects of the procedure and clinical features of the disease are discussed.

33. *(1C)* **Doppman JL** et al. Distinction between hyperaldosteronism due to bilateral hyperplasia and unilateral aldosteronoma: Reliability of CT. Radiology 1992;184:677–682.

    This study compared the efficacy of CT and adrenal vein sampling in 24 patients with primary hyperaldosteronism. CT diagnosed unilateral adenoma in 19 patients and hyperplasia in seven patients. After adrenal venous sampling, unilateral adenoma was diagnosed in 22 patients. In their study, six of seven patients with bilateral nodules were found to have unilateral adenoma after venous sampling.

34. *(1C)* **Nocaudie-Calzada M** et al. Efficacy of iodine-131 6-beta-methyl-iodo-19-norcholesterol scintigraphy and computed tomography in patients with primary aldosteronism. Eur J Nucl Med 1999;26:1326–1332.

    This article reports on 41 patients who underwent CT and adrenal scintigraphy. Correct diagnosis was made in 92% of cases compared with only 58% by using CT alone.

35. *(2C)* **Weigel RJ** et al. Surgical treatment of primary hyperaldosteronism. Ann Surg 1994;219: 347–352.

    This article summarizes the surgical care of a patient with an aldosteronoma and describes long-term results of resection.

36. *(1C)* **Celen O** et al. Factors influencing outcome of surgery for primary hyperaldosteronism. Arch Surg 1996;131:646–650.

    This article summarizes the role and predictive factors of successful surgery for primary hyperaldosteronism. The study of 42 patients who underwent adrenalectomy for primary hyperaldosteronism between the years 1970 and 1993 showed that the main determinants of a surgical cure of hypertension in primary hyperaldosteronism were presence of adenoma and preoperative response to spironolactone. The authors favored CT as the initial modality to establish preoperative diagnosis of adenoma because of its reproducibility and high specificity.

Cushing Syndrome

37. **Raff H** et al. A physiologic approach to diagnosis of the Cushing syndrome. Ann Intern Med 2003;138:980–991.

    This article provides an excellent overview of Cushing syndrome.

38. **Lacroix A** et al. Bilateral adrenal Cushing's syndrome: Macronodular adrenal hyperplasia and primary pigmented nodular adrenocortical disease. Endocr Metab Clin North Am 2005;34: 441–458.

    Detailed review of in vitro and in vivo evidence of ectopic abnormal adrenal membrane receptors causing ACTH-independent CS. Strategies for the investigation, as well as opportunities of new pharmacologic therapies, are discussed.

39. **Pivonello R** et al. The metabolic syndrome and cardiovascular risk in Cushing's syndrome. Endocr Metabol Clin North Am 2005;34:327–339.

    In-depth review of metabolic syndrome in setting of Cushing syndrome, including changes after remission of the disease.

40. *(1C+)* **Putignano P** et al. Midnight salivary cortisol versus urinary free and midnight serum cortisol as screening tests for Cushing's syndrome. J Clin Endocrinol Metab 2003;88:4153–4157.

    Authors compare diagnostic performance of urinary free cortisol with that of midnight serum cortisol and midnight salivary cortisol in differentiating 41 patients with Cushing syndrome from 33 with pseudo-Cushing syndrome, 199 with simple obesity, and 27 healthy normal-weight volunteers. Overall diagnostic accuracy for urinary free cortisol was 95.3%, sensitivity 90.2 %, specificity 96% (using a cutoff of ≥120 μg/24 h) and similar to the two other screening tests.

41. *(1C)* **Invitti C** et al. Diagnosis and management of Cushing's syndrome: Results of an Italian multicenter study: Study Group of the Italian Society of Endocrinology on Pathophysiology of the Hypothalamic-Pituitary-Adrenal Axis. J Clin Endocrinol Metab 1999;84:440–448.

    This retrospective analysis of 426 patients with Cushing syndrome (288 with Cushing disease, 80 with adrenal adenoma, 24 with adrenal carcinoma, 25 with ectopic CRH, and nine with ACTH-independent nodular adrenal hyperplasia) showed that overnight low-dose suppression test that is considered as a screening test for Cushing syndrome was as reliable (95% accuracy) as the standard 2-day low-dose dexamethasone suppression test.

42. *(1C)* **Findling J** et al. The low-dose dexamethasone suppression test: A reevaluation in patients with Cushing's syndrome. J Clin Endocrinol Metab 2004;89:1222–1226.

Authors assess diagnostic utility of overnight 1-mg dexamethasone suppression test and the 2-day, low-dose dexamethasone suppression test in 103 patients with Cushing syndrome. Fourteen patients suppressed serum cortisol to less than 5 μg/dl, whereas six patients actually suppressed it to less than 2 μg/dl after a 1-mg test. In addition, the 2-day, low-dose dexamethasone suppression test yielded false-negative results in 38% of patients when urine cortisol was used.

43. **Liu H** et al. Update on the diagnosis of Cushing syndrome. Endocrinologist 2005;15:165–180.

Detailed, practical description and literature analysis of definitive diagnosis, as well as special challenges in diagnosis and differential diagnosis of Cushing syndrome.

44. *(1C)* **Yanowski JA** et al. Corticotropin-releasing hormone stimulation following low-dose dexamethasone administration: A new test to distinguish Cushing's syndrome from pseudo-Cushing's states. JAMA 1993;269:2232–2238.

Fifty-eight adults with mild hypercortisolism (24-h urine free cortisol level, 1,000 nmol/day; surgically confirmed Cushing syndrome in 39 patients, pseudo-Cushing in 19) were given 0.5 mg dexamethasone orally every 6 hours for 2 days, followed 2 hours later by ovine CRH (1-μg/kg intravenous bolus). Using 24-h urinary free cortisol criterion for Cushing syndrome diagnosis on the second day of dexamethasone administration of greater than 100 nmol/day, the test had 100% specificity, 56% sensitivity, and 71% diagnostic accuracy. A plasma cortisol concentration above 1.4 μg/dl measured 15 minutes after CRH administration correctly identified all cases of Cushing syndrome and all cases of pseudo-Cushing states (100% specificity, sensitivity, and diagnostic accuracy).

45. *(1C)* **Avgerinos P** et al. The metyrapone and dexamethasone suppression tests for the differential diagnosis of the ACTH-depended Cushing's syndrome: A comparison. Ann Intern Med 1994; 121:318–327.

Retrospective cohort of 186 patients with ACTH-dependent Cushing syndrome. Criteria of more than 90% urinary cortisol suppression after 2-day high-dose dexamethasone suppression test had sensitivity of 59%, specificity of 73%, and diagnostic accuracy of 61% for diagnosis of pituitary-dependent Cushing disease. Similar values (54%, 73%, and 58%, respectively) were achieved when criteria of more than 69% 24-h urinary suppression of 17-hydroxysteroids was applied.

46. *(1C)* **Dichek HL** et al. A comparison of the standard high dose dexamethasone suppression test and the overnight 8 mg dexamethasone supression test for the differential diagnosis of adrenocorticotropin dependent Cushing's syndrome. J Clin Endocrinol Metab 1994;78:418–422.

A direct comparison of the standard high-dose dexamethasone suppression test and the overnight dexamethasone supression tests performed in 41 patients (34 with Cushing disease and seven with ectopic ACTH syndrome).The sensitivity of the tests was comparable: 79% versus 71% with a specificity of 100%; however, a post-dexamethasone cortisol decline of more than 68% for the latter was used. The diagnostic performance of combining both tests was better than either test alone.

47. *(1C)* **Aron DE** et al. Effectiveness versus efficacy: The limited value in clinical practice of high-dose dexamethasone suppression test in differential diagnosis of ACTH dependent Cushing's syndrome. J Clin Endocrinol Metab 1997;82:1780–1785.

The sensitivity and specificity of HDDS for the diagnosis of pituitary-dependent Cushing syndrome are reported to be 81% and 66.7%, respectively, based on standard criteria of more than 50% suppression of baseline plasma or 24-h urinary cortisol.

48. *(1C+)* **Assalia A** et al. Laparoscopic adrenalectomy. Br J Surg 2004;91:1259–1274.

Meta-analysis of 20 comparative case–control studies comparing laparoscopic adrenalectomy with open adrenalectomy (2,550 procedures, including 225 patients with Cushing syndrome). The results of laparoscopic adrenalectomy were reproducible, associated with lower morbidity (10.9% vs. 35%), less blood loss (154 vs. 309 ml), similar hormonal outcome, and shorter hospital stay (12 vs. 18.2 days).

49. *(2C)* **Engelhardt D** et al. Therapy of Cushing's syndrome with steroid biosynthesis inhibitors. J Steroid Biochem Mol Biol 1994;49:261–267.

Meta-analysis of 82 patients with Cushing disease treated with ketoconazole. Daily doses of 400 to 1,600 mg effectively reduce plasma cortisol in 70% of patients. Long-term follow-up data were not included. Results in 26 patients with Cushing syndrome are presented as well.

50. *(2C)* **Luton JP** et al. Treatment of Cushing's disease by O,p'DDD: Survey of 62 cases. N Engl J Med 1979;300:459–464.

Retrospective review of cases treated with up to 12 g of mitotane daily, which achieved remission in 83% of patients. One third continued to be in remission after therapy discontinuation.

51. **Nieman L**. Medical therapy of Cushing's disease. Pituitary 2002;5:77–82.

Concise review of available medications for medical therapy of Cushing disease. Limitations of various agents are described in detail.

Adrenal Incidentalomas

52. *(1C+)* **Herrera MF** et al. Incidentally discovered adrenal tumors: An institutional perspective. Surgery 1991;110:1014–1021.

Some 2,066 patients with adrenal masses were analyzed from a total of 61,054 CT scans done from 1985 through 1989. Excluding patients with previous or concurrent malignancies, adrenal tumors localized after biochemical documentation of disease, and adrenal nodules smaller than 1 cm, 342 patients were analyzed, including 136 men and 206 women with a mean age of 62 years. Tumor diameter ranged from 1 to 11 cm (mean, 2.5 cm). Histologic diagnosis was available in 55 patients at the time of adrenalectomy; malignancy was discovered in five patients (four primary and one metastatic); the smallest malignant tumor detected measured 5 cm.

53. **Grumbach M** et al. Management of clinically inapparent adrenal mass ("incidentaloma"): NIH conference. Ann Intern Med 2003;138:424–429.

    The NIH Consensus Development Program convention of experts in field report to address prevalence, causes, evaluation, and treatment of adrenal masses. Panel recommendation included 1-mg dexamethasone suppression tests and measurement of plasma-free metanephrines for patients with adrenal incidentalomas, serum potassium, plasma aldosterone/renin values in hypertension.

54. *(1C+)* **Mantero F** et al. A survey on adrenal incidentaloma in Italy: Study Group on Adrenal Tumors of the Italian Society of Endocrinology. J Clin Endocrinol Metab 2000;85:637–644.

    This was a multicenter retrospective study of 1,096 incidentalomas from 1980 to 1995. Questionnaires were obtained from 1,004 patients (420 men and 584 women), with a median age of 58 years. Mass size ranged from 0.5 to 25 cm (median, 3.0 cm). Some 85% of the masses were nonfunctional; 9.2% were defined as representing subclinical Cushing syndrome; 4.2% were pheochromocytomas; and 1.6% were aldosteronomas. Patients with subclinical Cushing syndrome showed low baseline ACTH in 79%, cortisol unsuppressibility after 1 mg dexamethasone in 73%, above-normal urinary free cortisol in 75%, disturbed cortisol rhythm in 43%, and blunted ACTH response to CRH in 55%. Adrenalectomy was performed in 380 patients; 198 cortical adenomas (52%), 47 cortical carcinomas (12%), 42 pheochromocytomas (11%), and other less-frequent tumor types were found. Patients with carcinoma were significantly younger (median, 46 years; range, 17–84 years) than patients with adenoma (median, 57 years, range, 16–83 years; $p = 0.05$) and adenomas were significantly smaller than carcinomas (3.5, 1–15 vs. 7.5, 2.6–25 cm; $p < 0.001$). A cutoff of 4 cm had the highest sensitivity (93%) in differentiating between benign and malignant tumors. Only 43% of patients with pheochromocytomas were hypertensive, and 86% showed elevated urinary catecholamines. All patients with aldosteronomas were hypertensive and had suppressed upright PRA.

55. *(1C)* **Lenders J** et al. Biochemical diagnosis of pheochromocytoma: Which is the best test? JAMA 2002;287:1427–1434.

    Multicenter cohort study of 214 patients with pheochromocytomas (large proportion with hereditary disease) and 644 patients without pheochromocytomas. Sensitivities and specificities of various tests were as follows: 99% and 89% for plasma free metanephrines, 97% and 69% for urinary fractionated metanephrines, 84% and 81% for plasma catecholamines, 77% and 93% for urinary total metanephrines, and 64% and 95% for urinary vanillylmandelic acid, respectively.

56. *(1C)* **Sawka AM** et al. A comparison of biochemical tests for pheochromocytoma: measurement of fractionated plasma metanephrines compared with the combination of 24-hour urinary metanephrines and catecholamines. J Clin Endocrinol Metab 2003; 88:553–558.

    Retrospective analysis of 31 patients with catecholamine-secreting tumors and 261 patients without pheochromocytoma. The sensitivity of fractionated plasma metanephrines and 24-hour urinary total metanephrines and catecholamines (either test positive) were 97% and 90%, respectively; however, the specificity for these were 85% and 98%, respectively. Authors' recommendation is that plasma metanephrine collection is the test of choice in high-risk patients (adrenal vascular mass, familiar syndromes).

57. **Terzolo M** et al. Subclinical Cushing's syndrome in adrenal incidentalomas. Endocrinol Metab Clin North Am 2005;34:423–439.

    Excellent up-to-date review of the topic.

58. *(2C)* **Tauchmanova L** et al. Patients with subclinical Cushing's syndrome due to adrenal adenoma have increased cardiovascular risk. J Clin Endocr Metab 2002;87:4872–4878.

    Cross-sectional study of 28 consecutive SCS patients compared with 100 matched controls. Systolic and diastolic pressure, fasting glues, insulin, total cholesterol, triglycerides, fibrinogen, and mean carotid artery intima–media thickness were higher in patients. Of the patients, 60.7% had hypertension, 71% had lipid abnormalities, 29% had impaired glucose tolerance, and 54% had impairment in hemostatic parameters. Eight patients underwent surgical removal of the adenoma, and on median follow-up of 44 months, a significant decrease of body mass index (BMI), systolic and diastolic blood pressures, and fibrinogen levels occurred ($p < 0.005$).

59. *(1C+)* **Assalia A, Gagner M.** Laparoscopic adrenalectomy. Br J Surg 2004;91:1259–1274.

    Meta-analysis of 20 comparative case–control studies comparing laparoscopic adrenalectomy with open adrenalectomy (2,550 procedures, including 225 patients with Cushing syndrome). The results of laparoscopic adrenalectomy were reproducible, associated with lower morbidity (10.9% vs. 35%), less blood loss (154 vs. 309 ml), similar hormonal outcome, and shorter hospital stay (12 versus 18.2 days).

60. *(1C)* **Icard P** et al. Adrenocortical carcinomas: Surgical trends and results of a 253-patient series from the French association of Endocrine Surgeons study group. World J Surg 2001;25: 891–897.

Results of a large cohort of patients with adrenal cortical cancer are presented. Adjuvant mitotane after complete resection has not shown to provide survival benefit.

Adrenal Insufficiency

61. **Arlt W** et al. Adrenal insufficiency. Lancet 2003;361:1881–1893.

   This is an excellent review of the etiology, pathogenesis, clinical presentation, and diagnostic workup of adrenal insufficiency. Therapy for adrenal insufficiency is discussed in detail as well.

62. *(1C)* **Falorni A** et al. Italian Addison Network study: Update on diagnostic criteria for the etiological classification of primary adrenal insufficiency (PAI). J Clin Endocrinol Metab 2004;89: 1598–1604.

   Results of Italian Society of Endocrinology specific study group regarding etiological classification of PAI are presented. Two-hundred-twenty-two participants were tested for the presence of 21OHAb and adrenal cortex autoantibodies in two independent laboratories. Both antibodies were positive in 57%, 21OHAb only in 8%, and ACA were present in 12% of patients. Fifty patients had negative adrenal antibodies; of these, six had idiopathic etiology of insufficiency (falsely negative antibodies). A comprehensive flowchart for the classification of PAI was developed by authors.

63. *(2A)* **Annane D** et al. Effect of treatment with low doses of hydrocortisone and fludrocortisone on mortality in patients with septic shock. JAMA 2002;288:862–868.

   Authors report results of French multicenter placebo-controlled, randomized, double-blinded trial of 300 adults with septic shock who were enrolled after undergoing a short corticotropin test. Patients were randomized to receive either hydrocortisone (50 mg i.v. every 6 hours) and fludrocortisone (50-μg tbl once a day) or matching placebos all for 7 days. Twenty-eight–day survival was analyzed. Of 229 nonresponders (defined as change of cortisol of less than 9 μg/dl), 73 (63%) deaths occurred in the placebo group and 60 (53%) deaths in the intervention group (hazard ratio, 0.67; p = 0.02). No significant difference between groups was found in responders.

64. *(1B)* **Minneci P** et al. Meta-analysis: The effect of steroids on survival and shock during sepsis depends on the dose. Ann Intern Med 2004;141:47–56.

   This meta-analysis includes five randomized double-blinded controlled trials published after 1997 of 5- to 7-day courses of physiologic stress doses of hydrocortisone i.v., regardless of adrenal function. The results showed a beneficial effect on survival (relative benefit, 1.23; p = 0.036) and shock reversal (relative benefit, 1.71; p < 0.001). These data are in contrast to those of eight previous studies in which glucocorticoids were used in higher doses, earlier in the course of septic shock and for a shorter time. Authors recognized the limitations of time-related improvements in medical care and potential bias secondary to nonreporting of negative study results.

65. *(1C+)* **Erturk E** et al. Evaluation of the integrity of the hypothalamic-pituitary-adrenal axis by insulin hypoglycemia test. J Clin Endocrinol Metab 1998;83:2350–2354.

   Retrospective review of ACTH and cortisol responses to insulin hypoglycemia in 193 subjects with suspected ACTH deficiency. Of these, 133 subjects were classified as having an intact hypothalamic–pituitary–adrenal axis, and 60 subjects were determined to have ACTH deficiency based on a cutoff value for peak cortisol of 18 mg/dl. Baseline and peak cortisol concentrations were strongly correlated (r = 0.63; p < 0.0001). Basal cortisol values more than 17 mg/dl or less than 4 mg/dl were highly predictive of an intact or impaired hypothalamo–pituitary–adrenal axis, respectively, but intermediate values had only limited sensitivity and specificity. An increase in plasma cortisol of more than 7 mg/dl above baseline or doubling of the baseline cortisol value had high false-positive and false-negative rates in predicting integrity of the hypothalamic–pituitary–adrenal axis.

66. *(1C)* **Kong WM** et al. The midnight to morning urinary cortisol increment is an accurate, noninvasive method for assessment of the hypothalamic-pituitary-adrenal axis. J Clin Endocrinol Metab 1999;84:3093–3098.

   Forty patients with pituitary disease and 40 controls collected double-voided urine samples at midnight and on awakening. Cortisol/creatinine (Cort/Cr) ratios were calculated. The Cort/Cr increment was defined as the morning Cort/Cr ratio minus the midnight Cort/Cr ratio. The Cort/Cr increment of the patients was compared with the results of their insulin tolerance test or short Synacthen test. Using the results from the 40 controls, a normal Cort/Cr increment was defined as greater than 9. The positive predictive value of a Cort/Cr increment for the diagnosis of hypothalamopituitary–adrenal insufficiency was 95%. These findings suggest that the midnight-to-morning Cort/Cr increment is a reliable, noninvasive alternative to the ITT/SST for assessment of the hypothalamic–pituitary–adrenal axis.

67. *(1C)* **Oelkers WS** et al. Diagnosis and therapy surveillance in Addison's disease: Rapid adrenocorticotropin (ACTH) test and measurement of plasma ACTH, renin activity, and aldosterone. J Clin Endocrinol Metab 1992;75:259–264.

   In 45 patients with primary adrenal insufficiency (PIA), results of the rapid ACTH test and single measurements of plasma cortisol, ACTH, aldosterone, and PRA taken between 8:00 and 9:00 a.m. were compared with measurements in 55 normal subjects and 46 patients with pituitary disease (cortisol and ACTH only). The rapid ACTH test result was abnormal in all 41 patients who underwent PAI testing. Plasma ACTH, PRA, and the ratios of ACTH to cortisol and PRA to plasma or urinary aldosterone were clearly elevated in all of patients with PAI. The ACTH/cortisol ratio distinguished 100% of patients with PAI from secondary adrenal insufficiency (SAI), but not control subjects from those with SAI. PRA measurements during treatment with hydrocortisone and fludrocortisone correlated better with the mineralocorticoid dose than did plasma potassium and sodium levels. PRA measurement is a valuable tool in assessing mineralocorticoid therapy.

68. *(1C)* **Abdu T** et al. Comparison of the low dose short Synacthen test (1 μg), the conventional dose short Synacthen test (250 μg), and the insulin tolerance test for the assessment of the hypothalamo-pituitary-adrenal axis in patients with pituitary disease. J Clin Endocrinol Metab 1999;84:838–843.

Authors prospectively studied 42 patients with suspected or proven pituitary disease and compared results of three tests as described in the title. The low-dose Synacthen test was slightly more sensitive than the standard Synacthen test (6% of patients had false reassurance with the standard test; with a 30-min cortisol cutoff as 500 nmol/L (18 μg/dl).

69. *(1C+)* **Dorin RI** et al. Diagnosis of adrenal insufficiency. Ann Intern Med 2003;139:194–201.

Authors generated summary receiver-operating characteristic (ROC) curves from 20 various published studies for standard cosyntropin test and for nine published low-dose cosyntropin test studies (all identified on MEDLINE database). They further provided sensitivity and specificity results. At a specificity of 95%, sensitivities for secondary adrenal insufficiency diagnosis were 57% and 61% for summary ROC curves in tests for standard-dose test and low-dose test, respectively. The area under the curve did not differ significantly ($p > 0.5$).

70. *(1C)* **Alonso N** et al. Evaluation of two replacement regiments in primary adrenal insufficiency patients: Effect on clinical symptoms, health-related quality of life (HRQL) and biochemical parameters. J Endocr Invest 2004;27:449–454.

Authors prospectively studied two different regiments of hydrocortisone in PAI (20 mg−0 mg−10 mg and 10 mg−5 mg−5 mg), each maintained for 3 months and compared with healthy controls. Patients with adrenal insufficiency had a worse HRQL in the energy dimension compared with the general population, regardless of the treatment regimen. However, the thrice-daily hydrocortisone regimen showed a more physiologic cortisol profile.

71. *(2A)* **Arlt W** et al. Dehydroepiandrosterone replacement in women with adrenal insufficiency. N Engl J Med 1999;341:1013-1016.

Prospective double-blinded randomized trial in 24 women with PAI regarding dehydroepiandrosteone replacement (50 mg orally daily) for 4 months with 1-month washout. Treatment with dehydroepiandrosterone improved overall well-being as well as scores for depression and anxiety and sexuality.

72. *(2A)* **Dhatariya K** et al. Effect of dehydroepiandrosterone replacement on insulin sensitivity and lipids in hypoadrenal women. Diabetes 2005;54:765–770.

This was a randomized, double-blind, placebo-controlled, crossover study in 28 hypoadrenal women receiving a 50-mg dose of dehydroepiandrosterone. After 12 weeks, insulin sensitivity (assesed by hyperinsulinemic–euglycemic clamp) was increased ($p < 0.05$), and levels of total cholesterol, triglycerides, LDL cholesterol, and HDL cholesterol were reduced ($p < 0.05$).

73. *(2A)* **Lovas K** et al. Replacement of dehydroepiandrosterone in adrenal failure: No benefit for subjective health status and sexuality in a 9-month, randomized, parallel group clinical trial. J Clin Endocrinol Metab 2003;88:112–1117.

Prospective randomized trial of dehydroepiandrosterone replacement (25 mg orally daily) in 39 women with adrenal failure. No difference in subjective health scales was found between the placebo and treatment groups. Androgenic side effects were seen in 89% of the dehydroepiandrosterone group.

Pheochromocytoma

74. *(1A)* **Young WF Jr**. Pheochromocytoma and primary aldosteronism: Diagnostic approaches. Endocrinol Metab Clin North Am 1997;26:801–827.

This is an excellent overview of the current diagnosis and treatment of pheochromocytoma.

75. *(1A)* **Januszewicz W, Wocial B**. Pheochromocytoma: The catecholamine-dependent hypertension. J Physiol Pharmacol 1995;46:285–295.

A comprehensive review of the physiology of catecholamine synthesis and pheochromocytoma.

76. *(1B)* **Pacak K** et al. Recent advances in genetics, diagnosis, localization, and treatment of pheochromocytoma. Ann Intern Med 2001;134:315–329.

This reference provides an excellent summary of the recent advances in genetic testing for pheochromocytoma.

77. *(1C)* **Manger WM, Gifford RW Jr**. Pheochromocytoma: Current diagnosis and management. Cleve Clin J Med 1993;60:365–378.

The reference reviews the current patient evaluation of pheochromocytoma. Pheochromocytoma can mimic several other diseases, making recognition difficult. Hypertension may be paroxysmal or sustained. The signs and symptoms of pheochromocytoma are mostly due to hypercatecholaminemia, hypertension, complications, or coexisting diseases; however, measurements of catecholamines and their metabolites in the plasma and urine may be normal between attacks, and other conditions can elevate these values. The clonidine suppression test confers specificity to the clinical and laboratory findings, and MRI is the most reliable method of locating a tumor. Surgical resection is successful in

90% of patients; however, the disease is fatal if it is not detected and treated. Pheochromocytoma should be suspected in patients with paroxysmal or sustained hypertension, particularly if symptoms are present.

78. *(1C)* **Omura M** et al. Prospective study on the prevalence of secondary hypertension patients visiting a general outpatient clinic in Japan. Hypertens Res 2004;27:193–202.

This study investigates the incidence of pheochromocytoma in random patients with hypertension.

79. *(1C)* **Lo CY** et al. Adrenal pheochromocytoma remains a frequently overlooked diagnosis. Am J Surg 2000;179:212–215.

This study documents the delay in diagnosis of pheochromocytoma in many patients and incidence of these tumors in autopsy series.

80. *(1C)* **Mansmann G** et al. The clinically inapparent adrenal mass: Update in diagnosis and management. Endocr Rev 2004;25:309–340.

This review focuses on the detection and incidence of pheochromocytoma in incidentally discovered adrenal masses. It provides a logical strategy for the evaluation and management of these tumors in this clinical setting.

81. *(1C)* **Lairmore TC** et al. Management of pheochromocytoma in patients with multiple endocrine neoplasia type 2 syndromes. Ann Surg 1993;217:595–601.

This article provides advice and recommendations for the treatment of pheochromocytoma in the context of the MEN 2 syndrome. The results of unilateral or bilateral adrenalectomy were studied in 58 patients (49 with MEN 2A and nine with MEN 2B). Recurrence of disease was evaluated by measuring 24-hour urinary excretion rates of catecholamines and metabolites and by CT scanning. In a mean postoperative follow-up of 9.4 years, no operative mortality occurred; malignant or extra-adrenal pheochromocytomas were not present. Twenty-three patients with a unilateral pheochromocytoma and a macroscopically normal contralateral gland underwent unilateral adrenalectomy. A pheochromocytoma developed in the remaining gland a mean duration of 11.87 years after the primary adrenalectomy in 12 (52%) patients. Conversely, pheochromocytoma did not develop in 11 (48%) patients during a mean interval of 5.18 years. In the interval after unilateral adrenalectomy, no patient experienced hypertensive crises or other complications related to an undiagnosed pheochromocytoma. Ten (23%) of 43 patients who earlier had both adrenal glands removed (either at a single operation or sequentially) experienced at least one episode of acute adrenal insufficiency or addisonian crisis, including one patient who died during an episode of influenza. Based on these data, the treatment of choice for patients with MEN 2A or MEN 2B and a unilateral pheochromocytoma is resection of only the involved gland. Substantial morbidity and significant mortality are associated with the addisonian state after bilateral adrenalectomy.

82. *(1C+ *)* **Modigliani E** et al. Pheochromocytomas in multiple endocrine neoplasia type 2: European study: The European Study Group. J Intern Med 1995;238:363–367.

This reference describes the unique characteristics and genetic testing of pheochromocytomas occurring in patients with the MEN II syndrome.

83. *(1C*)* **Sheps SG** et al. Recent developments in the diagnosis and treatment of pheochromocytoma. Mayo Clin Proc 1990;65:88–95.

This reference describes the clinical presentation of a patient with pheochromocytoma. Recent clinical developments include the detection of asymptomatic paroxysms of hypertension by 24-hour ambulatory monitoring, detailed characterization of catecholamine cardiomyopathy by echocardiography, and further experience with Carney's triad and other polyglandular and multiple neoplasia syndromes associated with pheochromocytoma. Refinement in interpretation of catecholamine measurements and the development of radionuclide scanning with m-[^{131}I]iodobenzylguanidine, CT, and MRI have greatly enhanced clinicians' diagnostic acumen. Developments in antihypertensive drug therapy and chemotherapy have improved management of catecholamine hypersecretion and tumor growth, respectively, in inoperable patients and in the preparation of patients for anesthesia and surgical treatment. Flow cytometry to detect abnormal DNA histograms may prove particularly useful in predicting the malignant nature of the tumors.

84. *(1C+)* **Nativ O** et al. The clinical significance of nuclear DNA ploidy pattern in 184 patients with pheochromocytoma. Cancer 1992;69:2683–2687.

This article describes aspects of malignancy determination in patients with pheochromocytoma by using flow cytometry. Flow-cytometric nuclear DNA analysis was performed on paraffin-embedded tissue samples taken from 184 patients with pheochromocytoma and paraganglioma treated between 1960 and 1987. Hedley's technique was used for measurement of nuclear DNA content. About 35% of the tumors were DNA diploid, 33% showed a DNA tetraploid pattern, and 32% had a DNA aneuploid pattern. Familial pheochromocytoma and associated endocrine or neoplastic disorders were more common among patients with DNA nondiploid tumors. Eighty-four percent of the tumors that invaded blood vessels and all patients with regional or distant metastases were associated with tumors that were classified as DNA tetraploid or DNA aneuploid. Of 22 patients who had disease progression, 21 (95%) had tumors with abnormal DNA ploidy pattern ($p < 0.001$). All 12 patients who died of cancer-related disease had abnormal DNA ploidy; none of the 64 patients with DNA diploid tumor has died as a result of pheochromocytoma ($p < 0.01$). These results suggest that nuclear DNA ploidy pattern is an important and independent prognostic variable for patients with pheochromocytoma and paraganglioma.

85. *(1C)* **Batide-Alanore A** et al. Diabetes as a marker of pheochromocytoma in hypertensive patients. J Hypertens 2003;21:1703–1707.

    This study focuses on the incidence of pheochromocytoma in patients with diabetes and hypertension.

86. *(1C+)* **Lenders JWM** et al. Plasma metanephrines in the diagnosis of pheochromocytoma. Ann Intern Med 1995;123:101–109.

    This reference reviews the methods of detecting catecholamine excess by measuring urinary and plasma catecholamines. Results show that normal plasma concentrations of metanephrines rule out the diagnosis of pheochromocytoma, whereas normal plasma concentrations of catecholamines and normal urinary excretion of metanephrines do not. Tests for plasma metanephrines are more sensitive than tests for plasma catecholamines or urinary metanephrines for the diagnosis of pheochromocytoma.

87. *(1C)* **Lenders JW** et al. Biochemical diagnosis of pheochromocytoma: Which test is best? JAMA 2002;287:1427–1434.

    In this multicenter cohort study, findings in 214 patients with confirmed pheochromocytoma were compared with those of 644 normal patients. The sensitivities and specificities of the tests undertaken were plasma free metanephrines, 99% and 89%; urinary fractionated metanephrines, 97% and 69%; plasma catecholamines, 84% and 81%; urinary catecholamines, 86% and 88%; and urinary total metanephrines, 77% and 93%, respectively.

88. *(1A)* **Lenders JWM** et al. Phaeochromocytoma. Lancet 2005;366:665–675.

    This reference is an excellent review of all the most recent articles published from 2000 to 2005 on the subject of pheochromocytoma. The information was extracted from a database review of PubMed and EMBASE and includes book chapters, review articles, and commonly referenced new and older publications.

89. *(1C)* **Bravo EL** et al. Clonidine-suppression test: A useful aid in the diagnosis of pheochromocytoma. N Engl J Med 1981;305:623–626.

    This study provides the details and usefulness of the clonidine-suppression test to identify patients with pheochromocytoma.

90. *(1C)* **Varghese JC** et al. MR differentiation of phaeochromocytoma from other adrenal lesions based on qualitative analysis of T2 relaxation times. Clin Radiol 1997;52:603–606.

    This article reviews the imaging of pheochromocytoma and describes specific techniques using MRI to distinguish pheochromocytomas from other functional and nonfunctional adrenal tumors. It concludes that considerable overlap exists between the MRI appearance of pheochromocytoma and other adrenal lesions. A pheochromocytoma cannot be excluded on the basis of a lack of high signal intensity on T2-weighted MRI.

91. *(1C)* **van der Harst E** et al. [(123)I] metaiodobenzylguanidine and [(111)In] octreotide uptake in benign and malignant pheochromocytomas. J Clin Endocrinol Metab 2001;86:685–693.

    This study compares the use of MIBG and octreotide in the detection of pheochromocytomas. Some patients appear to have pheochromocytomas that concentrate radiolabled octreotide after MIBG imaging is negative.

92. *(1C)* **Shulkin BL** et al. Pheochromocytomas: Imaging with 2-[fluorine-18]fluoro-2-deoxy-D-glucose PET. Radiology 1999;212:35–41.

    Thirty-five FDG-PET and MIBG scans obtained from 29 patients with confirmed pheochromocytoma were compared. With FDG, 22 of 29 patients had positive scans, and four of 29 patients had negative MIBG and positive FDG scans. Most of these tumors (16 of 29) were seen by using both techniques, but the FDG images were judged to be superior to those of MIBG in 56% of cases.

93. *(1C)* **Gagner M** et al. Is laparoscopic adrenalectomy indicated for pheochromocytoma? Surgery 1996;120:1076–1080.

    This study examined the safety and efficacy of laparoscopic adrenalectomy for patients with pheochromocytoma. Based on 90 laparoscopic adrenalectomies performed in 82 patients, the authors concluded that laparoscopic adrenalectomy for pheochromocytoma is difficult because tumors are larger, and more complications are seen related to their hormonal secretions, despite adequate pharmacologic blockade. However, metastatic extensions can be diagnosed and laparoscopic ablation can be performed in most instances without recurrence. It is not, therefore, a contraindication for this approach.

94. *(1C)* **Amar L** et al. Year of diagnosis, features at presentation, and risk of recurrence in patients with pheochromocytoma or secreting paraganglioma. J Clin Endocrinol Metab 2005;90:268–2075.

    This study outlines the demographics of patients found to have a pheochromocytoma and focuses on the significant delay in diagnosis in many patients with this disorder.

95. *(1C)* **Rose B** et al. High-dose ^{131}I-metaiodobenzylguanidine therapy for 12 patients with malignant pheochromocytoma. Cancer 2003;98:239–248.

    This reference provides information regarding a small group of patients treated with high-dose radiolabeled MIBG in patients with extensive metastatic disease from malignant pheochromocytoma. The use of this agent is modestly successful in controlling catecholamine production for these patients over a short period in a palliative setting.

Metabolic Bone Disorders

Stephanie E. Painter and Pauline M. Camacho

EVALUATION OF METABOLIC BONE DISORDERS

As with any disease, the workup of metabolic bone disorders starts with a comprehensive history and physical examination. Diagnosis of these disorders is usually made based on the results of biochemical tests and radiologic studies.

Serum Calcium, Phosphate, and Magnesium

In patients with normal albumin concentrations, serum calcium is usually accurate. However, with abnormal albumin levels, the formula for their correction may be inaccurate in 20% to 30% of cases. In this case, one should obtain an ionized calcium measurement. Phosphate levels are useful in the evaluation of hypocalcemia and hypercalcemia. Magnesium levels should be checked in the workup of hypocalcemia, because low magnesium may decrease parathyroid hormone (PTH) secretion or lead to resistance to its effects.

Intact Parathyroid Hormone

The most reliable measure of PTH status is the intact molecule. Radioimmunoassay (RIA) is most commonly used, but two-site immunologic assays using immunoradiometric assay (IRMA) or colorimetric/chemiluminescence detection also are available. A new assay, bio-intact PTH, eliminates the effect of PTH fragments that build up in renal failure.

Vitamin D Metabolites

The two clinically useful metabolites are 25(OH)D, or calcidiol, and 1,25(OH)D, or calcitriol. Both tests are quantitated by using ^{125}I-based RIA. 25(OH)D, the major circulating hormone, is used to determine vitamin D status. 1,25(OH)D is the active form of vitamin D. Levels may not be reliable in vitamin D–deficiency states, because stimulation of 1α-hydroxylation of 25(OH)D in secondary hyperparathyroidism can increase this concentration.

Parathyroid Hormone–Related Protein

Compared with PTH, PTHrP is a larger molecule. They share many N-terminal, but few C-terminal sequence homologues. In addition, both share the same receptor.

lignancy.

Calcitonin

This is used mainly for diagnosis and follow-up of medullary carcinoma. Sensitivity for calcitonin increases with stimulation by pentagastrin or calcium.

Urinary Calcium Excretion

Normal calcium excretion usually falls in the range of 1.5 to 3.0 mg of calcium per kilogram body weight per 24 hours. A simultaneous urine creatinine should be measured to ensure complete collection. The fractional excretion of calcium is calculated by using the following formula: (Urinary calcium × Serum creatinine)/(Urinary creatinine × Serum calcium).

Biochemical Markers of Bone Turnover

Bone-Formation Markers

Osteocalcin and bone-specific alkaline phosphatase (BSAP) are the most commonly used measures of bone formation. Of note, osteocalcin also reflects bone resorption, because it is released into the circulation from the matrix during this process. BSAP is produced by osteoblasts and is an enzyme necessary for bone mineralization. Other markers of bone formation are carboxy and amino terminal propeptide of type 1 collagen (PICP and PINP); however, the presence of type 1 collagen in other tissues makes these markers less clinically helpful.

Osteoprotegerin has become better understood regarding its role in bone formation. It inhibits RANKL and subsequent osteoclast production. Estrogen and raloxifene enhance its concentration, whereas corticosteroids inhibit it. However, osteoprotegerin is not specific for bone, and its concentration is affected by disease processes such as renal failure; this limits its clinical utility as a bone marker [1].

Bone-Resorption Markers

Urinary levels of N- and C-telopeptide of collagen cross-links (NTX and CTX), free and total pyridinolines (Pyd), deoxypyridinolines (Dpd), and hydroxyproline are used as markers of bone resorption. Urinary NTX and CTX are the most commonly used in clinical practice. RANKL, briefly mentioned earlier, is a ligand that, on binding to its receptor RANK, stimulates osteoclast production and inhibits osteoclast destruction. A negative association between RANKL and 17β-estradiol and a positive correlation between RANKL and bone-resorption markers has been noted. However, clinical utility is still limited [1].

Clinical Use

Because of the diurnal variation and technical variability of these markers, controversy remains as to their routine use in osteoporosis management. Long-term variability can vary by as much as 20% to 30% for urine markers and 10% to 15% for serum markers [2,3]. Obtaining a 24-hour urine collection for bone markers may help avoid circadian variations.

Bone markers have an increasing role in the management of osteoporosis. They are useful in predicting fracture risk and response to therapy. In one study, baseline degrees of NTX elevation and the subsequent degrees of suppression predicted bone mineral density (BMD) gains in subjects receiving hormone replacement therapy (HRT) [4]. This association was also demonstrated in patients taking alendronate [5], as was a positive correlation between BSAP decline and decrease in fracture risk [6].

In a different application, they may be independent predictors of fracture risk [7,8]. The most widely accepted use of bone markers is in determining medication compliance and efficacy of antiresorptive therapy. For this purpose, they are usually obtained before and 3 to 6 months after initiation of treatment; declines of 30% to 50% in bone-resorption markers can be seen with antiresorptive agents and increases seen with anabolic therapy.

BONE IMAGING

Classic radiographic findings in common metabolic bone diseases are shown in Table 4.1.

Bone Densitometry

Bone mineral density can be measured with different techniques. The most commonly used method is dual energy x-ray absorptiometry (DXA), which gives a precise measure of a real density of bone (expressed in grams per square centimeter). DXA scans compare bone density with the mean for younger controls (T score) or the mean for the gender- and age-matched population (Z score). T scores are used for defining osteoporosis, and Z scores provide an idea of the "age-appropriateness" of bone loss.

The World Health Organization (WHO) classification is widely used for the diagnosis of osteoporosis (Table 4.2). For each standard deviation (SD) decrease in BMD, fracture risk increases 1.5- to threefold [9]. The National Health and Examination BMD III (NHANES III) database provides standardized total hip and femoral neck

Table 4.1. Features of Common Metabolic Bone Diseases

Disease	Radiograph	Bone Scan
Osteoporosis	Decreased bone density, cortical thinning, end-plate vertebral deformities, wedging, and compression fractures	Useful in differentiating old and new vertebral fractures. New fractures appear as hot areas
Osteomalacia	Decreased bone density, indistinct borders between cortex and trabeculae, widened growth plates, bowing deformities, and stress fractures	Increased activity in axial skeleton, long bones, mandible and calvaria, costochondral junction
Primary hyperparathyroidism	Subperiosteal resorption, thinning of distal third of the clavicle, salt-and-pepper appearance of the skull, brown tumors, osteitis fibrosa cystica, and decreased bone density	Most show no abnormalities. Fractures may be detected. There can be increased activity in the axial skeleton
Paget disease	Increased cortical thickness, irregular areas of bony sclerosis	Increased uptake in affected areas, flame- or V-shaped in the advancing edge; involvement of whole bone

Table 4.2. WHO Criteria for the Diagnosis of Osteoporosis

Classification	T score
Normal	−1 to 1
Osteopenia	−1 to −2.4
Osteoporosis	−2.5 or less
Severe osteoporosis	−2.5 or less, with fragility fractures

BMD values for men, white women, and nonwhite women. It is now the default database for most machines. The use of the NHANES database eliminates manufacturer-specific database variabilities.

The DXA scan also provides a reliable and objective means with which to monitor the response to osteoporosis therapy. The precision error of most DXA machines ranges from 0.5% to 2.5%, and the "least significant change" (LSC), or the change in bone density considered to be statistically significant, is at least 2.8 times the precision error of the machine. Abnormalities of the bone, such as degenerative joint disease and vertebral compression fractures, can falsely elevate the BMD. This is commonly seen in the spines of elderly individuals.

A possible alternate viewpoint is the lateral spine. One study found more bone loss on the lateral view with respect to the traditional posteroanterior (PA) view [10]. The International Society of Clinical Densitometry (ISCD) does not recommend using the lateral spine for diagnosing osteoporosis because it is thought to overestimate the disease. The lateral view, however, is useful in assessing for vertebral fragility fractures, and it may have a role in monitoring. A study of 342 patients who underwent DXA scanning with lateral vertebral views found compression fractures in 14.6% of these patients. In this trial, 73 (21.3%) of the 342 patients were at least 60 years old and osteopenic, and almost 28% of these subjects had compression fractures [11]. Lateral vertebral analysis is increasingly being used to identify prevalent vertebral fractures and to guide clinicians in the initiation of therapy. In addition, degenerative changes that are commonly seen in the PA view are usually absent from the lateral view. The lateral spine DXA may have some utility in the initial assessment and follow-up of bone loss in such cases.

Scintigraphy

The most commonly used radiolabeling compound is technetium 99m (^{99m}Tc). The availability of single-photon emission computed tomography (SPECT) has improved detection of vertebral fractures, but it is most useful in the detection of metastatic bone disease and in the localization of Paget disease.

Bone Biopsy

Rarely used in clinical practice, bone biopsies can help in the diagnosis of osteomalacia, and they are useful in renal osteodystrophy. They are also used in trials evaluating new osteoporosis drugs, allowing measurement of changes in cortical and trabecular thickness and estimates of structural competence.

OSTEOPOROSIS

Definition

Osteoporosis is a disease characterized by decreased bone strength due to decreased bone density and bone quality, leading to increased bone fragility. The WHO definition of osteoporosis is outlined in Table 4.2.

Epidemiology

The prevalence of low bone mass in the United States among individuals at least 50 years old was approximately 44 million in 2002, according to the National Osteoporosis Foundation (NOF). Women are most often affected, but men comprise an estimated 14 million of those with low bone mass. The prevalence of osteoporosis is projected to double by the year 2040. About 1.3 million fragility fractures occur each year in the United States, accounting for a significant cost burden to the country.

Pathophysiology

The disease results from an imbalance of bone resorption and bone formation. Some factors that can lead to predominance of bone resorption include estrogen deficiency, hyperthyroidism, hyperparathyroidism, and use of certain medications (e.g., glucocorticoids and other immunosuppressants). It is highly probable that as yet unknown hereditary factors contribute to the disease.

Diagnosis

Initial history and physical examination should include assessment of risk factors for fractures as well as secondary causes of osteoporosis. Those factors involved in fracture-risk analysis are listed in Table 4.3. Of those in this table, the National Osteoporosis Risk Assessment (NORA) found that age, history of fracture, maternal history of osteoporosis or fracture, Hispanic or Asian ethnicity, and smoking significantly increased one's chance of osteoporosis. In addition, body mass index, African-American ethnicity, estrogen use, diuretic ingestion, alcohol use, and exercise decreased this chance [12]. The most commonly encountered secondary causes of osteoporosis are detailed in Table 4.4. General recommendations for obtaining a screening DXA scan are outlined in Table 4.5.

Treatment

For postmenopausal osteoporosis, the NOF recommends the treatment of women with T scores less than -1.5 in the presence of at least one risk factor, and T scores less than -2.0 in the absence of risk factors. It must be emphasized that the decision to treat should not be based on the bone density result alone, because individuals can have significant risks for fractures even if they do not fulfill densitometric criteria for osteoporosis. A fracture risk-assessment scheme, which will help clinicians quantify patients' risk of fractures and determine the need for therapy, is currently being developed by the WHO.

Secondary causes of osteoporosis should be sought and corrected. Preventive therapy, with calcium and vitamin D supplements, and antiresorptive therapy are warranted

Table 4.3. Fracture Risk Assessment for Osteoporosis

Postmenopausal state	Recurrent falls
Advanced age*	Decreased vision
Family history of osteoporosis or fractures*	Poor balance
Low femoral neck BMD*	Need for hands to stand up from sitting position
History of fractures*	Dementia
Corticosteroid use*	Poor calcium intake
Cigarette smoking*	Low body mass index (BMI)*
Alcohol intake >2 units/day*	Limited exercise
Asian and white races	Caffeine intake

*Risk factors included in the WHO model.

Table 4.4. Secondary Causes of Osteoporosis

Primary hyperparathyroidism
Vitamin D deficiency
Idiopathic hypercalciuria
Hypogonadism
Hyperthyroidism
Cushing syndrome
Liver and renal disease
Medications [glucocorticoids, cyclosporine, phenytoin (Dilantin), thyroid hormone]
Malabsorption (inflammatory bowel diseases, celiac sprue)
Multiple myeloma

Table 4.5.   Recommendations for Osteoporosis Screening

All postmenopausal women aged 65 years or older

All adult women with a history of fragility fractures

Postmenopausal women younger than 65 years but with clinical risk factors for fractures

Men and women with known secondary causes of osteoporosis (long-term glucocorticoid therapy, primary hyperparathyroidism)

among patients on chronic glucocorticoid therapy (>5 mg of prednisone daily, or its equivalent, for >3 months).

Bisphosphonates

These pyrophosphate analogues bind to hydroxyapatite crystals in the bone, inhibit function and recruitment of osteoclasts, and increase osteoclast apoptosis. Oral bioavailability is only 1% to 3%, but they have prolonged skeletal retention. Patients must be advised to take this medication in the morning, to withhold food and drinks to ensure good absorption, and to remain upright for at least 30 minutes. Erosive esophagitis and gastric ulcers can be caused by these agents.

The three oral bisphosphonates that are approved for the management of osteoporosis are alendronate (Fosamax), risedronate (Actonel), and ibandronate (Boniva).

Alendronate

This drug is available in 5-, 10-, 35-, and 70-mg tablet forms. Prevention dose is 5 mg once daily or 35 mg once weekly, and treatment dose is 10 mg once daily or 70 mg once weekly. The Fracture Intervention Trial (FIT) was the landmark study that established the efficacy of alendronate for the treatment of postmenopausal osteoporosis [13,14]. After 3 years taking alendronate, those without prior vertebral fractures had a 47% reduction in new radiographic vertebral fractures, a 55% reduction in clinical vertebral fractures, a 90% reduction in multiple vertebral fractures, and a 51% reduction in hip fractures [13]. Those with prior vertebral fractures experienced a 44% reduction in new radiographic vertebral fractures [14]. Mean increases in BMD were 6% to 8% for the lumbar spine (LS) and 4% to 5% for the hip [13,14]. Similar fracture-reduction and BMD benefits were seen in two meta-analyses on alendronate for postmenopausal osteoporosis [15,16]. Follow-up of postmenopausal osteoporotic women taking 10 mg of alendronate for 10 years revealed the following BMD increases: lumbar spine, 13.7%; trochanter, 10.3%; femoral neck, 5.4%; and proximal femur, 6.7% [17].

The BMD benefit of alendronate was found to decline gradually years after its discontinuation, as shown in the 10-year study [17]. In addition, another trial showed that after 1 year of alendronate therapy, discontinuation led to a rate of bone loss that was similar to that of the group that did not receive alendronate. However, at the end of 15 months, a 3% difference in mean LS BMD was found between the groups, but the femoral neck BMD went back to baseline [18]. It is not known whether fracture protection was indeed lost as bone mass declined.

A comparison study of 70 mg weekly, 35 mg twice weekly, and 10 mg daily doses of alendronate over a 1-year period revealed similar increases in LS BMD (range, 5.1% to 5.4%) in these three groups without observed differences in the side-effect profile [19].

One recent concern raised about bisphosphonate therapy is the possibility of oversuppression of bone turnover, which might lead to bone fragility. A case series of nine patients taking alendronate for 3 to 8 years described fractures and delayed or no healing. Bone biopsy showed minimal bone formation. More studies must be done regarding this potential risk and the optimal duration of therapy with bisphosphonates [20].

Alendronate has also been found to be beneficial in men: 241 men with osteoporosis were studied in a 2-year double-blind, placebo-controlled trial. The men who received alendronate had a mean increase in BMD of 7.1% at the LS, 2.5% at the femoral neck, and 2.0% for the total body. Vertebral-fracture incidence was lower in the treated versus the placebo group (0.8% vs. 7.1%), and height loss was significantly greater in the placebo than in the alendronate group (2.4 vs. 6 mm) [21].

The efficacy of alendronate on glucocorticoid-induced osteoporosis has been established. A 2-year trial of 477 men and women taking glucocorticoids showed significant increases in mean LS BMD by 2.1% and 2.9%, respectively, with 5 and 10 mg of alendronate per day. The femoral neck bone density significantly increased by 1.2% and 1.0% in the respective alendronate groups [22].

A head-to-head study comparing weekly alendronate, 70 mg, with risedronate, 35 mg, for 1 year revealed small but significantly greater increases in BMD at 6 and 12 months and greater degrees of bone suppression in the alendronate group, with similar tolerability [23]. This study was not powered to detect differences in fracture rates.

Risedronate

This drug is available in a 5-mg once daily or a 35-mg weekly dose for prevention and treatment of osteoporosis. Two large randomized placebo-controlled studies showed a reduction in radiographic vertebral fractures by 41% to 49% after 3 years with risedronate [24,25]. One of these trials was extended to 7 years. This follow-up revealed persistence of BMD gains and fracture risk reductions through the seventh year of follow-up [26]. In the largest trial conducted, with hip fracture as the primary end point [27], risedronate significantly reduced the risk of these fractures by 30%. In the subgroup of patients with known osteoporosis, a significant 40% risk reduction for fracture was seen.

A meta-analysis on the use of risedronate for postmenopausal osteoporosis [28] showed a pooled risk reduction (RR) of 0.64 for vertebral and 0.73 for nonvertebral fractures. The pooled estimate of the differences in percentage of change between risedronate (5 mg) and placebo were 4.54% at the LS and 2.75% at the femoral neck.

The efficacy of once-weekly risedronate was shown in a randomized placebo-controlled study of 1,456 postmenopausal women with T scores less than -2.5 or less than -2.0 with a prevalent vertebral fracture taking 5 mg daily, 35 mg weekly, or 50 mg weekly doses. Mean percentage changes in LS BMD after 12 months were similar, as were mean increases in femoral neck BMD in the three groups [29].

Risedronate is also effective in prevention and treatment of glucocorticoid-induced osteoporosis, as evidenced by two major prospective studies [30,31].

Both of these bisphosphonates are alkaline substances that have been reported to cause esophageal and gastric ulcers. An initial Mayo Clinic study reported esophagitis among alendronate-treated patients [32]. This is the reason that patients are advised to remain upright after taking the bisphosphonates. Which oral bisphosphonate is more erosive remains controversial. Head-to-head endoscopy studies have shown conflicting results [33,34]. A meta-analysis of eight trials that included 10,086 patients showed no difference in gastrointestinal adverse events, clinically or endoscopically, in patients treated with risedronate versus placebo [35].

Ibandronate

Ibandronate is another bisphosphonate recently approved by the Food and Drug Administration (FDA) for the treatment and prevention of postmenopausal osteoporosis. This medication is available in two oral forms, 2.5 mg daily and 150 mg monthly, as well as an i.v. form, 3 mg quarterly. With a monthly option, this bisphosphonate has the advantage of less-frequent dosing. The Monthly Oral Pilot Study was a randomized, double-blind, multicenter, placebo-controlled study of 144 postmenopausal women who were given 50, 100, or 150 mg of ibandronate or placebo. No significant differences in adverse events compared with placebo were observed. Ibandronate also significantly decreased serum C-telopeptide cross-links (CTXs) in those taking 100- or 150-mg dosages [36]. The MOBILE study was a 2-year, randomized, double-blind trial that searched for the appropriate ibandronate dose for the treatment of osteoporosis. The 1,609 women in the study were assigned to four groups: 2.5 mg daily, 50 mg once a month, 100 mg once a month, or 150 mg once a month. Those taking monthly ibandronate experienced increases in lumbar spine (3.9%, 4.3%, 4.1%, and 4.9%, respectively) and hip (about 2% to 3%) BMD. The 150-mg group had a small but significantly greater increase in LS BMD than did those on the daily regimen. In addition, when the groups were evaluated for those who achieved BMD gains above baseline as well as more than 6% at the LS or 3% at the hip, the 150-mg and 100-mg groups had significantly more patients at these goals than with the daily regimen (only 150 mg at the LS with respect to gains above baseline). Regarding side effects, the frequency of gastrointestinal symptoms with each dose was similar, but a small increase in flu-like symptoms was noted with the monthly regimens [37].

In a noninferiority study, two regimens (2 mg i.v. every 2 months and 3 mg i.v. every 3 months) were found to be similar in efficacy to daily ibandronate (2.5 mg) in terms of mean increases in lumbar spine and hip BMD at 1 and 2 years. Safety profiles were similar [38].

Osteonecrosis of the Jaw
There have been recent reports of patients who have suffered from osteonecrosis of the jaw while on bisphosphonates therapy. The exact pathogenesis is not clear, but having recent dental work appeared to be a risk factor. The vast majority of the patients were on IV bisphosphonates (monthly zoledronic acid and q 3 month pamidronate for cancer indications) and only a small proportion of patients were on alendronate and risedronate for osteoporosis [38a].

Raloxifene
Raloxifene is a selective estrogen-receptor modulator, with agonistic effects on bone. The major efficacy trial for raloxifene was the Multiple Outcomes of Raloxifene Evaluation (MORE) Trial [39]. The LS BMD increase over the 3-year study period was 2–3%, and vertebral fracture–reduction rates in women with and without preexisting fractures were 50% and 30%, respectively. No significant difference in nonvertebral and hip fracture reduction was observed. Efficacy of raloxifene was sustained through 4 years of treatment [40]. A meta-analysis of seven trials comparing raloxifene and placebo showed a similar BMD increase at the LS and a 2% increase for the combined hips [41]. This drug has other potential benefits, including reduction in breast cancer risk and improvement in lipids and markers of cardiovascular disease, but these are not discussed in this section.

Calcitonin
Because of its modest effect on BMD, its fracture reduction, and its systemic analgesic effects, this drug is useful as an alternative agent after an acute vertebral fracture. However, the authors believe that it should be used with a stronger antiresorptive when possible. The major efficacy trial was the PROOF study, which demonstrated a 1.2% increase in LS BMD and a 33% reduction in vertebral fractures with 200 international units of intranasal calcitonin [42]. No significant reduction was seen in the 100- or 400-IU groups. No significant reduction in nonvertebral and hip fractures was demonstrated in this trial. In a meta-analysis of 30 trials that compared calcitonin with placebo, the smaller studies were found to have more impressive results than the PROOF study [43]; the authors of that meta-analysis suggested a possible bias in the smaller studies.

Hormone Replacement Therapy
Hormone replacement therapy (HRT) was the initial antiresorptive therapy for osteoporosis. However, current controversies centered on increased breast cancer and cardiovascular risks have resulted in a marked decline in use for osteoporosis. A meta-analysis of 57 randomized studies that compared at least 1 year of HRT in postmenopausal women with controls showed a trend toward reduction of vertebral and nonvertebral fracture incidence. BMD increased by 6.76% at 2 years in the LS and 4.12% in the femoral neck [44]. Perhaps the best prospective data to date that showed

fracture reduction with combined HRT were those established in the Women's Health Initiative study. The incidence of clinical vertebral fractures was reduced by 34%, hip fractures by 34%, and all fractures by 24%. However, increased breast cancer and cardiovascular risk led to discontinuation of this treatment arm. Absolute excess risks per 10,000 person-years attributable to estrogen plus progestin were eight more coronary heart disease events, eight more strokes, eight more pulmonary emboli, and eight more invasive breast cancers, whereas absolute RRs per 10,000 person-years were six fewer colorectal cancers and five fewer hip fractures [45].

Combination

Combined HRT and alendronate have demonstrated superiority in BMD benefit over either agent alone. In a 2-year study of 425 postmenopausal women who were randomly assigned to receive estrogen, alendronate, a combination of the two, or placebo, the mean change in LS BMD was statistically higher with combination therapy than with either agent alone [46]. Another trial gave alendronate, 10 mg/day, or placebo to 428 postmenopausal women receiving HRT for at least 1 year. After 12 months, alendronate produced significantly greater BMD increases in the LS (3.6% vs. 1.0%) and the hip trochanter (2.7% vs. 0.5%) than did placebo [47].

A study comparing raloxifene, 60 mg per day, and alendronate, 10 mg per day, in combination or alone, in 331 postmenopausal women with femoral neck T scores less than −2 found a significantly greater LS BMD increase in the combination group than in those with alendronate or raloxifene alone (3.7% vs. 2.7% vs. 1.7%, respectively) [48].

Teriparatide

Synthetic human PTH (1-34), or teriparatide, is an anabolic agent that has been approved for postmenopausal and male osteoporosis treatment. The landmark trial in postmenopausal women was the Fracture Prevention Trial (FPT). In this study, 1,637 postmenopausal women received 20 or 40 µg of teriparatide for a mean of 21 months. Vertebral fractures decreased by 65% and 69%, respectively, and nonvertebral fractures were reduced by 53% and 54%. Mean increases in LS BMD of 9% and 13%, as well as 3% and 6% at the femoral neck, were seen. The most common side effects were nausea and headaches [49].

Teriparatide is approved for only 2 years of use; therefore it is of interest to see what happens to the bone mass of patients who discontinue the drug. Extensions of the FPT have looked at changes in BMD and fracture risk after discontinuation of teriparatide. One study found that 30 months after discontinuation of teriparatide, the hazard ratio for nonvertebral fragility fractures was still significantly lower than with placebo but only in the 40-µg group. BMD decreased over those months in both groups, except in those who received bisphosphonates for at least 2 years during the trial [50]. Another study looked at vertebral BMD changes and fractures 1.5 years after discontinuing teriparatide. There continued to be a statistically significant increase in BMD and a decrease in fractures in those who had been taking teriparatide. Those who used bisphosphonates for at least 1 year continued to gain BMD, whereas those who did not lost BMD [51].

The role of PTH as combination or monotherapy has been addressed. The results have not been consistent, and conclusions have mostly been drawn from BMD and bone marker data. A study comparing PTH (1-84), 100 µg daily alone, alendronate alone, and the PTH–alendronate combination found no significant difference in LS BMD between PTH and the combination, but a significantly higher increase in hip BMD was seen in the combination therapy group compared with the PTH group. [52]. A randomized double-blind trial compared teriparatide, 40 µg, with alendronate, 10 mg daily. By 3 months, and through the 14 months of the study, those in the teriparatide group experienced significantly greater increases in LS and hip BMD than with alendronate. Nonvertebral fractures were significantly less in the teriparatide group [53].

The effects of teriparatide after administration of alendronate or raloxifene have been assessed. The prior raloxifene group had higher gains in BMD at the LS and the hip. The difference in LS BMD was largely due to an increase in the first 6 months [54]. Bone-formation markers had a lesser and later peak in the alendronate group.

Teriparatide also has been shown to increase bone mass by 13% in the LS and 2.9% in the femoral neck in men with idiopathic osteoporosis [55]. A randomized trial of 83 men, with an LS or femoral neck T score of at least -2, compared teriparatide, alendronate, and their combination over a 2.5-year period (teriparatide was started at month 6). The teriparatide group had significant increases in BMD at the LS and the femoral neck, which were greater than those in the alendronate and combination groups [56]. In a study that assessed BMD and fractures for 30 months after a year of exposure to teriparatide, LS and total hip BMD remained significantly higher in the PTH group than in the placebo group, even though the BMDs decreased after discontinuation. When the subjects were divided according to bisphosphonate use, those who took bisphosphonates had an increase in spine and hip BMD, although significant intergroup differences were lost. Among those who did not take bisphosphonates, the BMD decreased. A significant decrease in moderate to severe spine fractures was seen at 18 months of follow-up [57].

The frequency of transient hypercalcemia within 4 to 6 hours after administration is 10-fold higher among patients who received teriparatide compared with placebo, and in one third of these, the transient hypercalcemia was reverified on consecutive measurements. The occurrence of leg cramps was also significantly higher in the teriparatide group than in the placebo group [49]. The drug carries a black-box warning about osteosarcoma in rats. Teriparatide caused a dose- and duration-dependent increase in this condition among rats treated with the drug. For this reason, children, patients with prior radiation therapy, and those with high bone turnover, such as bone metastasis or Paget's disease of bone, should not receive the drug.

In a large clinical trial, in 2.8% of patients, antibodies to the drug developed, generally within 12 months of treatment. In these patients, no evidence of hypersensitivity or allergic reactions was seen [49].

Calcium and Vitamin D Supplementation

In a meta-analysis of 15 trials comparing calcium with placebo, the pooled increase in percentage change from baseline was 2.05% for the total body BMD, 1.66% for the LS, and 1.64% for the hip in patients who received calcium. Vertebral fracture risk decreased by 23%, and nonvertebral fracture risk, by 14% in the calcium group [58].

The recommended intake of elemental calcium is 1,200 to 1,500 mg/day for adults older than 50 years. Intake more than 2,000 to 2,500 mg is not recommended, as it may cause hypercalciuria (please see section on calcium in Hypocalcemia). Vitamin D supplementation has been found to reduce vertebral fractures by 37% in a meta-analysis of 25 trials. A trend was noted toward reduction in nonvertebral fractures as well (RR, 0.72; $p = 0.09$). Patients who received hydroxylated forms of vitamin D had larger increases in BMD than did those who received vitamin D_2 [59]. For patients who are not found to be vitamin D insufficient or deficient, the current recommended dose of vitamin D_2 (ergocalciferol) is at least 400 to 800 IU/day (also refer to section on Vitamin D deficiency).

Other Therapies

The use of hip protectors may reduce hip fractures in those at high risk; however, adherence is only about 40% [60]. Weight-bearing and back-strengthening exercises are also helpful adjunctive measures in the management of osteoporosis.

Future Therapies

Zoledronic Acid

In a 1-year randomized, double-blind, placebo-controlled trial, a once-a-year zoledronic acid infusion (4- and 2-mg doses) increased LS BMD (4%–5%) and femoral neck BMD (3%–3.5%) compared with placebo. Three other groups that received varying doses of the drug at 3-month intervals had similar increases in BMDs [61].

Strontium Ranelate

Strontium ranelate is a natural element that is normally present in very small amounts in bone [62]. In recent years, it has emerged as a possible new therapy for osteoporosis. One study assessed spine-fracture risk in osteoporotic women taking strontium ranelate for 3 years and found a relative risk reduction of about 40%. The most common gastrointestinal side effect was diarrhea, but this abated after 3 months. No abnormal bone mineralization was seen [63]. The Treatment of Peripheral Osteoporosis study (TROPOS) assessed nonvertebral fractures and found a decrease in risk here as well, albeit less than that in the vertebrae [64].

Denosumab (AMG 162)

A human antibody has been developed against RANKL (Receptor Activator of Nuclear kappyB ILigand) that results in inhibition of osteoclast differentiation, activation, function and increased apoptosis. Phase 1 and 2 studies have shown promising results and a fracture study is underway [64a].

Monitoring Therapy

Most experts would agree that DXA scans should be obtained annually after initiation of treatment until bone stability has been demonstrated. Therapy should not be changed if BMD decline is seen after 1 year of treatment, because it has been found that some patients who "lose" bone after 1 year tend to gain bone later. This was demonstrated in a post hoc analysis of data from the Fracture Intervention Trial and the Multiple Outcomes of Raloxifene Evaluation Trial. In examining the baseline, 1-year, and 2-year BMDs of the patients in these studies, the investigators found that the degree of BMD decline the first year on treatment was associated with a gain in BMD the next year. This phenomenon is known as "regression to the mean"; that is, outlying results may be due to random or technical error that may not represent true biologic change and, subsequently, these changes revert to the mean. If loss continues in succeeding DXAs, therapy can be altered at that time [65]. Furthermore, one study showed significant fracture protection while taking bisphosphonate therapy among patients who lost up to 4% in the spine or the hip [66].

Bone-turnover markers are helpful in determining efficacy of therapy and patient compliance. The most commonly used bone-resorption markers include urinary NTX and serum CTX. Markers of bone formation often used include bone-specific alkaline phosphatase and serum osteocalcin (see earlier section on evaluation of metabolic bone disorders). Fracture protection being the primary end point, it is important for clinicians to monitor patients for the occurrence of new fractures. Repeated fractures while receiving therapy may warrant a change in therapy or reevaluation for secondary causes of osteoporosis. The majority of vertebral compression fractures are asymptomatic, however. A recent study assessed the correlation between height loss and vertebral fractures. The investigators found that height loss of greater than 2 cm in 3 years had the sensitivity for new vertebral fractures of only 36%, but a specificity of almost 94%. The positive predictive value for this degree of height loss was about 35%, and the negative predictive value was about 92% [67]. Thus height measurement should be accurately performed during patient visits.

PAGET DISEASE OF BONE

Paget disease is a metabolic bone disorder resulting from exaggerated osteoclastic bone resorption and formation of architecturally disrupted and weak bone. This causes skeletal pain, deformity, and fractures.

Epidemiology

The estimated prevalence, based on autopsies and review of radiographs, is about 3%. The disease is commonly seen in Britain, Australia, New Zealand, and the United States. Rare in people younger than 20 years, it is most commonly diagnosed at age 50 years.

Pathophysiology

The exact etiology of Paget disease is currently unknown. Family history of the disease is identified in 12%–23% of patients, and environmental factors, such as measles, exposure to lead, and previous dog ownership, have been linked to the disease.

The primary disturbance seems to be increased activation of the osteoclasts. Large, multinucleated osteoclasts can be seen in the borders of the lesion that apposes normal bone.

Diagnosis

Most affected patients have no symptoms, so diagnosis is based on serendipitous findings of a high alkaline phosphatase or abnormal radiographs. Some patients, however, have symptoms, or they may have already had complications at the time of diagnosis. Common complaints include dull achy bone pain and various bony deformities, such as enlargement of the skull or bowing of the long bones. Fractures, arthritis in the nearby joints, hearing loss, nerve impingement, high-output heart failure, and osteosarcoma are complications of Paget disease.

Biochemically, an elevated total or bone-specific alkaline phosphatase suggests the presence of the disease. Serum and urine calcium levels are rarely elevated unless the patient becomes immobilized. Markers of bone resorption such as urinary CTX and NTX and osteocalcin values are usually high.

Pagetic areas are visualized as areas of intense uptake on bone scan. Usually, the whole bone is involved, such as in the pelvis, vertebrae, or scapula. A leading edge shaped like a flame or the letter V may be seen in the appendicular bones. Plain radiographs of the affected areas will show cortical thickening and irregular areas of lucency and sclerosis. Pagetic involvement of the skull usually shows enlargement due to cortical thickening and areas of sclerosis and lucencies giving an appearance of cottonwool. Bowing deformities of the long bones, particularly the tibia, may be appreciated.

Treatment

Treatment is targeted toward slowing osteoclastic bone resorption. Indications are outlined in Table 4.6. Oral and intravenous bisphosphonates are the most commonly used agents for treatment of Paget disease, particularly risedronate, alendronate, and pamidronate.

Bisphosphonates

Risedronate

The recommended dose is 30 mg/day for 2 months, with an optional third month if no decline in alkaline phosphatase is seen 1 month after the end of treatment. In an open-label study of 162 patients, 30 mg of risedronate was given for 84 days, followed by 112 days without therapy. The cycle was repeated if the alkaline phosphatase remained high or increased by 25%. Normalization of alkaline phosphatase was seen in 54% of patients after 7 to 14 months of therapy. A significant decrease in bone pain also occurred [68].

A randomized controlled trial comparing risedronate (30 mg/day for 60 days) with etidronate (400 mg/day for 6 months) showed better efficacy with risedronate than

Table 4.6.   Indications for Treatment of Paget Disease

Serum alkaline phosphatase ≥3 or 4 times upper limit of normal

Fractures or pain in involved bone

Involvement of critical sites that may lead to complications such as arthritis or
   fractures or nerve compression

Skull involvement associated with hearing loss or headache

Monostotic disease of weight-bearing bones

Pretreating patients before surgery to reduce hypervascularity and blood loss etidronate. At 12 months, alkaline phosphatase normalized in 73% of risedronate-treated patients, compared with only 15% in the etidronate group. This value also normalized faster in the risedronate group (3 months vs. 1 year) [69].

Alendronate
Alendronate is administered at 40 mg/day, typically for 6 months. In a double-blind, randomized, placebo-controlled study of 55 patients, 40 mg/day of alendronate resulted in normalization of alkaline phosphatase in 48% of patients. Declines in urine NTX and alkaline phosphatase were seen in 86% and 73% of patients, respectively. Radiographic improvement was noted in 48% of patients [70].

A head-to-head trial of alendronate (40 mg/day) and etidronate (400 mg/day), both administered for 6 months, showed higher rates of normalization of alkaline phosphatase (61% vs. 17%), and greater reduction in alkaline phosphatase (79% vs. 44%), with alendronate than with etidronate. No evidence of osteomalacia was seen on bone biopsies of patients in the alendronate group, whereas one patient taking etidronate was found to have osteomalacia, a known complication of large doses of this drug [71].

Pamidronate
Intravenous pamidronate is ideal for patients who are unable to tolerate oral bisphosphonates. It also may be used as a therapeutic trial in those who have pain of indeterminate nature in an area involved with Paget disease. Dosing is determined by disease severity. The recommended dose is a 30 mg IV infusion over a 4-hour period (in 500 ml saline or 5% dextrose) for 3 consecutive days. However, most clinicians opt for higher doses such as 60 or 90 mg given once, followed by alkaline phosphatase monitoring. Biochemical remissions are usually sustained for 12 to 18 months, depending on disease severity.

A prospective, nonrandomized study of 80 patients with Paget disease investigated the use of 180 mg IV over a 3- or 6-week period. Alkaline phosphatase declined by 63% compared with baseline, and 62% achieved normalization of alkaline phosphatase [72].

Common side effects include flulike symptoms or mild fever for a few days after the infusion and, more rarely, iritis.

Calcitonin
Calcitonin is available as salmon or human preparations for subcutaneous administration. Calcitonin nasal spray has not been approved for this disease. The starting dose for the subcutaneous injection is 100 MRC of salmon calcitonin at bedtime. After clinical improvement, which can generally be expected in a few weeks to months, the dose can be reduced to half every other day.

Other Therapies
Nonsteroidal anti-inflammatory agents and analgesics play supportive roles in the management of Paget disease. Patients who need fracture repairs, joint replacements, and osteotomies for severe bowing deformities are usually co-managed with orthopaedic surgeons. Neurosurgeons may be involved when evidence of compressive neurologic damage is present.

Newer-generation bisphosphonates, such as ibandronate and zoledronic acid, are currently being investigated as treatment options for Paget disease. Zoledronic acid has been studied in this disease. In two randomized, double-blind, active controlled trials, patients were given either one dose of 5 mg of zoledronic acid or 30 mg of risedronate for 2 months. After 6 months, more subjects taking zoledronic acid experienced a disease response (96% vs. 74%), alkaline phosphatase normalized more often in the zoledronic acid group (89% vs. 58%), the quality of life in those who received zoledronic acid was higher, and fewer patients in the zoledronic acid group had a relapse [73].

PRIMARY HYPERPARATHYROIDISM
Primary hyperparathyroidism is one of the most common causes of hypercalcemia, occurring in about 1 in 800 persons. Before the advent of autoanalyzers, most patients

Table 4.7.   Clinical Manifestations of Primary Hyperparathyroidism

Musculoskeletal	Cardiovascular
Osteoporosis	Hypertension
Fractures	Left ventricular hypertrophy
Muscle weakness and fatigue	Valvular calcifications
	Increased vascular stiffness
Renal	
Nephrolithiasis	**Rheumatologic**
Renal insufficiency	Gout
Mild hypomagnesemia	Chondrocalcinosis
Hypophosphatemia	Pseudogout
Neuropsychiatric	**Hematologic**
Anxiety	Normochromic, normocytic anemia
Depression	**Ocular**
Cognitive dysfunction	Band keratopathy

with this condition were first seen with severe hypercalcemia and classic manifestations of "stones, bones, abdominal moans, and groans with psychic overtones." The classic radiologic findings in advanced disease are nephrolithiasis, subperiosteal bone resorption, thinning of the distal third of the clavicle, and osteitis fibrosa cystica (Table 4.7). Today, asymptomatic hyperparathyroidism accounts for most cases encountered by clinicians.

Epidemiology

This disease is more frequent among women, with a predilection of 3:1, and it usually occurs among people in their sixth or seventh decade. Ten percent of hyperparathyroidism is familial, inherited in an autosomal dominant manner in syndromes such as familial hyperparathyroidism and multiple endocrine neoplasia (MEN) 1 and 2A. Onset is much younger among those with familial hyperparathyroidism and MEN. Because of this, consideration should be given to measurement of serum calcium concentration in primary relatives of those patients with confirmed primary hyperparathyroidism.

Pathogenesis

The disease arises from proliferation of parathyroid cells that have decreased ability to sense calcium. This proliferation has been attributed to various genetic alterations, such as those in parathyroid adenomatosis 1 (PRAD-1) or MEN 1 genes, and loss of function of a tumor-suppressor gene on chromosome 1p. Such other chromosomal sites as 1q, 6q, 9p, 15q, and retinoblastoma gene, have been investigated as probable causes of the clonal proliferation. It seems logical that a mutation in the calcium-sensing receptor would lead to primary hyperparathyroidism, but this has not been proven. Of note, an association between head and neck irradiation and primary hyperparathyroidism has been reported. Thiazide diuretics may exaggerate or unmask the hypercalcemia in many cases.

Primary hyperparathyroidism is due to parathyroid adenomas in 80%, parathyroid hyperplasia in 15%, a "double adenoma" in 1% to 2%, and parathyroid carcinoma in 1% of cases. In the hands of an experienced surgeon, parathyroid adenomas can be successfully identified and resected in more than 90% of cases. However, ectopic adenomas may be seen in unusual locations such as in the tracheoesophageal groove, the carotid bifurcation, or the thymus. Hyperplasia of multiple glands is more common in those with familial or MEN syndromes.

Diagnosis

Because most patients have asymptomatic hyperparathyroidism, the history and physical examination rarely clinch the diagnosis. They are considered in ruling out other causes of hypercalcemia. A family history of hypercalcemia should be sought, and a careful review of the patient's medication list should be undertaken.

Biochemical features include hypercalcemia and a high or inappropriately elevated intact PTH. Urinary calcium excretion is high in fewer than 50% of cases, but it is usually greater than 200 mg/24 hr. The urine calcium/creatinine ratio is usually more than 0.01. The challenge arises in patients with normocalcemia and mild elevations of intact PTH. In these cases, 25(OH)D and creatinine levels should be checked to rule out secondary hyperparathyroidism. On long-term follow-up of these patients, hypercalcemia, albeit mild, eventually manifests. Phosphate levels are typically in the low-normal range; they are frankly low in fewer than 25% of cases.

Lithium and thiazide use can mimic primary hyperparathyroidism, occurring with mild hypercalcemia and elevated intact PTH levels. If it is clinically safe, these drugs should be discontinued and reevaluation performed in 2 to 3 months.

Initial evaluation should include a DXA scan of the spine and hip. If available, distal radius bone density should be done as well. The radius area, composed primarily of cortical bone, is affected to a greater degree by primary hyperparathyroidism. Serum creatinine should be obtained and a renal ultrasound performed to screen for nephrolithiasis and nephrocalcinosis. Familial benign hypocalciuric hypercalcemia (FBHH), which typically occurs with asymptomatic hypercalcemia, is usually associated with a 24-hour urinary calcium excretion of less than 100 mg and a fractional excretion of calcium less than 0.01.

Treatment

Surgical Management

Surgery by an experienced endocrine surgeon is the definitive treatment. The National Institutes of Health Consensus Development Conference on the Management of Asymptomatic Primary Hyperparathyroidism in 2002 recommended these guidelines for surgery [74]:

- Serum calcium level higher than 1 mg/dl above the upper limit of normal
- Presence of complications, such as osteoporosis, renal insufficiency, nephrolithiasis
- Urinary calcium excretion more than 400 mg/24 hr
- An episode of life-threatening hypercalcemia
- *T* score less than −2 at the LS, hip, or distal radius
- Age younger than 50 years
- Creatinine clearance reduced by 30% compared with age-matched persons
- Patients for whom medical surveillance is not desirable or possible

One group reported their 10-year follow-up experience with 121 patients with asymptomatic primary hyperparathyroidism [75]. During the study, 61 patients underwent parathyroidectomy, and 60 patients were observed without surgery, as they had remained asymptomatic with no evidence for complications of the disease. All patients who underwent parathyroidectomy saw normalization of their serum calcium concentrations. LS BMD in the postsurgical patients increased significantly by 8% after 1 year and 12% after 10 years. Femoral neck BMD also significantly increased by 6% after 1 year and 14% after 10 years. No changes were observed in serum calcium concentrations, urinary calcium excretions, or BMDs in those who did not undergo surgery. In 14 of those patients who initially did not undergo surgery, disease progression developed, requiring parathyroidectomy.

Minimally invasive surgery requires the use of preoperative localization studies. This can be done by using noninvasive techniques such as ultrasound, CT, MRI, and ^{99m}Tc sestamibi scan. ^{99m}Tc has a sensitivity ranging from 80% to 100%. In cases of failed primary surgery and negative localization studies, invasive techniques such as arteriography and selective venous sampling with PTH measurement may be necessary, but these should be done by highly experienced individuals.

Intraoperative PTH monitoring has increased surgical success rates for primary hyperparathyroidism.

Medical Management

In patients with mild, uncomplicated primary hyperparathyroidism, many will need no therapy at all. Scholz et al. [76] showed that in roughly 25% of such patients, a need for operation developed within 10 years. Two other groups (Henry Ford Hospital and Columbia University) reported similar results [77,78]. Individuals who meet criteria for surgery but are not surgical candidates or who refuse surgery should be treated medically. Patients are advised about maintaining adequate hydration and avoidance of thiazide diuretics. Moderate oral calcium intake (750–1,000 mg/day) also is advised.

Bisphosphonates may be useful agents in patients with primary hyperparathyroidism. However, data on long-term use for this purpose is limited. In a pilot study of 26 postmenopausal osteopenic women with primary hyperparathyroidism [79], alendronate, 10 mg once a day, decreased serum calcium and urinary calcium excretion for 3 to 6 months. However, these levels increased afterward. Statistically significant increases were noted in LS, total hip, and total body BMD compared with baseline and controls. A more recent, small trial also assessed the effect of alendronate in primary hyperparathyroidism. Those in the treatment group experienced significant increases in BMD at the LS, the total hip, and the femoral neck compared with those taking placebo. Bone-turnover markers NTX and BSAP declined by at least half. The calcium, PTH, and urine calcium concentrations remained stable [80].

Estrogen therapy in this disease has been associated with mild declines in serum calcium levels and increases in BMD. A small, randomized, placebo-controlled trial compared estrogen/progesterone with placebo in 33 patients with asymptomatic primary hyperparathyroidism [81]. Total body, LS, femoral neck, and forearm BMD increased at 4 years. Serum ionized calcium was stable for 2 years and then mildly declined in the fourth year. An increase in intact PTH was found in the placebo group. The risks of estrogen therapy for this purpose must be carefully discussed with patients.

The newest therapeutic agent for this disease is the calcimimetic, cinacalcet. This drug targets calcium-sensing receptors, which reduce PTH production directly. A multicenter, randomized, double-blind, placebo-controlled trial studied patients with mild hyperparathyroidism (serum calcium between 10.3 and 12.5 mg/dl on enrollment, with a PTH of >45 pg/ml) for about 1 year. They received placebo or 30 mg cinacalcet twice a day, with the cinacalcet dose being increased to 40 mg and then 50 mg twice a day at weeks 4 and 8 if hypercalcemia persisted. More women taking cinacalcet experienced normalization of calcium levels, with a decrease in the calcium concentration of at least 0.5 mg/dl. The mean calcium levels in the treatment group decreased to normal within 2 weeks of therapy initiation. PTH also significantly decreased. No BMD difference was noted [81]. Other studies on this agent are reviewed in the sections on parathyroid carcinoma and hypercalcemia.

PARATHYROID CARCINOMA

Epidemiology

This disease is a rare entity of the parathyroid glands. It is seen in fewer than 1% of those with primary hyperparathyroidism [82]. Parathyroid carcinoma has no gender preference; men and women are affected equally [82,83]. Patients are usually diagnosed in their 40s [82].

Pathogenesis

The cause of parathyroid carcinoma is as yet unknown. Mutations of the cyclin D1 gene and of chromosome 13 may play a role. Several links have been reported with other diseases and conditions, such as renal failure, neck radiation, and other abnormalities of the parathyroid glands. Those with hereditary hyperparathyroidism–jaw tumor syndrome have a higher chance of developing this cancer [82].

Clinical Manifestations

Parathyroid carcinoma secretes increased amounts of PTH, which results in hypercalcemia. Patients may complain of the symptoms of hypercalcemia. They may also develop hoarseness, due to damage to the recurrent laryngeal nerve. Up to three fourths of those with parathyroid carcinoma will have a neck mass that is palpated on examination [82].

In addition to symptoms and signs, this elevated parathyroid hormone secretion can result in metabolic, skeletal, and organ derangements. These are similar to that seen in primary hyperparathyroidism, although usually to more pronounced degrees. Hypercalcemia develops, but the calcium concentration is usually at least 14 mg/dl [82]. PTH also is markedly elevated, and it can increase to 10 times normal. Patients with this carcinoma can have high alkaline phosphatase levels as well. The proportion with renal stones or insufficiency can range from approximately 30% to 80%. Such bony changes as fractures, osteitis fibrosa cystica, absent lamina dura, subperiosteal bone resorption, and decreased BMD have been reported in 40% to 90% of these patients [82,83]. In addition, they can develop pancreatitis, anemia, and ulcers [82].

This carcinoma often recurs at the resection site and via contiguous spread [82]. Recurrence occurs in about 33% to 78% of patients [83], usually about 3 years after resection. Metastases occur later by way of the lymphatic and hematologic systems. When the carcinoma does spread, the lungs and the cervical nodes are affected more often, and the liver is involved in about 10% of cases. The 5-year survival rate can range from 40% to 86% [82].

Diagnosis

The diagnosis may be suspected when patients have the biochemical findings described earlier or neck masses. Technetium scans may aid in the localization of the abnormal gland [82,83]. Ultrasound can help assess the features of the abnormal parathyroid gland; such aspects associated with parathyroid carcinoma include being lobular and heterogeneous [83]. However, diagnosis is made on pathological review [82].

Treatment

The mainstay of treatment is resection of the primary tumor and of recurrence. Given the likelihood of recurrence, such other treatments as radiation and chemotherapy have been investigated, with limited results. Several options are available to control the hypercalcemia that can ensue with unresectable disease. Intravenous bisphosphonate infusions can reduce the calcium concentration. Calcitonin is less effective. Calcimimetics have been studied as therapies for the hypercalcemia [82], and one such medication, cinacalcet, is approved for this use [84].

HYPERCALCEMIA

The most common causes of hypercalcemia are primary hyperparathyroidism and malignancy. Together they account for about 90% of cases. Other causes of serum calcium elevation are outlined in Table 4.8. Most patients with primary hyperparathyroidism are asymptomatic, whereas those with malignancies and hypercalcemia usually have advanced and readily apparent disease. Signs and symptoms of hypercalcemia are reviewed in Table 4.9.

Diagnosis

With the advent of routine biochemical screening, hypercalcemia is detected earlier, and most patients are asymptomatic or have few clinical symptoms. It is prudent to repeat the serum calcium test or confirm hypercalcemia with measurement of an ionized calcium level before embarking on an expensive workup. Because the most

Table 4.8.   Common Causes of Hypercalcemia

Increased bone resorption
Primary hyperparathyroidism
Malignancy: PTHrP, ectopic PTH
production, cytokine production,
osteolytic bone metastasis
Hyperthyroidism
Vitamin A intoxication
Paget disease with immobilization

Increased intestinal calcium absorption or exogenous administration
Vitamin D intoxication
Granulomatous and lymphoproliferative
diseases
Milk-alkali syndrome
Hemodialysis
Hyperalimentation

Downregulation of parathyroid calcium sensor receptor
Familial hypocalciuric hypercalcemia
Lithium

Decreased renal excretion of calcium
Thiazide diuretics
Acute renal failure

Others
Adrenal insufficiency

Table 4.9.   Clinical Manifestations of Hypercalcemia

Gastrointestinal
Constipation
Anorexia
Abdominal pain
Peptic ulcer due to increased gastrin
production

Renal
Nephrolithiasis, nephrocalcinosis
Renal insufficiency
Nephrogenic diabetes insipidus
Renal tubular acidosis

Neuropsychiatric
Depression, anxiety, decreased
cognitive function
Psychosis, hallucination, lethargy,
coma with higher calcium levels

Cardiovascular
Shortened QT interval
Calcium deposition in coronary arteries,
myocardium, and heart valves
Hypertension

Musculoskeletal
Muscle weakness
Chondrocalcinosis

Others
Band keratopathy, limbic calcification

common cause is primary hyperparathyroidism, the first step is to obtain an intact PTH to determine whether the hypercalcemia is mediated by PTH.

Primary hyperparathyroidism usually is initially seen with mild to moderate hypercalcemia (usually <11 mg/dl), and high or inappropriately normal PTH values. Serum phosphate values may be normal or low, and 24-hour urinary calcium excretion may be normal or high. Mild hyperchloremia can be seen.

Rapid onset of hypercalcemia points to humoral hypercalcemia of malignancy. PTHrP levels are elevated in 60% to 80% of cases.

If hypercalcemia is not mediated by PTH or PTHrP, 25(OH)D and 1,25(OH)$_2$D should be measured. If elevated, the first step is to rule out exogenous intake. Granulomatous diseases or lymphomas cause hypercalcemia by increasing 1α-hydroxylation of 25(OH)D. Phosphate levels and urinary calcium excretion may be normal or high.

Familial hypocalciuric hypercalcemia (FBHH) is first seen with hypercalcemia and low urinary calcium excretion. The fractional excretion of calcium is usually less than 0.01. Family history of hypercalcemia should be elicited.

Intact PTH is usually suppressed in hypercalcemia due to hyperthyroidism, milk-alkali syndrome, immobilization experienced by patients with Paget disease, vitamin A and D toxicities, and rarely adrenal insufficiency.

Treatment

Address the Primary Cause

Surgery is the treatment of choice for primary hyperparathyroidism, if the patient meets criteria. Treatment should be directed at the primary malignancy after it has been identified. Medications likely contributing to the hypercalcemia should be discontinued and the patient retested in 2 to 3 months. No treatment is required for FBHH.

Decrease Intestinal Absorption

In chronic granulomatous diseases or lymphoma, glucocorticoids, such as prednisone, 20 to 40 mg/day, effectively reduce calcium levels. Of note, higher doses may be required for lymphoma. Although rarely used, antimalarial agents such as chloroquine and hydroxychloroquine reduce endogenous calcitriol production, and they may be used as well. Exogenous calcium, vitamin D, and oxalate intake should be limited.

Oral phosphates (250–500 mg 4 times daily) may be used to limit intestinal calcium absorption by forming calcium phosphate complexes. However, when the calcium-phosphorus product is too high, ectopic calcifications may result.

Increase Urinary Calcium Excretion

Hydration is the most important first step. This can be achieved through infusion of intravenous 0.9% NaCl, which increases delivery of calcium to the loop of Henle. The rate of saline infusion must be adjusted in patients with congestive heart failure or renal insufficiency. Electrolytes should be carefully monitored and replaced. If normocalcemia is not achieved, patients may be carefully given diuretics, such as furosemide, to facilitate calcium excretion. This must be done only once the patient is fluid replete.

Inhibit Bone Resorption

Bisphosphonates

Intravenous bisphosphonates are effective in reducing serum calcium values. The effect is not achieved until a few days after administration, but it is more sustained than with intravenous hydration, furosemide, or calcitonin.

Zoledronic acid is approved for the treatment of hypercalcemia of malignancy. It is a third-generation bisphosphonate that is 100 to 800 times more potent than pamidronate. In a randomized, double-blind study of 287 patients with hypercalcemia of malignancy, zoledronic acid (4 and 8 mg) or pamidronate (90 mg) were given to patients with serum calcium levels exceeding 12 mg/dl. Both doses of zoledronic acid were superior to pamidronate, with response rates by day 10 of 88.4% (4 mg zoledronic acid), 86.7% (8 mg zoledonic acid), and 69.7% (90 mg pamidronate) for zoledronic acid, 4 and 8 mg, and pamidronate, 90 mg, respectively. Normalization of serum calcium by day 4 was approximately 45% to 55% in the zoledronic acid groups and only 33.3% in the pamidronate-treated patients [85].

Pamidronate was widely used before the introduction of zoledronic acid. The recommended dose depends on the severity of hypercalcemia, ranging from 30 to 90 mg infused over a 2- to 4-hour period. A study comparing pamidronate with clodronate in 41 patients with hypercalcemia of malignancy had more favorable results for pamidronate than in this trial. In this investigation, pamidronate normalized calcium levels in all patients by a median of 4 days, and the normocalcemia lasted for 28 days [86]. The optimal frequency of pamidronate administration can be variable. One small prospective randomized trial found that infusion of pamidronate every 2 weeks conferred less hypercalcemia than that every 3 weeks (10% vs. 50%) [87]. Given that bisphosphonates are excreted by the kidneys, dosage should be adjusted in cases of renal insufficiency.

Calcitonin
The dose of calcitonin is 4 IU/kg intramuscularly or subcutaneously every 12 hours. This dose works rapidly, reducing calcium levels by 1 to 2 mg/dl over that achieved with hydration only; however, tachyphylaxis is frequently seen after 2 or 3 days. Thus the drug is a useful adjunct while waiting for the intravenous bisphosphonate to take effect.

Mithramycin
This drug is given intravenously at a dose of 25 mg/kg over a 3- to 6-hour period. Serum calcium decreases within 12 hours, and this effect lasts for several days. However, a small, randomized prospective study in patients with hypercalcemia of malignancy demonstrated serum calcium normalization in only three of the 11 patients taking mithramycin [88]. Contraindications to the drug include liver, kidney, or bone marrow disease. Because of numerous hematologic side effects and the effectiveness of previously described drugs, it is infrequently used now.

Dialysis
This is useful in severe, life-threatening hypercalcemia, or in cases in which immediate serum calcium reduction is needed and intravenous infusion of saline or bisphosphonates are contraindicated. However, hypercalcemia recurs quickly after dialysis stops.

Hypercalcemic Emergencies
Symptomatic individuals with hypercalcemia should be admitted to the hospital for immediate treatment. Aggressive hydration with IV fluids should be initiated regardless of the etiology of hypercalcemia. If the cause is increased bone resorption, such as primary hyperparathyroidism or metastatic bone disease, or immobilization of a Pagetic patient, IV bisphosphonates (i.e., pamidronate at 60–90 mg IV over a 4-to 6-hour period or zoledronic acid at 4 mg IV over a 15-min period can be given). If the etiology is due to vitamin D toxicity or excess states (lymphoma, sarcoidosis, milk-alkali), bisphosphonates do not have a significant impact, as bone resorption is usually not the main mechanism. Hydration would be the main modality. Steroids can be tried for sarcoidosis.

It takes a few days for IV bisphosphonates to have an effect. Calcitonin, 100 IU subcutaneously, can be used for a few days while waiting for the bisphosphonates to work. Diuresis can be tried with IV or oral furosemide, but only after significant reduction in calcium is not achieved with any of these measures, and only once the patient is volume replete.

Future Therapy
Among calcimimetic agents, cinacalcet has been shown to reduce calcium levels in primary [89] or secondary hyperparathyroidism in hemodialysis patients [90] and parathyroid carcinoma [91].

22-Oxocalcitriol and EB 1089, an analogue of calcitriol, were found during in vitro studies to suppress parathyroid hormone–related protein gene expression [92,93].

HYPOCALCEMIA

Diagnosis
The diagnosis of hypocalcemia should be confirmed by measurement of ionized calcium. Other tests that are useful in determining the etiology include intact PTH, phosphate, 25(OH)D, 1,25(OH)$_2$D, magnesium, creatinine, ALT, and total or bone-specific alkaline phosphatase. Common causes are shown in Table 4.10.

In adults, hypoparathyroidism is frequently a result of thyroid or parathyroid surgery. Presentation during childhood raises the possibility of congenital hypoparathyroidism or pseudohypoparathyroidism (Table 4.10). Whether congenital or acquired, hypoparathyroidism is first seen with a low serum calcium and a low or inappropriately normal PTH level (Table 4.11). Phosphate levels may be normal or high. A syndrome of hypocalcemia with hypercalciuria due to an abnormal calcium-sensing receptor gene has been reported [94].

If vitamin D metabolite levels are low, the cause should be determined by history and examination. One should look for rickets, osteomalacia, malabsorption, hepatic disease, renal insufficiency, and medications that interfere with vitamin D metabolism, such as phenytoin. Serum phosphate levels may be low or low normal, and urinary excretion of calcium may be low. A bone biopsy is the gold standard for diagnosing osteomalacia; however, an elevation in bone-specific alkaline phosphatase in an individual with vitamin D or calcium deficiency and secondary hyperparathyroidism usually suggests the disease.

Hypomagnesemia causes hypocalcemia through failed PTH secretion or bone resistance to PTH at exceedingly low concentrations. Serum levels may be normal despite low tissue levels seen in association with chronic malabsorption and alcoholism.

In hospitalized patients, hypocalcemia can develop from diuretics, blood transfusions, chemotherapy, and other concomitant illnesses such as sepsis, pancreatitis, acute renal failure, and hemodialysis.

Table 4.10. Common Causes of Hypocalcemia

Hypoparathyroidism	Hungry-bone syndrome following parathyroidectomy
Pseudohypoparathyroidism	
Nutritional hypovitaminosis D	Bisphosphonates
Malabsorption	Fluoride poisoning
Hypomagnesemia	Concomitant illnesses: sepsis, surgery, chemotherapy, tumor lysis syndrome, renal failure
Vitamin D–dependent rickets type 1 and 2	
Intravascular and extravascular calcium deposition	

Table 4.11. Clinical Manifestations of Hypocalcemia

Musculoskeletal	**Ocular**
Tetany, muscle cramps and spasms, myopathy, circumoral and acral paresthesia	Cataracts
	Keratoconjunctivitis
	Papilledema with severe hypocalcemia
Trousseau sign: carpal spasm with inflation of blood pressure cuff to above systolic	**Cardiovascular**
	Hypotension
Chvostek sign: facial muscle contraction when the facial nerve is tapped on the ipsilateral side, anterior to the ear	Myocardial dysfunction
	Congestive heart failure
	Prolonged QT interval
	Decreased digitalis effect
Neuropsychiatric	
Seizures, fatigue, depression, anxiety, lethargy, mental retardation in children	**Gastrointestinal**
	Steatorrhea
	Decreased gastric acid secretion
Movement disorders	**Skin**
Dystonia, hemiballismus	Dry and coarse skin and hair, brittle hair, and nails
Basal ganglia calcifications	

Treatment

Hypocalcemic Emergencies

Symptomatic hypocalcemia, particularly in those patients with tetany, seizures, electrocardiographic changes, and decreased cardiac function, should be treated with intravenous calcium. Calcium gluconate, as a bolus of 1 to 2 g, provides 100 to 200 mg elemental calcium, followed by a continuous drip at 0.5 to 1.5 mg/kg/hr. Calcium gluconate is preferred over highly alkaline calcium chloride because it produces less local tissue necrosis. Calcitriol should be started immediately at a loading dose of 1.0 μg, followed by 0.5 μg daily with reduction, generally to 0.25 μg over a few days as the calcium deficiency is resolved. Once stabilized and able to take oral medications, the patient may be started on calcium supplements and calcitriol continued.

Oral Calcium Supplements

The goal of treatment in chronic hypocalcemia is to maintain serum calcium in the low-normal range. The elemental calcium dose required is quite variable and generally ranges from 1.5 to 3.0 g daily in divided doses (TID or QID), usually with an active vitamin D analogue. In hypoparathyroidism, the absorption of oral calcium is very low (thus the reason for large amounts described earlier). Various preparations of oral calcium are available. Calcium carbonate (250 mg elemental calcium per 600-mg tablet) is the least expensive, but it has poor absorption in patients with low gastric acid production. Ultradense calcium citrate (315–500 mg elemental calcium per tablet) is preferred except in patients with renal failure. One must remember that the elemental calcium content of calcium lactate and gluconate tablets is very low. Because most of these patients will be taking supraphysiologic doses of vitamin D, the authors caution readers that hypercalciuria, usually in the setting of normocalcemia, may exist [24]. Urine calcium excretion should be monitored frequently; even biannually in very stable patients. Should hypercalciuria be found, defined as more than 300 mg/24 hours, it is important to reduce the supplementation, particularly of the vitamin D.

Vitamin D

Various forms of vitamin D are available—ergocalciferol (vitamin D_2), cholecalciferol (vitamin D_3), dihydrotachysterol, 1-α-hydroxyvitamin D_3, and calcitriol (1-25 dihydroxyvitamin D_3). Ergocalciferol and calcitriol are the most frequently used. Ergocalciferol is available in 50,000-IU capsules, an 8,000-IU/ml liquid form, or a 500,000 IU/ml infusion. Because this form of vitamin D must be activated, intact hepatic and kidney function are necessary. Patients with renal failure and hypoparathyroidism need to receive supplementation with calcitriol. This is available in 0.25- and 0.5-μg capsules. It is the most rapid-acting metabolite of vitamin D. Hypercalcemia and hypercalciuria can occur, more commonly with calcitriol. Thus urinary and serum calcium levels should be monitored at least biannually. The goal is to maintain a low normal serum calcium concentration and normal calcium excretion.

Calcidiol [25(OH)D] is available in 20- and 50-mg capsules. Action is more rapid, but it is not as prolonged as with vitamin D dihydrotachysterol (the equivalent of $1(OH)_2D$), which requires 25-hydroxylation in the liver.

One study that compared the calcium-absorptive effects of calcitriol, calcidiol, and cholecalciferol found the potency of calcitriol and calcidiol to be 100:1. Vitamin D_3, or cholecalciferol, was the least potent in increasing calcium absorption [95]. However, a meta-analysis showed greater beneficial effects of hydroxylated vitamin D on BMD than of nonhydroxylated vitamin D [59].

Newer analogues of vitamin D, paricalcitol and doxercalciferol, have become available. They are both indicated for patients with advanced renal insufficiency, both providing the advantage of avoiding increases in the calcium/phosphorus product that may lead to deleterious effects. Both products effectively reduce PTH levels without causing significant hypercalcemia and hypercalciuria [94,95]. However, in situations in which the goal is to improve calcium absorption and increase calcium levels, calcitriol, ergocalciferol, or cholecalciferol would be preferred over these two newer analogues.

Magnesium

Concomitant magnesium deficiency should be corrected, provided that renal function is normal. The starting dose may be 2 g of magnesium sulfate given as an intravenous bolus over a 10-minute period, followed by 1 g/hr if necessary. Once the patient is replete, maintenance therapy may be initiated with oral magnesium supplements.

Parathyroid Hormone

It seems logical that PTH would be beneficial in treating hypoparathyroidism. However, few studies are available that have looked at this treatment possibility. One such trial randomized 20 patients with hypoparathyroidism to PTH twice a day or calcium and calcitriol. The patients taking PTH required about 37 μg, and those taking calcitriol needed 0.91 μg to attain normal calcium concentrations. Calcium, phosphorus, and magnesium levels did not differ between the groups. PTH normalized urine calcium levels, whereas calcitriol did not. No significant changes were seen in BMD between the groups. Bone-turnover markers increased more in the PTH group. Many subjects preferred injection to the pills [96]. PTH, however, does not have the FDA indication for hypoparathyroidism.

OSTEOMALACIA

Osteomalacia refers to a defect in mineralization of bone matrix or osteoid, which can have various causes. Congenital deficiencies typically demonstrate classic findings during infancy and childhood. In contrast, osteomalacia in adults is frequently detected as low bone mass and as biochemical abnormalities (elevated alkaline phosphatase; low calcium, phosphate, or 25(OH)D levels; secondary elevation in intact PTH).

One study showed a vitamin D–deficiency prevalence of approximately 50% among hospitalized individuals [97]. Increasingly, it is being more often discovered in ambulatory patients as well. About half of nonhospitalized women with osteoporosis were found to have a 25(OH)D concentration of less than 30 ng/ml in one study [98].

Most adults have no symptoms, and the disease is usually detected as part of a workup for osteoporosis. Those with more severe disease may have bone pain, spontaneous pelvic fractures, pseudofractures, and muscle weakness. Common causes of the deficiency include lack of sunlight exposure, inadequate nutritional intake, malabsorption due to celiac sprue or inflammatory bowel disease, and chronic renal insufficiency. Laboratory evaluation reveals low 25(OH)D concentrations and frequently decreased serum calcium, phosphate, and 24-hour urinary calcium. Most patients have secondary hyperparathyroidism, and in general, the lower the vitamin D concentration, the higher the PTH concentration [98,99].

The exact concentrations of 25(OH)D that are seen with various bone changes, such as osteoporosis and osteomalacia, although still not entirely clear, have begun to be more defined. Concentrations over approximately 30 ng/ml are generally considered sufficient. Those between approximately 8 and 30 ng/ml are insufficient, with increased fracture risk and decreased calcium absorption. Concentrations less than 8 ng/ml may be associated with osteomalacia. One issue plaguing this is the lack of standardization and the variability of 25(OH)D assays [100].

Vitamin D deficiency is treated with supplementation of vitamin D and calcium. Treatment recommendations for vitamin D repletion vary. Most experts use calcitriol in these situations because of the shorter half-life and rapid action. Usual starting dose is 0.5 μg oral calcitriol BID, monitoring serum calcium, intact PTH regularly, every 2 weeks until normocalcemic. Then dose adjustment should occur. Urinary calcium should be monitored as well, every 3 months and less frequently as the patient stabilizes. A gluten-free diet in celiac sprue usually improves calcium and vitamin D absorption, leading to reduced requirements for these agents.

Other modalities for lesser degrees of vitamin D deficiency include 50,000 IU once a week for 2 to 3 months, as well as 100,000 IU once, followed by maintenance doses of

800 to 1,200 IU daily. 25 (OH) D, serum calcium, and PTH levels should be rechecked after 3 months of therapy and at regular intervals thereafter, as hypercalcemia and hypercalciuria can happen. Replacement has been shown to decrease fracture rate [101]. Controversy exists regarding vitamin D replacement in hyperparathyroid patients. One recent small study of patients with hyperparathyroidism and mild hypercalcemia revealed a decrease in PTH with replacement and no increase in mean calcium concentrations. Of note, increases in urine calcium concentrations were seen in several patients [102].

Vitamin D–Dependent Rickets (Type 1 and Type 2)

These are rare congenital errors of vitamin D metabolism. Type 1 rickets is commonly an autosomal recessive disorder that results in a defect in renal tubular 25(OH)D-1α-hydroxylase. It usually appears during the first 2 years of life. Calcium and 1,25(OH)$_2$D levels are low, 25(OH)D levels may be normal or low, and intact PTH levels are elevated. Calcitriol in the dose of 0.25 to 1 μg/day is usually enough to correct the deficit. Careful monitoring of serum calcium, urinary calcium, and intact PTH should be used to titrate the dose.

Type 2 rickets, however, is a hereditary condition that results in resistance to the effects of 1,25(OH)$_2$D. Usually, the disease is first seen during infancy, before age 2 years, but reports have been made of the disorder in adults [103,104]. Calcium levels have been normal in patients with the first appearance later in life. It can be distinguished from type 1 rickets by normal or elevated 1,25(OH)$_2$D levels. Similarly, 25(OH)D levels may be normal, or low and intact PTH levels are elevated. Large doses of calcitriol (30–60 mg/day) are necessary to correct hypocalcemia and to induce mineralization of bones.

Oncogenic Osteomalacia

This osteomalacia is induced by a mesenchymal tumor and remits after the tumor's excision. The cause is thought to be overexpression of FGF23 by the mass. Support for this exists in several reports. Elevated serum concentrations of the FGF23 protein have been measured before removal of the tumor causing oncogenic osteomalacia, and these levels have then normalized after resection of the tumor. In addition, the FGF23 protein and its mRNA have been reportedly seen in the offending mass. Finally, a defect in phosphate reabsorption in the kidney has not only been noted before surgical resection, with subsequent improvement in these laboratory data after surgery, but it was also seen in the tumors [105,106]. Patients can have symptoms for months to years, with complaints of muscle weakness, bone pain, or recurrent fractures. Biochemical findings include hypophosphatemia and low tubular reabsorption of phosphorus [107,108]. A thorough search for the tumor must be undertaken with radiographs or MRI. In a recent case series, technetium scanning was found to be useful in localizing the tumors [109]. Treatment consists mainly of excision of the tumor. Some investigators have also found improvement of the disease with calcitriol and phosphorus supplementation [110].

Hypophosphatemic Rickets

This X-linked disorder results in decreased renal tubular reabsorption of phosphorus. So-called classic cases involve male patients with low phosphorus levels, stunted growth, and lower limb deformities. However, cases of mild isolated hypophosphatemia have been seen in women who are heterozygous for the gene known as PHEX. Optimal treatment involves phosphorus and calcitriol [110].

Growth hormone therapy has had positive effects on growth in children afflicted with the disorder [111,112]. Twelve months of growth hormone supplementation has improved height and growth velocity standard deviation scores compared with those with placebo [111].

Hypophosphatasia

This rare disorder results from decreased tissue-nonspecific alkaline phosphatase activity. Presentation may be severe during childhood or mild during adulthood. Adult hypophosphatasia can be first seen with recurrent stress fractures, painful hips, or pseudofractures. Clinical presentation can vary [113]. Diagnosis is made via low alkaline phosphatase levels, normal or high levels of calcium and phosphate, high phosphoethanolamine, and high inorganic pyrophosphate (Ppi). Measurement of pyridoxal 5'-phosphate (PLP) is the most sensitive and specific test for hypophosphatasia. No approved medical treatment is known for this condition. Vitamin D and calcium supplementation could produce more harm than good, because associated calcium and vitamin D levels are not low. Use of teriparatide has been reported in a few cases [114,115]. Further studies should be conducted regarding the benefits and risks of this application of teriparatide.

Drug-Induced Osteomalacia

Commonly used drugs that can cause osteomalacia include anticonvulsants (inhibition of 25-hydroxylation), cholestyramine (reduced absorption), glucocorticoids (inhibition of the vitamin D action), aluminum-containing antacids (inhibition of phosphate absorption), and etidronate (inhibition of osteoblast activity). Treatment consists of discontinuation of the offending agents.

REFERENCES

Evaluation of Metabolic Bone Disorders

1. **Hofbauer L, Schoppet M.** Clinical implications of the osteoprotegerin/RANKL/RANK system for bone and vascular diseases. JAMA 2004;292:490–495.

   This article comprehensively reviews osteoprotegerin, RANKL, and RANK. Their actions, the interplay among each other, effects on bone metabolism, and regulation are explained. Their roles in diseases other than those affecting bone are also detailed. Finally, possible uses of these markers in diagnostics and therapy are described.

2. *(1C)* **Panteghini M, Pagani F.** Biological variation in bone-derived biochemical markers in serum. Scand J Clin Lab Invest 1995;55:609–616.

   This small study of 10 patients examined intrasubject and intersubject variability of several bone markers. Total alkaline phosphatase (ALP) and its bone isoform had the lowest intrasubject variability (most of the observed variability was biologic), whereas osteocalcin and tartrate-resistant acid phosphatase (TR-ACP) had relatively high analytic variability and showed the lowest intersubject fluctuation.

3. *(1C+)* **Gertz BJ** et al. Monitoring bone resorption in early postmenopausal women by an immunoassay for cross-linked collagen peptides in urine. J Bone Miner Res 1994;9:135–142.

   Urinary excretion of cross-linked N-telopeptides of type 1 collagen was obtained from 65 early postmenopausal women who participated in a placebo-controlled trial of the aminobisphosphonate, alendronate sodium. Intersubject variability for cross-linked peptide excretion was 20.2% over the 9 months in placebo-treated subjects, substantially lower than that observed for other biochemical markers of bone resorption: 45%, 53%, and 63% for fasting urinary calcium and hydroxyproline and 24-hour urinary lysylpyridinoline (by high-performance liquid chromatography assay), respectively. Baseline cross-linked peptide excretion correlated significantly ($p < 0.001$) with baseline total urine lysylpyridinoline and serum osteocalcin, but not with other biochemical markers. Initial peptide excretion also correlated inversely with LS BMD at entry ($r = -0.26$; $p < 0.05$). Alendronate treatment for 6 weeks produced a dose-dependent suppression of cross-linked peptide excretion (0 ± 8, 29 ± 6, 56 ± 5, and $64 \pm 3\%$ for 0, 5, 20, and 40 mg, respectively; $p < 0.01$ vs. placebo for treatment effect), with a return toward pretreatment values during follow-up.

4. *(1A)* **Chesnut CH III.** Hormone replacement therapy in postmenopausal women: Urinary N-telopeptide Urinary of type I collagen monitors therapeutic effect and predicts response of bone mineral density. Am J Med 1997;102:29–37.

   This was a 2-year randomized controlled study of 236 healthy women at 1 to 3 years after menopause. Women received estrogen plus progesterone plus calcium (treated group) or calcium alone (control group). In the treated group, NTX significantly decreased ($p < 0.0001$), and spine and hip BMD significantly increased ($p < 0.00001$ and $p < 0.005$, respectively); in the control group, NTX did not change but BMD decreased significantly ($p < 0.01$). Subjects in the highest quartiles for baseline NTX (67–188 units) or decreasing NTX (−66%–87%) through 6 months demonstrated the greatest gain in BMD in response to HRT ($p < 0.05$ and $p < 0.005$). For every increase of 30 units in baseline NTX, the odds of gain in BMD in response to HRT increased by a factor of 5.0 (CI, 1.9–13.3); for every 30% decrease in NTX through 6 months, the odds of gaining BMD in response to HRT increased by a factor of 2.6 (CI, 1.6–4.4). In the control group, an increase of 30 units in NTX across the study indicated higher odds of losing BMD by a factor of 3.2 (CI, 1.6–6.5). A high baseline NTX (67 units) indicated a 17.3 times higher risk of BMD loss if not treated with HRT.

5. *(1A)* **Greenspan S** et al. Early changes in biochemical markers of bone turnover are associated with long-term changes in bone mineral density in elderly women on alendronate, hormone

replacement therapy, or combination therapy: A three-year, double-blind, placebo-controlled, randomized clinical trial. J Clin Endocrinol Metab 2005;90:2762–2767.

In this trial, 373 women who were 65 years of age and older were randomized to alendronate, hormone replacement therapy, a combination of the two, or placebo, and then followed up for 3 years, with NTX, BSAP, and osteocalcin levels determined every 6 months. A positive correlation was demonstrated between a decrease in the bone markers at month 6 and an increase in BMD at the spine and hip at the end of the study, in the patients taking the active medications. Those taking alendronate had greater decreases in bone markers and increases in BMD than did those receiving hormone replacement therapy. With respect to specific bone markers, the tertile that had the greatest decrease in NTX was associated with BMD increases of 10.1% at the hip and 6.1% at the hip as compared with the lowest tertile, which had BMD increases of 5.9% at the spine and 2.1% at the hip

6. *(1C)* **Bauer D** et al. Change in bone turnover and hip, nonspine, and vertebral fracture in alendronate-treated women: The Fracture Intervention Trial. J Bone Miner Res 2004;19:1250–1258.

   BSAP, PINP, and PICP were measured in the 6,186 participants of the Fracture Intervention Trial after 1 year of exposure to alendronate or placebo, and the results were analyzed with respect to fractures that occurred during the trial. A significant positive association was seen. A decrease in BSAP by one standard deviation was linked to less spine (26% reduction; CI, 12%–37%), nonspine (14% reduction; CI, 2%–24%), and hip fractures (40% reduction; CI, 21%–55%).

7. *(1C+)* **Melton LJ III** et al. Relationship of bone turnover to bone density and fractures. J Bone Miner Res 1997;12:1083–1091.

   Serum levels of osteocalcin, BSAP, and carboxy-terminal propeptide of type I procollagen (PICP), as well as 24-hour urine levels of NTX and the free pyridinium cross-links (pyridinoline and deoxypyridinoline) were measured in 351 randomly selected Minnesota women. PICP, NTX, and deoxypyridinoline were negatively associated with age among the 138 premenopausal women. All biochemical markers were positively associated with age among the 213 postmenopausal women, and the prevalence of elevated turnover (>1 SD above the premenopausal mean) varied from 9% (PICP) to 42% (pyridinoline). After adjusting for age, a negative correlation was found between the markers and BMD of the hip, spine, or forearm as measured by DXA, and women with osteoporosis were more likely to have a high bone turnover. A history of osteoporotic fractures of the hip, spine, or distal forearm was associated with reduced hip BMD and with elevated pyridinoline levels.

8. *(1C+)* **Garnero P** et al. Markers of bone resorption predict hip fracture in elderly women: The EPIDOS Prospective Study. J Bone Miner Res 1996;11:1531–1538.

   This is a prospective cohort study of 7,598 healthy women 75 years and older. The group comprised 126 women who sustained a hip fracture during a mean 22-month follow-up who were age-matched with three controls who did not experience fracture. Elderly women had higher markers of bone formation and resorption than did healthy premenopausal women. CTX and free deoxypyridinoline, but not other markers, were higher in patients with hip fracture (p = 0.02 and 0.005, respectively). CTX and free deoxypyridinoline excretion above the premenopausal range was associated with an increased hip fracture risk with an odds ratio of 2.2 (CI, 1.3–3.6) and 1.9 (CI, 1.1–3.2), respectively, whereas markers of formation were not. Increased bone resorption was an independent predictor of hip fracture. Women with both a femoral T score of −2.5 or less and either high CTX or high free deoxypyridinoline levels were at greater risk of hip fracture, with ORs of 4.8 and 4.1, respectively, than were those with only low BMD or high bone resorption.

Bone Imaging

9. *(1C+)* **Johnell O** et al. Predictive value of BMD for hip and other fractures. J Bone Miner Res 2005;20:1185–1194.

   This is a meta-analysis of 12 studies, consisting of 9,891 men and 29,082 women in total. It sought to find the correlation between BMD and fracture risk, as well as the influence of such factors as age, gender, and initial BMD. At age 65 years, an SD decrease in BMD increased the risk ratio for hip fracture by 2.94 (CI, 2.02–4.27) in men and 2.88 (CI, 2.31–3.59) in women. In addition, the risk for all fragility fractures increased by 1.41 (CI, 1.33–1.51) in men and 1.38 (CI, 1.28–1.48) in women.

10. *(1C)* **Zmuda J** et al. Posterior-anterior and lateral dual-energy x-ray absorptiometry for the assessment of vertebral osteoporosis and bone loss among older men. J Bone Miner Res 2000;15:1417–1424.

    This was an observational study of 193 men who were aged 51 to 81 years. BMD at the supine lateral, posteroanterior (PA), and proximal femur views were measured via DXA scan. One hundred two of these subjects had repeated DXAs 4 years later. BMD decreased with increasing age at the midlateral (r = −0.27) and lateral (r = −0.24) positions, but not the PA view (r = 0.04). Mean T scores were significantly less at the midlateral and lateral sites than at the PA site (p < 0.0001). T scores were in the osteoporotic range in 11% of cases at the femoral neck, 22.5% at the lateral view, 24.6% at the midlateral spine, and only 2.6% at the PA view.

11. *(1C)* **Schousboe J** et al. Prevalence of vertebral compression fracture deformity by x-ray absorptiometry of lateral thoracic and lumbar spines in a population referred for bone densitometry. J Clin Densitom 2002;5:239–246.

This observational study assessed the lateral spines of 342 subjects by DXA. Fifty of the 342 patients (14.6%; CI 11%–18.8%) had at least one vertebral compression deformity. 21.3% of the study population (73 of 342) were at least 60 years old and osteopenic by T score criteria; 27 of these 73 subjects (27.4%) had at least one vertebral deformity.

Osteoporosis

12. **(1C+) Siris E** et al. Identification and fracture outcomes of undiagnosed low bone mineral density in postmenopausal women; Results from the National Osteoporosis Risk Assessment. JAMA 2001;286:2815–2822.

This observational study observed 200,160 postmenopausal women at least 50 years old, who were newly diagnosed with osteoporosis, for about 1 year. Here, 39.6% had osteopenia by T score, and 7.2% had osteoporosis. Analysis of the BMDs and osteoporosis risk factors of the subjects revealed that certain risks (age, history of fracture, family history of fracture, Asian ethnicity, Hispanic ethnicity, tobacco use, and cortisone ingestion) increased the chance of osteoporosis. In addition, other factors (increased body mass index, African-American ethnicity, estrogen use, diuretic ingestion, exercise, and alcohol use) decreased this risk. Finally, 163,979 of the original cohort had fracture data over the year; analysis of these data reveal a fourfold increase in fractures in the osteoporotic population over those with normal BMD and a 1.8-fold increase in osteopenic patients. Of patients who had fractures, 50% did not meet densitometric criteria for osteoporosis.

13. **(1A) Black DM** et al. Randomised trial of effect of alendronate on risk of fracture in women with existing vertebral fractures: Fracture Intervention Trial Research Group. Lancet 1996;348:1535–1541.

This is a randomized placebo-controlled trial of 2,027 postmenopausal women aged between 55 and 81 years with low femoral neck BMD who were assigned to receive placebo ($n = 1005$) or daily alendronate ($n = 1022$) and were observed during a follow-up for 36 months. Alendronate reduced the risk of new radiographic fractures by 47%. Clinically apparent vertebral fractures were reduced in the alendronate group (2.3% vs. 5.0%; relative hazard [RH], 0.45; CI, 0.27–0.72). The risk of any clinical fracture was lower in the alendronate group than in the placebo group (139 [13.6%] vs. 183 [18.2%]; relative hazard 0.72 [0.58–0.90]), including a 51% reduction in hip fractures. No significant differences in the number of adverse events in the two groups were seen.

14. **(1A) Cummings SR** et al. Effect of alendronate on risk of fracture in women with low bone density but without vertebral fractures: Results from the Fracture Intervention Trial. JAMA 1998; 280:2077–2082.

A prospective, double-blind, randomized, placebo-controlled study of 4,432 postmenopausal women aged between 54 to 81 years without preexisting vertebral fractures who were randomly assigned to receive alendronate or placebo and followed up for 4 years. Similar to FIT 1, alendronate was initially given at 5 mg/day for 2 years followed by 10 mg/day. Alendronate increased BMD at all sites studied ($p < 0.001$). Risk of radiographic vertebral fracture was reduced by 44% (relative risk, 0.56; 95% CI, 0.39–0.80; treatment–control difference, 1.7%; number needed to treat [NNT], 60). Clinical vertebral fracture reduction was not significantly different; however, in the subset of patients with femoral neck T scores of -2.5 or less, alendronate reduced clinical vertebral fractures by 36% (RH, 0.64; 95% CI, 0.50–0.82; treatment–control difference, 6.5%; NNT, 15).

15. **(1C+) Cranney A** et al. Meta-analysis of alendronate for the treatment of postmenopausal women. Endocr Rev 2002;23:508–516.

This was a meta-analysis of 11 randomized, placebo-controlled trials of alendronate for postmenopausal osteoporosis. The pooled RR for vertebral fracture for the 5-mg dose was 0.52 (95% CI, 0.43–0.65), and for the nonvertebral fracture RR for 10 mg or more was 0.51 (CI, 0.38–0.69). Results for nonvertebral fractures were similar. Two- to 4-year percentage increases in BMD between alendronate and placebo were 7.48% (CI, 6.12–8.85) for the LS, 5.6% (CI, 4.8–6.39) for the hip, 2.08% for the forearm (CI, 1.53–2.63), and 2.73% (CI, 2.27–3.2) for the total body. Pooled RR for gastrointestinal side effects was 1.03 (0.81–1.3; $p = 0.83$).

16. **(1A) Papapoulos S** et al. Meta-analysis of the efficacy of alendronate for the prevention of hip fractures in postmenopausal. Osteoporos Int 2005;16:468–474.

This was a meta-analysis of six randomized trials of alendronate that lasted from 1 to 4.5 years. At least 95% received 5 to 10 mg of alendronate daily. The subjects with a vertebral fracture or T scores ≥ -2.0 who were taking alendronate had a hip-fracture risk reduction of 45% (CI, 16%–64%; $p = 0.007$); those with osteoporosis by T score had a 55% reduced risk (CI, 29%–72%; $p = 0.0008$).

17. **(1A) Bone H** et al. Ten years' experience with alendronate for osteoporosis in postmenopausal women. N Engl J Med 2004;350:1189–1190.

This extension of a multicenter, randomized, double-blind study, originally of 994 postmenopausal women, assessed the BMD changes in 804 of them over a 10-year period. The original cohort was divided into four dosage groups: 20 mg for 2 years and then 5 mg for the third year, and 5 mg, 10 mg, or placebo for 3 years. In the extension period, those in the 5-mg and 10-mg groups remained on their respective doses. The group originally taking 20 mg and then 5 mg remained on 5 mg for 2 more years, and then they were given placebo. The placebo group received 10 mg for the first 2 years of the extension, after which they did not take any further study medication. The most significant BMD changes were seen in those taking 10 mg for

10 years. This group's BMD at the lumbar spine increased by a mean of 13.7% (CI, 12%–15.5%), at the trochanter by a mean of 10.3% (CI, 8.1%–12.4%), at the femoral neck by a mean of 5.4% (CI, 3.5%–7.4%), and by a mean of 6.7% at the proximal femur (CI, 4.4%–9.1%).

18. *(1A)* **Uusi-Rasi K** et al. Effect of discontinuation of alendronate treatment and exercise on bone mass and physical fitness: 15-month follow-up of a randomized, controlled trial. Bone 2004;35: 799–805.

These investigators conducted a 15-month extension of a 1-year trial examining the effect of alendronate and exercise on BMD and physical-fitness parameters. Of the 152 original postmenopausal female subjects, 102 of them participated in the follow-up trial. After 1 year, alendronate was discontinued. Over the next 15 months, those in the prior alendronate group lost bone mass at a rate similar to that of those in the placebo group. Although a difference in mean BMD of 3.2% (CI, 1%–5.4%) persisted in the lumbar spine between the treatment and placebo groups, no difference was found at the femoral neck at the end of the follow-up phase.

19. *(1A)* **Schnitzer T** et al. Therapeutic equivalence of alendronate, 70 mg, once weekly and alendronate, 10 mg daily, in the treatment of osteoporosis: Alendronate Once-Weekly Study Group. Aging (Milano) 2000;12:1–12.

The efficacy and safety of treatment with oral once-weekly alendronate, 70 mg, twice-weekly alendronate, 35 mg, and daily alendronate, 10 mg, were compared in a 1-year, double-blind, multicenter study of postmenopausal women with osteoporosis by T score or previous vertebral or hip fracture. Mean increases in LS BMD at 12 months were 5.1% (CI, 4.8–5.4) in the 70-mg once-weekly group, 5.2% (CI, 4.9–5.6) in the 35-mg twice-weekly group, and 5.4% (CI, 5.0–5.8) in the 10-mg daily treatment group. Increases in BMD at the total hip, femoral neck, trochanter, and total body were similar for the three groups. Reduction in markers of bone resorption (urinary NTX) and bone formation (serum BSAP) were similar across three groups into the middle of the premenopausal reference range. Upper gastrointestinal adverse experiences were similar, with a trend toward a lower incidence of esophageal events in the once-weekly dosing group.

20. *(1C)* **Odvina C** et al. Severely suppressed bone turnover: A potential complication of alendronate therapy. J Clin Endocrinol Metab 2005;90:1294–1301.

This is a case report of nine osteoporotic patients taking calcium and alendronate, 10 mg daily or 70 mg weekly, for 3 to 8 years. They each had a nonvertebral fragility fracture while taking this bisphosphonate, and two thirds either did not heal this fracture or healed it slowly. Bone biopsies in these patients revealed decreased bone volume and minimal bone formation. Seven of the nine patients demonstrated few, if any, osteoblasts. Of note, osteocalcin was low normal to low in these patients.

21. *(1A)* **Orwoll E** et al. Alendronate for the treatment of osteoporosis in men. N Engl J Med 2000; 343:604–610.

This is a 2-year double-blind placebo-controlled trial. The effect of daily alendronate (10 mg) or placebo on BMD in 241 men with osteoporosis was evaluated. About one third had low serum free testosterone concentrations at baseline; the rest had normal concentrations and no other secondary causes of osteoporosis. The men who received alendronate had a mean (±SEM) increase in BMD of 7.1% ± 0.3% at the LS, 2.5% ± 0.4% at the femoral neck, and 2.0% ± 0.2% for the total body ($p < 0.001$ for all comparisons with baseline). In contrast, men who received placebo had an increase in LS BMD of 1.8% ± 0.5% ($p < 0.001$ for the comparison with baseline) and no significant changes in femoral-neck or total-body BMD. Vertebral fracture incidence was lower in the alendronate group than in the placebo group (0.8% vs. 7.1%; $p = 0.02$), and height loss was significantly greater in the placebo than alendronate group (2.4 vs. 0.6 mm; $p = 0.02$).

22. *(1A)* **Saag K** et al. Alendronate for the prevention and treatment of glucocorticoid-induced osteoporosis: Glucocorticoid-Induced Osteoporosis Intervention Study Group. N Engl J Med 1998;339: 292–299.

Two 48-week, randomized, placebo-controlled studies of two doses of alendronate were conducted on 477 men and women taking glucocorticoids. The mean BMD of the LS increased by 2.1% ± 0.3% and 2.9% ± 0.3% in the groups that received 5 and 10 mg of alendronate per day, respectively ($p < 0.001$), and decreased by 0.4% ± 0.3% in the placebo group. The femoral neck bone density increased by 1.2% ± 0.4% and 1.0% ± 0.4% in the respective alendronate groups ($p < 0.01$) and decreased by 1.2% ± 0.4% in the placebo group ($p < 0.01$). The BMD of the trochanter and total body also increased significantly in the patients taking alendronate. There were proportionally fewer new vertebral fractures in the alendronate groups (overall incidence, 2.3%) than in the placebo group (3.7%; RR, 0.6; CI, 0.1–4.4). Markers of bone turnover decreased significantly in the alendronate groups ($p < 0.001$). There were no differences in serious adverse effects among the three groups, but there was a small increase in minor upper gastrointestinal effects in the 10 mg group.

23. *(1A)* **Rosen C** et al. Treatment with once-weekly alendronate 70 mg compared with once-weekly risedronate 35 mg in women with postmenopausal osteoporosis: A randomized double-blind study. J Bone Miner Res 2005;20:141–151.

This randomized, double-blind, active-controlled, multicenter trial assessed BMD and bone turnover–marker changes, as well as side effects, in 1,053 postmenopausal osteoporotic women who were randomized to alendronate, 70 mg weekly, or risedronate, 35 mg weekly, for 12 months. At 1 year, those taking alendronate had small but significant increases in BMD over the subjects taking risedronate, with treatment differences of 1.4% at the trochanter (CI, 0.8%–1.9%; $p < 0.001$), 1.1% at the hip (CI, 0.7%–1.4%; $p < 0.001$), 0.7% at the femoral neck (0.1%–1.2%; $p = 0.005$), and 1.2% at the lumbar spine (CI, 0.7%–1.6%; $p < 0.001$). Significant differences at all sites in BMD were seen at 6 months as well. More patients (10.3%) in the alendronate group demonstrated at least a 3% increase in trochanter BMD at 1 year (CI, 4%–16.7%; $p = 0.002$), and 16.7% more patients taking alendronate than risedronate exhibited a maintenance of or gain in trochanter BMD at 12 months ($p < 0.001$). CTX, NTX, BSAP, and PINP were all depressed more with alendronate ($p < 0.001$). No significant differences in adverse events were noted between the two groups.

24. *(1A)* **Harris ST** et al. Effects of risedronate treatment on vertebral and nonvertebral fractures in women with postmenopausal osteoporosis: A randomized controlled trial: Vertebral Efficacy with Risedronate Therapy (VERT) Study Group. JAMA 1999;282:1344–1352.

In this randomized, double-blind, placebo-controlled trial, 2,458 postmenopausal women younger than 85 years and with at least one vertebral fracture were randomly assigned to receive 3 years of rise-dronate (2.5 or 5 mg/day) or placebo. All subjects received calcium (1,000 mg/day), and cholecalciferol (≥500 IU/day) was provided if baseline levels of 25(OH)D were low. The 2.5 mg/day of the risedronate arm was discontinued after 1 year. Treatment with 5 mg/day of risedronate decreased the incidence of new vertebral fracture risk by 41% (CI, 18%–58%) over a 3-year period (11.3% vs. 16.3%; $p = 0.003$). Ver-tebral fracture reduction of 65% (CI, 38%–81%) was seen after the first year (2.4% vs. 6.4%; $p < 0.001$). Nonvertebral fracture incidence over a 3-year period was reduced by 39% (CI, 6%–61%) (5.2% vs. 8.4%; $p = 0.02$). BMD increased significantly compared with placebo at the LS (5.4% vs. 1.1%), femoral neck (1.6% vs. 21.2%), femoral trochanter (3.3% vs. 20.7%), and midshaft of the radius (0.2% vs. 21.4%). Bone biopsies obtained showed histologically normal bone.

25. *(1A)* **Reginster J** et al. Randomized trial of the effects of risedronate on vertebral fractures in women with established postmenopausal osteoporosis: Vertebral Efficacy with Risedronate Ther-apy (VERT) Study Group. Osteoporos Int 2000;11:83–91.

The design of this European arm of the VERT study was similar to that of the U.S. arm. The study in-cluded 1,226 postmenopausal women. Risedronate reduced the risk of new vertebral fractures by 49% over a 3-year period compared with placebo ($p < 0.001$). A significant reduction of 61% was seen within the first year ($p = 0.001$). The risk of nonvertebral fractures was reduced by 33% compared with placebo over a 3-year period ($p = 0.06$). Risedronate significantly increased BMD at the spine and hip within 6 months. The adverse-event profile of risedronate was not significantly different from that with placebo.

26. *(1A)* **Mellstrom DD** et al. Seven years of treatment with risedronate in women with post-menopausal osteoporosis. Calcif Tissue Int 2004;75:462–468.

This was the second 2-year extension of an originally 3-year randomized placebo-controlled trial that as-sessed the effect of risedronate on BMD and fractures. In this portion of the trial, 164 subjects enrolled, and 83% of them (136 subjects) completed the 2-year phase. All patients received 5 mg/day of rise-dronate. In those who had been receiving treatment before this extension, their BMD gains persisted or improved. The incidence of vertebral fractures remained similar in years 4 through 7. Those who were in the placebo group before this extension experienced significant BMD gains; they also noted decreases in fracture rates similar to those in the treatment group.

27. *(1A)* **McClung MR** et al. Effect of risedronate on the risk of hip fracture in elderly women: Hip Intervention Program Study Group. N Engl J Med 2001;344:333–340.

In this study, 5,445 postmenopausal women, 70 to 79 years old with osteoporosis (femoral neck T score −4 or less or below −3 with a nonskeletal risk factor for hip fracture, such as poor gait or a propensity to fall; group 1) and 3,886 women at least 80 years old who had at least one nonskeletal risk factor for hip fracture or low BMD at the femoral neck (T score below −4 or below −3 with a hip axis length ≤11.1 cm; group 2) were randomly assigned to receive oral risedronate (2.5 or 5.0 mg/day) or placebo for 3 years. The incidence of hip fracture among all the women in the risedronate group was reduced significantly (RR, 0.7; CI, 0.6–0.9; $p = 0.02$). In group 1, a significant reduction in hip fractures was found compared with the placebo group (RR, 0.6; CI, 0.4–0.9; $p = 0.009$). In group 2, the incidence of hip fracture was not significantly different between the two groups ($p = 0.35$).

28. *(1C+)* **Cranney A III** et al. Meta-analysis of risedronate for the treatment of postmenopausal osteoporosis. Endocr Rev 2002;23:517–523.

This was a meta-analysis of eight randomized trials that compared risedronate with placebo. The pooled RR of vertebral fractures in postmenopausal women given 2.5 mg or more of risedronate was 0.64 (CI, 0.54–0.77). The pooled RR of nonvertebral fractures was 0.73 (CI, 0.61–0.87). Mean percentage change difference between risedronate and placebo was 4.54% (CI, 4.12–4.97) in the LS, and 2.75% (CI, 2.32–3.17) in the femoral neck.

29. *(1A)* **Brown JP** et al. The efficacy and tolerability of risedronate once a week for the treatment of postmenopausal osteoporosis. Calcif Tissue Int 2002;71:103–111.

This study's design included a randomized double-blind active controlled group of 1,456 postmenopausal women 50 years and older with T score of less than −2.5 or of less than −2.0 with at least one prevalent fracture. Risedronate (35 mg once weekly, 50 mg once weekly, and 5 mg once daily) had similar efficacy and safety profiles. The mean percentage change in LS BMD after 12 months was 4.0% (0.2%) in the 5-mg daily group, 3.9% (0.2%) in the 35-mg group, and 4.2% (0.2%) in the 50-mg group.

30. *(1A)* **Eastell R** et al. Prevention of bone loss with risedronate in glucocorticoid-treated rheumatoid arthritis patients. Osteoporos Int 2000;11:331–337.

This was a 2-year, double-masked, placebo-controlled trial with a third year of nontreatment follow-up in which 120 women on long-term glucocorticoid therapy (>2.5 mg/day prednisolone) were randomly assigned to receive daily placebo, risedronate 2.5 mg/day, or cyclic risedronate (15 mg/day for 2 of 12 weeks). At the end of 97 weeks, BMD was maintained at the LS (1.4%) and trochanter (0.4%) in the daily 2.5-mg risedronate group, whereas significant bone loss occurred in spine and hip of the placebo group (−1.6%, *p* = 0.03; and −4.0%; *p* < 0.005, respectively). At the femoral neck, an insignificant bone loss was noted in the daily 2.5-mg risedronate group (−1.0%), whereas in the placebo group, bone density decreased significantly (−3.6%; *p* < 0.001). The difference between placebo and daily 2.5-mg risedronate groups was significant at the LS (*p* = 0.009) and trochanter (*p* = 0.02) but was not significant at the femoral neck. Although not significantly different from placebo at the LS, the overall effect of the cyclic regimen was similar to that of the daily 2.5-mg risedronate regimen. After treatment was withdrawn, significant bone loss occurred at the LS. Adverse events (including upper gastrointestinal events) were similar across treatment groups.

31. *(1A)* **Reid DM** et al. Efficacy and safety of daily risedronate in the treatment of corticosteroid-induced osteoporosis in men and women: A randomized trial: European Corticosteroid-Induced Osteoporosis Treatment Study. J Bone Miner Res 2000;15:1006–1013.

This was a multicenter, double-blind, placebo-controlled study of 290 men and women taking high-dose oral corticosteroid therapy (prednisone ≤7.5 mg/day or equivalent) for ≤6 months. Risedronate, 2.5 or 5 mg/day, or placebo was administered for 12 months. All patients received 1 g calcium and 400 IU vitamin D daily. The primary end point was LS BMD at month 12. Overall, statistically significant treatment effects were found on BMD at 12 months at the LS (*p* < 0.001), femoral neck (*p* = 0.004), and trochanter (*p* = 0.010). Risedronate, 5 mg, increased BMD at 12 months by an SEM of 2.9% (0.49%) at the LS, 1.8% (0.46%) at the femoral neck, and 2.4% (0.54%) at the trochanter, whereas BMD was maintained only in the control group. The incidence of vertebral fractures was reduced by 70% in the combined risedronate treatment groups, relative to placebo (*p* = 0.042). No difference in gastrointestinal adverse events was noted between the risedronate and placebo groups.

32. *(1C)* **De Groen PC** et al. Esophagitis associated with the use of alendronate. N Engl J Med 1996;335:1016–1021.

Report of three cases of severe esophagitis among alendronate-treated patients and review of postmarketing data.

33. *(1A)* **Lanza F** et al. An endoscopic comparison of the effects of alendronate and risedronate on upper gastrointestinal mucosae. Am J Gastroenterol 2000;95:3112–3117.

This was a multicenter, randomized, parallel-group, double-blind, placebo-controlled trial of 235 patients (men or postmenopausal women, aged 45–80 years) with normal upper gastrointestinal endoscopies at baseline. They received 28 days of the following therapy: alendronate, 40 mg/day, risedronate, 30 mg/day, placebo, or placebo with aspirin, 650 mg 4 times per day, for the last 7 days. Endoscopy was repeated on day 29. After 28 days of treatment, the alendronate and risedronate groups had comparable mean gastric and duodenal erosion scores, which were significantly lower than those of the aspirin group. Esophageal scores were comparable in all groups. Gastric ulcers alone, or combined with large numbers of gastric erosions, occurred in 3% of alendronate and risedronate patients versus 60% in those treated with aspirin and placebo.

34. *(1A)* **Lanza FL** et al. Endoscopic comparison of esophageal and gastroduodenal effects of risedronate and alendronate in postmenopausal women. Gastroenterology 2000;119:631–638.

Healthy postmenopausal women were randomly assigned to receive 5 mg risedronate or 10 mg alendronate for 2 weeks. Endoscopies were performed at baseline and on days 8 and 15. Gastric ulcers were observed during the treatment period in nine of 221 (4.1%) evaluable subjects on risedronate compared with 30 of 227 (13.2%) taking alendronate (*p* < 0.001). Mean gastric endoscopy scores for the risedronate group were lower than those for the alendronate group at days 8 and 15 (*p* ≥ 0.001). Mean esophageal and duodenal endoscopy scores were similar in the two groups at days 8 and 15. Esophageal ulcers were noted in three evaluable subjects in the alendronate group, compared with none in the risedronate group, and duodenal ulcers were noted in one evaluable subject in the alendronate group and two in the risedronate group.

35. *(1C+)* **Taggart H** et al. Upper gastrointestinal tract safety of risedronate: A pooled analysis of 9 clinical trials. Mayo Clin Proc 2002;77:262–270.

The nine included studies enrolled 10,068 men and women who received placebo or 5 mg of risedronate sodium for ≥3 years (intent-to-treat population). The treatment groups were similar with respect to baseline gastrointestinal tract disease and use of concomitant treatments during the studies. No significant difference was found in upper gastrointestinal tract adverse events in the risedronate and placebo groups (29.8% and 29.6%, respectively). Risedronate-treated patients with preexisting active upper gastrointestinal disease did not experience worsening of their underlying conditions or an increased frequency of upper gastrointestinal adverse events. Concomitant use of NSAIDs, requirement for gastric antisecretory drugs, or the presence of active gastrointestinal tract disease did not result in a higher frequency of upper gastrointestinal tract adverse events in the risedronate-treated patients compared with findings in controls. Endoscopy, performed in 349 patients, demonstrated no statistically significant differences across treatment groups.

36. *(1B)* **Reginster J** et al. Monthly oral ibandronate is well tolerated and efficacious in post-menopausal women: Results from the Monthly Oral Pilot Study. J Clin Endocrinol Metab 2005; 90:5018–5024.

In this randomized, double-blind, multicenter, placebo-controlled study, 144 postmenopausal women were given 50, 100, or 150 mg of ibandronate or placebo monthly. They were followed up for 3 months for tolerability and changes in the bone-turnover marker CTX. No significant differences in adverse events compared with placebo were discovered. CTX significantly decreased over these 3 months in those taking 100- and 150-mg dosages (serum, -40.7% and -56.7%, respectively, $p < 0.001$; urinary, -34.6% and -54.1%, respectively, $p < 0.001$).

37. *(1A)* **Miller P** et al. Monthly oral ibandronate therapy in postmenopausal osteoporosis: 1-year results from the MOBILE study. J Bone Miner Res 2005;20:1315–1322.

This was a randomized, double-blind trial that searched for the appropriate ibandronate dose for the treatment of osteoporosis. The 1,609 postmenopausal osteoporotic women in the study were assigned to four groups: 2.5 mg daily, 50 mg/50 mg once a month, 100 mg once a month, or 150 mg once a month, and they were followed up for 2 years. Those taking monthly ibandronate experienced increases in lumbar spine (3.9%, 4.3%, 4.1%, and 4.9%, respectively) and similar increases in hip BMD (2%–3%). The 150-mg group had small but significantly greater increases in lumbar spine BMD than did the group with the daily regimen ($p < 0.0001$). When the groups were evaluated for those who achieved BMD gains above baseline as well as >6% at the LS or 3% at the hip, the 150-mg and 100-mg groups had significantly more patients at these goals than did those with the daily regimen at the LS and at the hip (only 150 mg at the LS with respect to gains above baseline). Regarding side effects, the frequency of gastrointestinal symptoms with each dose was similar, but there was a small increase in flulike symptoms with the monthly regimens (6.6% in the 50/50-mg group, 6.8% in the 100-mg group, 8.3% in the 150-mg group, and 2.8% in the daily group).

38. **Emkey R** et al. Two year efficacy and tolerability of intermittent intravenous ibandronate injections in postmenopausal osteoporosis: The DIVA study: Presented at the Annual Scientific Meeting of ACR/ARHP, November 2005; San Diego, CA.

Two-year multinational, randomized, double-blind, double-dummy, phase III study in postmenopausal women with osteoporosis. Efficacy and safety of oral 2.5-mg ibandronate daily was compared with two IV ibandronate regimens (2 mg every 2 months and 3 mg every 3 months). At 1 and 2 years, IV ibandronate produced similar increases in BMD, 6.4%, 6.3%, and 4.8%, with the two IV regimens producing significantly higher BMD gain at the lumbar spine and proximal hip than did the daily dose ($p < 0.001$). All treatment arms had similar decreases in sCTX and similar safety profile.

38a. *(2C)* **Ruggiero SL, Mehrotra B, Rosenberg TJ**, et al: Osteonecrosis of the jaws associated with the use of bisphosphonates: A review of 63 cases. J Oral Maxillofac Surg 62:527-534, 2004.

Osteonecrosis of the jaw was first brought into focus by this descriptive study of 63 cases.

39. *(1A)* **Ettinger B** et al. Reduction of vertebral fracture risk in postmenopausal women with osteoporosis treated with raloxifene: Results from a 3-year randomized clinical trial: Multiple Outcomes of Raloxifene Evaluation (MORE) Investigators. JAMA 1999;282:637–645.

This is a multicenter, randomized, blinded, placebo-controlled trial of 7,705 postmenopausal women with osteoporosis. They were randomly assigned to receive 60 or 120 mg/day of raloxifene or placebo. At 36 months, the risk of vertebral fracture was reduced in both study groups receiving raloxifene (60 mg/day group: RR, 0.7, and CI, 0.5–0.8; 120 mg/day group: RR, 0.5, and CI, 0.4–0.7). Frequency of vertebral fracture was reduced both in women with (50% reduction) and without prevalent fractures (30% reduction). Nonvertebral fracture reduction was not significant. Raloxifene increased BMD in the femoral neck by 2.1% (60 mg) and 2.4% (120 mg) and in the spine 2.6% (60 mg) and 2.7% (120 mg) ($p < 0.001$ for all comparisons). Women receiving raloxifene had increased risk of venous thromboembolus compared with those taking placebo (RR, 3.1; CI, 1.5–6.2).

40. *(1A)* **Delmas PD** et al. Efficacy of raloxifene on vertebral fracture risk reduction in postmenopausal women with osteoporosis: Four-year results from a randomized clinical trial. J Clin Endocrinol Metab 2002;87:3609–3617.

This was a 4-year extension of the MORE trial. The 4-year cumulative RRs for one or more new vertebral fractures were 0.64 (CI, 0.53–0.76) with raloxifene, 60 mg/day, and 0.57 (CI, 0.48–0.69) with raloxifene, 120 mg/day. The nonvertebral fracture risk was not significantly reduced (RR, 0.93; CI, 0.81–1.06). The safety profile after 4 years was similar to that observed after 3 years.

41. *(1C+)* **Cranney A** et al. Meta-analysis of raloxifene for the prevention and treatment of postmenopausal osteoporosis. Endocr Rev 2002;23:524–528.

This was a meta-analysis of seven trials comparing raloxifene with placebo. Pooled mean percentage increase in LS BMD was 2.51% (CI, 2.21–2.82), hip was 2.11 (CI, 1.68–2.53), total body was 1.33% (CI, 0.37–2.30), and forearm was 2.05%(CI, 0.71–3.39). Vertebral fracture reduction was 40% (CI, 0.5–0.7). Nonvertebral fracture reduction was not significant.

42. *(1A)* **Chestnut CH** et al. A randomized trial of nasal spray calcitonin in postmenopausal women with established osteoporosis: The Prevent Recurrence of Osteoporotic Fractures Study. Am J Med 2000;109:267–276.

This was a 5-year, prospective, randomized placebo-controlled study of 1,255 postmenopausal women with one or more vertebral compression fractures and with an LS T score of -2 or lower. The incidence of new vertebral fractures decreased significantly by 33% (p = 0.05) only in the 200 IU calcitonin group but not the 100-IU or 400-IU dose. No significant difference was seen in nonvertebral fracture risk reduction between placebo and calcitonin.

43. *(1C+)* **Cranney A** et al. Meta-analysis of calcitonin for the treatment of postmenopausal osteoporosis. Endocr Rev 2002;23:540–551.

In this meta-analysis of 30 studies, calcitonin reduced the incidence of vertebral fractures by 54% (CI, 0.25–0.87) over placebo. In a large randomized trial, the RR was 0.79 (CI, 0.62–1.0). The pooled RR for nonvertebral fractures was 0.52 (CI, 0.22–1.23). In the largest trial, this was not significant. Pooled increases in weighted mean difference were 3.74 (CI, 2.04–5.43) for the lumbar spine, 3.02 (CI, 0.98–5.07) at the combined mean forearm, and 3.80 (p = 0.07) at the femoral neck.

44. *(1C+)* **Wells G** et al. Meta-analysis of the efficacy of hormone replacement therapy in treating and preventing osteoporosis in postmenopausal women. Endocr Rev 2002;23:529–539.

This meta-analysis of 57 randomized studies showed a trend toward reduction of incidence of vertebral fractures (RR, 0.66; CI, 0.41–1.07; five trials) and nonvertebral fractures (RR, 0.87; CI, 0.71–1.08; six trials) with HRT. BMD increase was 6.76% at 2 years in the LS (21 trials), 4.12% (nine trials) in the femoral neck, and 4.53% (14 trials) in the forearm.

45. *(1A)* **Writing Group for the Women's Health Initiative Investigators**. Risks and benefits of estrogen plus progestin in healthy postmenopausal women: Principal results from the Women's Health Initiative (WHI) randomized controlled trial. JAMA 2002;288:321–333.

In this randomized control study of >16,000 postmenopausal women, Prempro (a proprietary named for CEE, 0.625 mg, and medroxyprogesterone 2.5 mg) significantly reduced the risk of clinical vertebral fractures by 34%, hip fractures by 34%, and all fractures by 24% over placebo over a 5-year period. Increased breast cancer and cardiovascular risk led to discontinuation of this treatment arm. Estimated hazard ratios were as follows: congestive heart disease, 1.29 (CI, 1.02–1.63); breast cancer, 1.26 (CI, 1.00–1.59); stroke, 1.41 (CI, 1.07–1.85); pulmonary embolism, 2.13 (CI, 1.39–3.25); colorectal cancer, 0.63 (CI, 0.43–0.92); endometrial cancer, 0.83 (CI, 0.47–1.47); hip fracture, 0.66 (CI, 0.45–0.98); death due to other causes, 0.92 (CI, 0.74–1.14).

46. *(1A)* **Bone HG** et al. Alendronate and estrogen effects in postmenopausal women with low bone mineral density: Alendronate/Estrogen Study Group. J Clin Endocrinol Metab 2000;85:720–726.

This was a prospective, double-blind, placebo-controlled, randomized clinical trial in which 425 postmenopausal women who had previously undergone hysterectomy with low bone mass were randomly assigned to receive placebo, oral alendronate, 10 mg/day, conjugated estrogen, 0.625 mg/day, or a combination of the two drugs. At 2 years, mean percentage changes in LS BMD were 0.6% for placebo, 6% for alendronate (p < 0.001 vs. placebo), 6% for CEE (p < 0.001 vs. placebo), and 8.3% for combination therapy (p < 0.001 vs. placebo and CEE; p = 0.022 vs. alendronate). The corresponding changes in total proximal femur BMD were 4.0%, 3.4%, 4.7%, and 0.3% for the alendronate, estrogen, alendronate plus estrogen, and placebo groups, respectively. Greater reductions in urinary NTX and BSAP were seen in the combination therapy than with either one alone.

47. *(1A)* **Lindsay R** et al. Addition of alendronate to ongoing hormone replacement therapy in the treatment of osteoporosis: A randomized, controlled clinical trial. J Clin Endocrinol Metab 1999; 84:3076–3081.

In this randomized, placebo-controlled trial of 428 postmenopausal women with osteoporosis who had been receiving HRT for ≤1 year, alendronate, 10 mg/day plus HRT, produced significantly greater increases in BMD of the LS (3.6% vs. 1.0%; p < 0.001) and hip trochanter (2.7% vs. 0.5%; p < 0.001) compared with HRT alone; the intergroup difference in BMD at the femoral neck was not significant (1.7% vs. 0.8%; p = 0.072). Serum BSAP and urine NTX decreased significantly at 6 and 12 months with alendronate plus HRT, after which they remained within premenopausal levels. No differences in upper gastrointestinal adverse events or fractures were seen.

48. *(1A)* **Johnell O** et al. Additive effects of raloxifene and alendronate on bone density and biochemical markers of bone remodeling in postmenopausal women with osteoporosis. J Clin Endocrinol Metab 2002;87:985–992.

This study was a phase 3, randomized, double-blind 1-year trial that evaluated the effects of combined raloxifene and alendronate in 331 postmenopausal women with osteoporosis. Patients received placebo, raloxifene, 60 mg/day, alendronate, 10 mg/day, or a combination of the latter two. Mean LS BMD increases over baseline were 2.1%, 4.3%, and 5.3% in the raloxifene, alendronate, and combination groups, respectively (p < 0.05). The mean increase in femoral neck BMD in the combination group was 3.7% compared with the 2.7% and 1.7% increases in the alendronate (p = 0.02) and raloxifene (p < 0.001) groups, respectively. The changes from baseline to 12 months in bone markers ranged from −7.1% to −16.0% with placebo, −23.8% to −46.5% with raloxifene, −42.3% to −74.2% with alendronate, and −54.1% to −81.0% in the raloxifene–alendronate combination group. Although the alendronate group had changes in BMD and bone markers that were approximately twice the magnitude found in the raloxifene group, clinical correlation to fractures is not known. Combined therapy reduced markers of bone turnover to a greater degree than did either drug alone.

49. *(1A)* **Neer RM** et al. Effect of parathyroid hormone (1-34) on fractures and bone mineral density in postmenopausal women with osteoporosis. N Engl J Med 2001;344:1434–1441.

In this study, 1,637 postmenopausal women with prior vertebral fractures were randomly assigned to once-daily 20 or 40 μg SC of PTH (1-34) or placebo for a median of 21 months. RRs of fracture in the 20- and 40-μg groups, compared with placebo, were 0.35 (CI, 0.22–0.55) and 0.3 (CI, 0.19–0.50). Nonvertebral fracture RRs were 0.47 (CI, 0.25–0.88) and 0.46 (CI, 0.25–0.861). Compared with placebo, the 20- and 40-mg doses of PTH increased LS BMD by 9% and 13%, and by 3% and 6% in the femoral neck; the 40-mg dose decreased BMD at the shaft of the radius by 2%, but total body BMD was increased by 2%–4%.Most common side effects included nausea and headache.

50. *(1C+)* **Prince R** et al. Sustained nonvertebral fragility fracture risk reduction after discontinuation of teriparatide treatment. J Bone Miner Res 2005;20:1507–1513.

This observational study assessed nonvertebral changes in 1,262 of the FPT subjects for 30 months after discontinuation of teriparatide. Although the hazard ratios for nonvertebral fragility fractures remained significantly less in the treatment groups when the entire 50 weeks were analyzed, if the period after teriparatide discontinuation was solely assessed, only the 40-mg group had a significant decrease. BMD decreased after teriparatide discontinuation in both groups, except in those taking bisphosphonates for ≤2 years during the trial.

51. *(1C+)* **Lindsay R** et al. Sustained vertebral fracture risk reduction after withdrawal of teriparatide in postmenopausal women with osteoporosis. Arch Intern Med 2004;164:2024–2030.

This is an observational study of 1,262 FPT subjects who were followed up for 18 months after teriparatide discontinuation. The treatment groups continued to have a significantly decreased risk of vertebral fractures (41% for 20 μg; $p = 0.004$; and 45% for 40 μg; $p = 0.001$). The absolute vertebral fracture risk reduction was about 13% for both treatment groups. In addition, although LS BMD was still significantly greater in the treatment groups at the end of the follow-up study, those who used bisphosphonates for ≤1 year continued to gain BMD, whereas those not taking bisphosphonates lost BMD.

52. *(1B)* **Black D** et al. The effects of parathyroid hormone and alendronate alone or in combination in postmenopausal osteoporosis. N Engl J Med 2003;349:1207–1215.

This is a randomized, double-blind trial that placed 238 postmenopausal women (T score less than −2.5 or less than −2 with another osteoporosis risk factor) taking PTH (1-84), 100 μg daily, alendronate, 10 mg daily, or both for 1 year. BMD increases at the spine were not significantly different between the groups (6.3%, 6.1%, and 4.6%, respectively). At the hip, the combination therapy group gained significantly more than the PTH group (1.9% vs. 0.3%; $p = 0.02$).

53. *(1B)* **Body J** et al. A randomized double-blind trial to compare the efficacy of teriparatide [recombinant human parathyroid hormone (1-34)] with alendronate in postmenopausal women with osteoporosis. J Clin Endocrinol Metab 2002;87:4528–4545.

In this randomized trial, 146 postmenopausal women with osteoporosis were studied for a median of 14 months. They received either 40 μg of teriparatide and a placebo tablet or 10 mg of alendronate and a placebo injection. A significantly greater increase in LS BMD increase was seen in the teriparatide group by the third month ($p < 0.001$). At the study's end, significantly greater increases in LS, femoral neck, and total-body BMD were noted in the teriparatide group. However, a significant decrease in one-third distal radius BMD occurred in the teriparatide group ($p \geq 0.05$). The teriparatide group also experienced a significant decrease in nonvertebral fracture incidence (4.1% vs. 13.7%; $p < 0.05$).

54. *(1B)* **Ettinger B** et al. Differential effects of teriparatide on BMD after treatment with raloxifene or alendronate. J Bone Miner Res 2004;19:745–751.

This is an 18-month observational study of 59 postmenopausal women, with a T score of at least −2, taking 20 μg of teriparatide after 1.5–3 years of either alendronate or raloxifene. Those in the alendronate group started with lower bone-turnover markers. The markers in the raloxifene group tended to be higher, but the difference was not statistically significant except for BSAP, osteocalcin, and PINP at 1 month. At 3 and 6 months, those in the prior raloxifene group had significant LS BMD increases (2.1% at 3 months and 5.2% at 6 months), whereas the prior alendronate group did not. After the first 6 months, the rates of increase in both groups were similar. At 18 months, the raloxifene group had gained 10.2% in LS BMD, compared with 4.1% in the alendronate group ($p < 0.001$). At the hip during the first 6 months, BMD in the raloxifene group changed little, whereas that in the alendronate group decreased by 1.8%. After 6 months, both groups had an 1.5% increase in hip BMD.

55. *(1A)* **Bilezikian JP, Kurland ES.** Therapy of male osteoporosis with parathyroid hormone. Calcif Tissue Int 2001;69:248–251.

This was the first controlled, randomized, double-blind study of PTH in men with idiopathic osteoporosis. Twenty-three men, aged 30 to 64 years with Z scores less than −2.0, were assigned to placebo or treatment. After 18 months, significant increases in LS BMD (13.5% ± 3%) and femoral neck BMD (2.9% ± 1.5%) were noted. The distal radius site did not change. No further increase in BMD was found in the LS, but the femoral neck continued to show gains during the 12-month extension. Markers of bone formation and resorption increased in the PTH arm, reaching a peak between 9 and 12 months of therapy and declining thereafter.

56. *(1A)* **Finkelstein J** et al. The effects of parathyroid hormone, alendronate, or both in men with osteoporosis. N Engl J Med 2003;349:1216–1226.

This is a randomized trial of 83 men, with an LS or femoral neck T score of at least −2, that compared daily teriparatide, 40 μg, alendronate, 10 mg, and their combination over a period of 2.5 years (teriparatide was started at month 6). Significant increases in BMD at the LS (PA view, 7.9% vs. 18.1% vs. 14.8%, respectively; $p < 0.001$) and the femoral neck [3.2% vs. 9.7% ($p < 0.001$)] versus 6.2% ($p = 0.01$) in the teriparatide group were seen over those on either alendronate or the combination. The differences between the alendronate and the combination groups were not significantly different, except at the spine. Significant increases in alkaline phosphatase were noted in the teriparatide group ($p < 0.001$).

57. *(1C+)* **Kaufman J** et al. Teriparatide effects on vertebral fractures and bone mineral density in men with osteoporosis: Treatment and discontinuation of therapy. Osteoporos Int 2005;16:510–516.

This observational study of BMD and fractures over a 30-month period, in 355 men who were exposed to 1 year of teriparatide, showed LS and hip BMD remained significantly higher in the teriparatide group than placebo ($p \geq 0.001$), even though BMDs overall decreased. Those taking bisphosphonates had an increase in spine and hip BMD, although the significant intergroup difference was lost. In those not taking bisphosphonates, the BMD decreased. A significant decrease in moderate to severe spine fractures was seen (83%; $p = 0.01$) at 18 months.

58. *(1C+)* **Shea B** et al. Meta-analysis of calcium supplementation for the prevention of post-menopausal osteoporosis. Endocr Rev 2002;23:552–559.

This is a meta-analysis of 15 trials comparing calcium with placebo. The pooled difference in percentage change from baseline was 2.05% for the total body BMD, 1.66% for the LS, 1.64% for the hip in patients who received calcium. Vertebral fracture RR was 23%, and nonvertebral fracture reduction was 14%.

59. *(1C+)* **Papadimitropoulos E** et al. Meta-analysis of the efficacy of vitamin D treatment in preventing osteoporosis in postmenopausal women. Endcr Rev 2002;23:560–569.

This was a meta-analysis of 25 randomized trials of vitamin D with or without calcium versus control. The incidence of vertebral fractures was reduced (RR, 0.63; CI, 0.45–0.88; $p < 0.01$) and nonvertebral fracture incidence showed a trend toward reduction (RR, 0.77; CI, 0.57–1.04; $p = 0.09$). Hydroxylated vitamin D had a more profound effect on BMD than standard vitamin D. Total body BMD was increased by 2.06% in patients who received hydroxylated vitamin D compared with 0.4% in those who received standard vitamin D.

60. *(2A)* **Cameron ID** et al. Hip protectors in aged-care facilities: A randomized trial of use by individual higher-risk residents. Age Ageing 2001;30:477–481.

This was a randomized controlled trial of 174 women who lived in nursing homes or aged-care facilities and who had two or more falls or at least one fall that required hospital admission in the previous 3 months. During follow-up, a mean of 4.6 falls per person occurred. No difference in mortality was found. Eight hip fractures occurred in the intervention group, and seven, in the control group (HR, 1.46; CI, 0.53–4.51). No hip fractures occurred when hip protectors were being worn as directed. Adherence was ~57% over the duration of the study, and hip protectors were worn at the time of 54% of falls in the intervention group.

61. *(2A)* **Reid IR** et al. Intravenous zoledronic acid in postmenopausal women with low bone mineral density. N Engl J Med 2002;346:653–661.

In this 1-year, randomized, double-blind, placebo-controlled trial, 351 postmenopausal women with low BMD were randomized to placebo or IV zoledronic acid 0.25, 0.5, or 1.0 mg at 3-month intervals. In addition, one group received a 4-mg single dose intravenously, and another received two doses of 2 mg each, 6 months apart. Similar increases in LS BMD, 4.3–5.1%, were seen in all zoledronic acid groups compared with placebo ($p < 0.001$). In addition, mean percentage change in femoral neck BMD was 3.1%–3.5% higher ($p < 0.001$). Markers of bone resorption were significantly suppressed in all zoledronic acid groups. Side effects included myalgia and fever.

62. **Fogelman I, Blake G**. Strontium ranelate for the treatment of osteoporosis. BMJ 2005;330:1400–1401.

This reviewed strontium ranelate and the studies that assessed its efficacy in osteoporosis.

63. *(1B)* **Meunier P** et al. The effects of strontium ranelate on the risk of vertebral fracture in women with postmenopausal osteoporosis. N Engl J Med 2004;350:459–468.

This is a 3-year randomized, placebo-controlled trial that assessed 1,649 postmenopausal osteoporotic women with at least one vertebral fracture. They received either 2 g oral strontium ranelate or placebo daily. A decrease in the risk of vertebral fractures of 49% after the first year and 41% after 3 years was seen. The most common gastrointestinal side effect was diarrhea (6.1% with strontium vs. 3.6% with placebo; $p = 0.02$), but this abated after 3 months. No abnormal bone mineralization was seen.

64. *(1B)* **Reginster J** et al. Strontium ranelate reduces the risk of nonvertebral fractures in post-menopausal women with osteoporosis: Treatment of peripheral osteoporosis (TROPOS) study. J Clin Endocrinol Metab 2005;90:2816–2822.

In this randomized, double-blind, placebo-controlled trial, 5,091 postmenopausal osteoporotic women received strontium ranelate, 2 g per day, or placebo for 5 years (main statistical analysis after 3 years). Nonvertebral fragility fractures significantly decreased by 19% ($p = 0.031$), in the strontium group at 3 years. Those who were 74 years or older and had a femoral neck T score of at least -3 experienced a 36% RR reduction for hip fracture ($p = 0.046$). A significant RR reduction for vertebral fractures of 39% ($p < 0.001$) was seen in the strontium group at 3 years.

64a. *(2A)* **McClung MR, Lewiecki EM, Cohen SB**, et al., AMG 162 Bone Loss Study Group. Deno-sumab in postmenopausal women with low bone mineral density. N Engl J Med 2006;354(8): 821–831.

 412 postmenopausal women were enrolled in a one year study where the effects of denosumab, adminis-tered q 3 months and q 6 months at varying doses and the lumbar spine BMD compared to alendronate and a placebo group. There was an observed increase of 3.0 to 6.7 percent (as compared with an increase of 4.6 percent with alendronate and a loss of 0.8 percent with placebo) in lumbar spine BMD, total hip of 1.9 to 3.6 percent (as compared with an increase of 2.1 percent with alendronate and a loss of 0.6 percent with placebo), and at the distal third of the radius of 0.4 to 1.3 percent (as compared with decreases of 0.5 percent with alendronate and 2.0 percent with placebo). Serum CTX declined to near maximal levels at 3 days after the administration.

65. *(1C+)* **Cummings SR** et al. Monitoring osteoporosis therapy with bone densitometry: Mislead-ing changes and regression to the mean: Fracture Intervention Trial Research Group. JAMA 2000;283:1318–1321.

 This article evaluated BMD data from the FIT and the MORE trials. Women with the greatest loss of BMD during the first year of treatment were the most likely to gain BMD during continued treatment. Among women receiving alendronate whose hip BMD decreased by >4% during the first year, 83% (CI, 82%–84%) had increases in hip BMD during the second year, with an overall mean increase of 4.7%. In contrast, those who seemed to gain ≤8% during the first year lost an average of 1% (CI, 0.1%–1.9%) dur-ing the next year. Similar results were observed with raloxifene.

66. *(1C+)* **Chapurlat RD** et al. Risk of fracture among women who lose bone density during treat-ment with alendronate: The Fracture Intervention Trial. Osteoporos Int 2005;16:842–848.

 This observational study analyzed the 5,220 subjects in the Fracture Prevention Trial who took ≤70% of their study medication, focusing on end-of-study fracture reduction and BMD changes after 1 and 2 years of therapy. The investigators found that those who lost ≥4% of spine BMD after 1 year had a ver-tebral fracture risk reduction of 60%. In addition, the subjects who lost ≥4% of hip BMD after 1 year ex-perienced a 53% vertebral fracture risk reduction. However, the fracture benefit was not observed if spine and hip BMD were lost.

67. *(1C+)* **Siminoski K** et al. Accuracy of height loss during prospective monitoring for detection of incident vertebral fractures. Osteoporos Int 2005;16:403–410.

 This was an observational study of 985 osteoporotic postmenopausal women who were in the placebo group of the Vertebral Efficacy with Risedronate Therapy studies. Their heights were measured every 3 years, and spine films were taken. Height loss of >2 cm in 3 years had the sensitivity for new vertebral fractures of only 36%, but a specificity of almost 94%, with a PPV for this degree of height loss of 35%, and a NPV of 92%.

Paget Disease

68. *(1C+)* **Siris ES** et al. Risedronate in the treatment of Paget's disease of bone: An open label, mul-ticenter study. J Bone Miner Res 1998;13:1032–1038.

 In this open-label study of 162 patients, risedronate was administered cyclically (30 mg daily for 84 days, and then no treatment for 112 days), followed by a repeat of the cycle if alkaline phosphatase did not normalize or if it increased from its nadir by ≤25%. Alkaline phosphatase normalized in 54% of pa-tients after treatment (7–14 months). The mean percentage decreases in this marker after the cycles 1 and 2 were 66% and 70%, respectively.

69. *(1A)* **Miller PD** et al. A randomized, double-blind comparison of risedronate and etidronate in the treatment of Paget's disease of bone: Paget's Risedronate/Etidronate Study Group. Am J Med 1999;106:513–520.

 In a prospective, randomized, double-blind study, 123 patients were administered risedronate, 30 mg/day, or etidronate, 400 mg/day, for 6 months. After 12 months, serum alkaline phosphatase normal-ized in 73% of the patients in the risedronate group, compared with only 15% in the etidronate group ($p < 0.001$). Median time to normalize was shorter with risedronate (91 vs. >360 days; $p < 0.001$) and relapse rates at 18 months were lower (3% vs. 15%; $p < 0.05$) than placebo. Pain-reduction scores were significantly lower with risedronate.

70. *(1A)* **Reid IR** et al. Biochemical and radiologic improvement in Paget's disease of bone treated with alendronate: A randomized, placebo-controlled trial. Am J Med 1996;101:341–348.

 This is a double-blind, randomized trial comparing oral alendronate, 40 mg/day, and placebo over a 6-month period in 55 patients with Paget disease. NTX declined by 86%, and serum alkaline phosphatase, by 73% in patients taking alendronate but remained stable in those taking placebo ($p < 0.001$ between groups for both indices). Alkaline phosphatase normalized in 48% of alendronate-treated patients. About 48% of these patients showed radiologic improvement in osteolysis, whereas 4% improved on placebo ($p = 0.02$). No evidence of osteomalacia was seen in 12 patients after biopsies.

71. *(1A)* **Siris E** et al. Comparative study of alendronate versus etidronate for the treatment of Paget's disease of bone. J Clin Endocrinol Metab 1996;81:961–967.

 Eighty patients were randomly assigned to receive alendronate, 40 mg/day, or etidronate, 400 mg/day, for 6 months. Compared with etidronate, alendronate resulted in higher rates of normalization of alkaline phosphatase (61% vs. 17%, respectively) and greater reduction in alkaline phosphatase (79% vs. 44%, respectively). No osteomalacia was seen on bone biopsies in the alendronate groups.

72. *(1C+)* **Tucci JR, Bontha S**. Intravenously administered pamidronate in the treatment of Paget's disease of bone. Endocr Pract 2001;7:423–429.

This was a prospective nonrandomized study and review of literature in which 80 patients (52 women and 28 men; age range, 53–93 years; mean age, 76 years) were treated with a total of 180 mg of intravenous pamidronate over a 6- or 3-week period. The mean serum alkaline phosphatase level was 1,051 U/L before therapy and 386 U/L after treatment, a decrease of 63% ($p < 0.0001$). In 50 patients, the serum alkaline phosphatase level declined to normal range. Normalization was noted in 43 of 50 patients (86%) whose baseline alkaline phosphatase was <3 times the upper limit of normal, in five of 13 patients (38%) whose baseline alkaline phosphatase was 3 to 6 times the upper limit of normal, and in only two of 17 patients (12%) whose baseline alkaline phosphatase exceeded 6 times the upper limit of normal. Adverse events included hypocalcemia and flulike symptoms.

73. *(1B)* **Reid I et al**. Comparison of a single infusion of zoledronic acid with risedronate for Paget's disease. N Engl J Med 2005;353:898–908.

In two randomized, double-blind, active controlled trials, subjects with Paget disease were given either one dose of 5 mg of zoledronic acid intravenously over a 15-minute period or 60 mg of risedronate for 6 months. After 6 months, more subjects taking zoledronic acid experienced a disease response (96% vs. 74%; $p < 0.001$), alkaline phosphatase normalized more often in the zoledronic acid group (;88.6% vs. 57.9%; $p < 0.001$), the quality of life in those who received zoledronic acid was higher, and fewer patients in the zoledronic acid group had a relapse after ;6 months off therapy (one of 113 in the zoledronic acid group versus 21 of 82 in the risedronate group; $p < 0.001$).

Primary Hyperparathyroidism

74. **Bilezikian JP et al**. Summary statement from a workshop on asymptomatic primary hyperparathyroidism: A perspective for the 21st century. J Bone Miner Res 2002;17:M12–M17.

Summarizes recent advances and future directions for primary hyperparathyroidism.

75. *(1C)* **Silverberg SJ et al**. A 10-year prospective study of primary hyperparathyroidism with or without parathyroid surgery. N Engl J Med 1999;341:1249–1255.

This reported ten-year follow-up experience with 121 hyperparathyroid patients, 61 of whom underwent parathyroidectomy and 60 of whom did not. Parathyroidectomy led to normal serum calcium concentrations and a mean increase in LS BMD of 8% after 1 year ($p = 0.005$) and 12% after 10 years ($p = 0.03$). Femoral neck BMD increased by 6% after 1 year ($p = 0.002$) and 14% after 10 years ($p = 0.002$). No changes were observed in serum calcium concentration, urinary calcium excretion, or BMD in 52 patients who did not undergo surgery. Fourteen of these 52 patients had disease progression, which required parathyroidectomy.

76. *(1C)* **Scholz DA, Purnell DC**. Asymptomatic primary hyperparathyroidism: 10-year prospective study. Mayo Clin Proc 1981;56:473–478.

Ten-year prospective study of patients with asymptomatic primary hyperparathyroidism followed up at Mayo Clinic. The study was unable to come up with criteria that would predict need for surgery.

77. *(1C)* **Rao DS et al**. Lack of biochemical progression or continuation of accelerated bone loss in mild asymptomatic primary hyperparathyroidism: Evidence for biphasic disease course. J Clin Endocrinol Metab 1988;67:1294–1299.

One hundred seventy-seven patients with mild asymptomatic primary hyperparathyroidism were followed up for >10 years for disease progression. No changes in biochemical progression or bone loss based on forearm BMD were noted.

78. *(1C)* **Silverberg SJ et al**. A 10-year prospective study of primary hyperparathyroidism with or without parathyroid surgery. N Engl J Med 1999;341:1249–1255.

One hundred twenty-one patients with primary hyperparathyroidism were followed up for 10 years. Fifty-two patients did not undergo surgery; worsening hypercalcemia, hypercalciuria, or bone loss was noted in these patients. In 14 of 52, however, indications developed for surgery, and they had to undergo parathyroidectomy.

79. *(2A)* **Rossini M et al**. Effects of oral alendronate in elderly patients with osteoporosis and mild primary hyperparathyroidism. J Bone Miner Res 2001;16:113–119.

In a pilot-controlled study, 26 patients aged 67 to 81 years were randomly assigned to oral 10 mg alendronate on alternate-day treatment or no treatment for 2 years. Urine deoxypyridinoline excretion significantly decreased after 1 month of alendronate, and alkaline phosphatase and osteocalcin, after 3 months. After 2 years, the alendronate group had significant increases in BMD at LS, total hip, and total body (+8.6% ± 3.0%, +4.8% ± 3.9%, and +1.2% ± 1.4%) in comparison with patients at baseline and controls. Serum calcium, serum phosphate, and urinary calcium excretion significantly decreased during the first 3 to 6 months but increased to baseline afterward. Serum PTH level increased significantly during the first year of treatment.

80. *(1B)* **Khan A et al**. Alendronate in primary hyperparathyroidism: A double-blind, randomized, placebo-controlled trial. J Clin Endocrinol Metab 2004;89:3319–3325.

This was a randomized, placebo-controlled trial of 44 patients with primary hyperparathyroidism, taking 10 mg alendronate or placebo daily for 1 year, and then all taking alendronate, 10 mg, for the second year. The alendronate group experienced significant increases in BMD at the LS compared with placebo throughout the 2 years of the trial (6.85%; $p < 0.001$). BMD also significantly increased by 4.01% at the hip in the alendronate group ($p < 0.001$) at 12 months. BMD gains were seen at the femoral neck after 2 years (3.67%; $p = 0.038$). No significant change was noted in the treatment group at the one-third radius. Bone-turnover markers NTX and BSAP declined by 66% at 3 months and 49% at 6 months, respectively. The calcium, PTH, and urine calcium concentrations remained stable.

81. *(1B)* **Peacock M** et al. Cinacalcet hydrochloride maintains long-term normocalcemia in patients with primary hyperparathyroidism. J Clin Endocrinol Metab 2005;90:135–141.

   This multicenter, randomized, double-blind, placebo-controlled study studied 78 women with primary hyperparathyroidism taking either 30 mg cinacalcet or placebo twice a day, followed up for ;1 year. The patients had a serum calcium level of 10.3 to 12.5 mg/dl on enrollment, with a PTH of >45 pg/ml. More women taking cinacalcet experienced normalization of calcium levels with a decrease in calcium concentration of ≤0.5 mg/dl (73% vs. 5%; $p < 0.001$). The mean calcium levels in the treatment group decreased to normal within 2 weeks of therapy initiation. PTH also significantly decreased by 7.6%; $p < 0.01$. However, no BMD difference was noted.

Parathyroid Carcinoma

82. **Shane E**. Parathyroid carcinoma. J Clin Endocrinol Metab 2001;86:485–493.

   A thorough review of the aspects of parathyroid carcinoma.

83. **Beus K, Stack B**. Parathyroid carcinoma. Otolaryngol Clin North Am 2004;37:845–854.

   A good review of parathyroid carcinoma, which includes its epidemiology, pathogenesis, diagnosis, and treatment.

84. **Balfour J, Scott L**. Cinacalcet hydrochloride. Drugs 2005;65:271–281.

   An excellent review of the pharmacodynamics, pharmacokinetics, tolerability, dosage, and efficacy of cinacalcet. It includes descriptions of trials that have evaluated this medication.

Hypercalcemia

85. *(1A)* **Major P** et al. Zoledronic acid is superior to pamidronate in the treatment of hypercalcemia of malignancy: A pooled analysis of two randomized, controlled clinical trials. J Clin Oncol 2001;19:558–567.

   Two identical concurrent, parallel, multicenter, randomized, double-blind, and double-dummy trials compared the efficacy and safety of zoledronic acid and pamidronate for treating hypercalcemia of malignancy. The 275 study patients had moderate to severe hypercalcemia, with a corrected serum calcium of ≤3.0 mmol/L (12.0 mg/dl). They were treated with a 5-min infusion of zoledronic acid (4 or 8 mg) or a 2-h infusion of pamidronate (90 mg). The response rates by day 10 for zoledronic acid, 4 and 8 mg, and pamidronate, 90 mg, were 88.4% ($p = 0.002$), 86.7% ($p = 0.015$), and 69.7%, respectively. Serum calcium normalized by day 4 in ;50% of the patients treated with zoledronic acid and 33.3% of the pamidronate-treated patients. The median duration of normocalcemia was higher for zoledronic acid, 4 and 8 mg, than for pamidronate, 90 mg, with response durations of 32, 43, and 18 days, respectively.

86. *(1A)* **Purohit OP** et al. A randomised double-blind comparison of intravenous pamidronate and clodronate in the hypercalcaemia of malignancy. Br J Cancer 1995;72:1289–1293.

   This was a prospective, randomized, double-blind study in which 41 patients with hypercalcemia of malignancy received either pamidronate, 90 mg, intravenously or clodronate, 1,500 mg, intravenously. After a median time of 4 days, 100% of patients taking pamidronate achieved normocalcemia compared with 80% who received clodronate. Normocalcemia persisted for a median for 28 days after pamidronate and 14 days after clodronate ($p < 0.01$).

87. *(1A)* **Wimalawansa SJ**. Optimal frequency of administration of pamidronate in patients with hypercalcaemia of malignancy. Clin Endocrinol (Oxf) 1994;41:591–595.

   In this prospective randomized study, 34 patients with hypercalcemia of malignancy received IV pamidronate every 14th or 21st day for 16 weeks. Normocalcemia was achieved at 48 h and maintained for an average of 15 days. When the drug was administered every 3 weeks, recurrent hypercalcemia was seen in 50% of patients during the third week. The incidence of symptomatic hypercalcemia was significantly decreased (10%, eight separate episodes; $p < 0.01$) and survival was improved ($p < 0.05$) in patients who received pamidronate every second week.

88. *(1A)* **Ostenstad B, Andersen OK**. Disodium pamidronate versus mithramycin in the management of tumour-associated hypercalcemia. Acta Oncol 1992;31:861–864.

   In this prospective randomized study, 28 consecutive hypercalcemic patients with cancer were randomly assigned to receive pamidronate (30, 60, or 90 mg, depending on the serum calcium) or rehydration, mithramycin (repeatedly), and supportive care. Pamidronate normalized serum calcium in all patients, and 12 of 14 were still normocalcemic on day 12. In contrast, mithramycin was effective in only three of 11 patients, and in those patients, hypercalcemia recurred rapidly.

89. *(2A)* **Shoback DM** et al. An evaluation of the calcimimetic AMG 073 in patients with hypercalcemia and primary hyperparathyroidism: Abstract presented at ASBMR Annual Meeting, 2001, Phoenix, AZ.

    This was a prospective, double-blind, randomized, placebo-controlled study in which nine patients received either 65 mg AMG 073 or placebo, twice daily for 4 weeks. Four of the five subjects taking AMG 073 experienced normalization of serum calcium levels ($\geq$10.3 mg) on day 28, compared with only one of four patients who received placebo. Serum calcium levels returned to predosage levels 1 week after discontinuation of AMG 073. Mean PTH level at 12 h decreased by 14.5% in the calcimimetic group compared with 10.6% in the placebo group.

90. *(1A)* **Goodman WG** et al. The calcimimetic agent AMG 073 lowers plasma parathyroid hormone levels in hemodialysis patients with secondary hyperparathyroidism. J Am Soc Nephrol 2002;13: 1017–1024.

    In this randomized placebo-controlled study, 52 hemodialysis patients with secondary hyperparathyroidism were given AMG 073 as single oral doses ranging from 5 to 100 mg, or placebo. Plasma PTH levels decreased 2 h after 25-, 50-, 75-, or 100-mg doses, decreasing by a maximum of 43% $\pm$ 29%, 40% $\pm$ 36%, 54% $\pm$ 28%, or 55% $\pm$ 39%, respectively. Plasma PTH levels decreased in all patients given doses of $\leq$25 mg but did not change in those who received placebo. Plasma PTH levels declined for the first 3 to 4 days and remained below baseline values after 8 days of treatment in patients who received 25- or 50-mg AMG 073. Serum calcium concentrations also decreased by 5% to 10% from pretreatment levels on 50 mg of AMG 073 for 8 days, but values were unchanged in those who received lower doses.

91. *(2C)* **Collins MT** et al. Treatment of hypercalcemia secondary to parathyroid carcinoma with a novel calcimimetic agent. J Clin Endocrinol Metab 1998;83:1083–1088.

    This case report describes prolonged successful treatment of a 78-year-old man with parathyroid carcinoma by using a calcimimetic agent.

92. *(2C)* **Falzon M, Zong J.** The noncalcemic vitamin D analogs EB1089 and 22-oxacalcitriol suppress serum-induced parathyroid hormone-related peptide gene expression in a lung cancer cell line. Endocrinology 1998;139:1046–1053.

    This study aimed to determine whether $1,25(OH)_2D_3$ and two nonhypercalcemic analogues, EB1089 and 22-oxa-$1,25(OH)_2D_3$ (22-oxacalcitriol; OCT), suppress serum and epidermal growth factor–induced PTHrP gene expression in a human lung squamous cancer cell line, NCI H520. EB1089 and OCT suppressed the basal and the growth factor–stimulated levels of PTHrP in a cancer cell line associated with hypercalcemia.

93. *(2C)* **Inoue D** et al. 22-Oxacalcitriol, a noncalcemic analogue of calcitriol, suppresses both cell proliferation and parathyroid hormone-related peptide gene expression in human T cell lymphotrophic virus, type I-infected T cells. J Biol Chem 1993;268:16730–16736.

    This study was undertaken to determine whether $1,25(OH)_2D_3$ and its noncalcemic analogue, OCT, could suppress cell proliferation and PTHrP gene expression in an HTLV-infected T-cell line, MT-2. OCT as well as $1,25(OH)_2D_3$ inhibited the proliferation of MT-2 cells in a time- and dose-dependent manner. OCT reduced PTHrP concentration by 50%.

Hypocalcemia

94. *(1C)* **Pearce SH** et al. A familial syndrome of hypocalcemia with hypercalciuria due to mutations in the calcium-sensing receptor. N Engl J Med 1996;335:1115–1122.

    Six kindreds with hypoparathyroidism and hypercalciuria that worsened with vitamin D supplementation were found to have mutations in the calcium-sensing receptor gene. Five heterozygous missense mutations were detected (Asn118Lys, Phe128Leu, Thr151Met, Glu191Lys, and Phe612Ser).

95. *(1C+)* **Heaney RP** et al. Calcium absorptive effects of vitamin D and its major metabolites. J Clin Endocrinol Metab 1997;82:4111–4116.

    Healthy adult males were given graded doses of vitamin D_3, 25(OH)D, and $1,25(OH)_2D$ for 8, 4, and 2 weeks, respectively. All three vitamin D compounds significantly elevated ^{45}Ca absorption from a 300-mg calcium load. In addition, $1,25(OH)_2D$ was active even at the lowest dose (0.5 mg/day); 25(OH)D was also active in elevating absorption and did so without increasing total $1,25(OH)_2D$ levels. Per the dose–response curves for $1,25(OH)_2D$ and 25(OH)D, the potency of these two is ;100:1. The absorptive effect of vitamin D_3 was seen only at the highest dose level (1,250 mg, or 50,000 IU/day) and was apparently mediated by conversion to 25(OH)D.

96. *(1B)* **Winer K** et al. Long-term treatment of hypoparathyroidism: A randomized controlled study comparing parathyroid hormone-(1-34) versus calcitriol and calcium. J Clin Endocrinol Metab 2003;88:4214–4220.

    In this 3-year randomized, open-label trial, 27 patients with hypoparathyroidism were given either PTH twice a day or calcitriol and calcium. The patients taking PTH required ;37 μg, and those taking calcitriol, ~0.91 μg to attain normal calcium concentrations. Those in each therapy group did not have different calcium, phosphorus, and magnesium levels. PTH normalized urine calcium levels, whereas calcitriol did not. No significant changes were seen in BMD in the groups. The bone-turnover markers alkaline phosphatase, osteocalcin, urinary deoxypyridinoline, and pyridinoline excretion increased more in the PTH group ($p < 0.001$).

Osteomalacia

97. *(1C+)* **Thomas MK** et al. Hypovitaminosis D in medical inpatients. N Engl J Med 1998;338:777–783.

    Of 290 consecutive patients admitted to a general medicine ward, 57% had 25(OH)D levels ≥15 ng/ml, and of these patients, 28% had levels <8 ng/ml. This included 43% of the patients who consumed more than the recommended dietary allowance of vitamin D.

98. *(1C)* **Holick M** et al. Prevalence of vitamin D inadequacy among postmenopausal North American women receiving osteoporosis therapy. J Clin Endocrinol Metab 2005;90:3215–3224.

    In this study, 1,536 nonhospitalized postmenopausal osteoporotic women were observed for vitamin D insufficiency risks. 25(OH)D concentrations <30 ng/ml were found in 52%, and <20 ng/ml in 18%. Decreased 25(OH)D levels were more frequent in women taking <400 U of vitamin D daily [25(OH)D <30 ng/ml in 63% taking <400 U per day and in 45% taking ≤400 U). 25(OH)D and PTH exhibited a negative association.

99. *(1C)* **Chapuy M** et al. Prevalence of vitamin D insufficiency in an adult normal population. Osteoporos Int 1997;7:439–443.

    This was an observational study of 1,569 French adults between November and April. 14% had 25(OH)D concentrations ≥12 ng/ml, and 75% had levels <31 ng/ml. Vitamin D concentrations varied with location. A negative association between PTH and 25(OH)D was found, and 25(OH)D levels ≥31 ng/ml were associated with the initiation of an increase in PTH.

100. **Heaney R**. Functional indices of vitamin D status and ramifications of vitamin D deficiency. Am J Clin Nutr 2004;80:1706S–1709S.

    Review of vitamin D, its role in disease, its measurement, and suboptimal levels.

101. **Rao D, Alqurashi S**. Management of vitamin D depletion in postmenopausal women. Curr Osteoporos Rep 2003;1:110–115.

    This is a review of decreased vitamin D. It explains assessment of this depletion, its prevalence, its effects, and treatment.

102. *(1C)* **Grey A** et al. Vitamin D repletion in patients with primary hyperparathyroidism and coexistent vitamin D insufficiency. J Clin Endocrinol Metab 2005;90:2122–2126.

    Twenty-one patients with primary hyperparathyroidism and hypercalcemia of <12 mg/dl with vitamin D insufficiency (<20 ng/ml) were given cholecalciferol, 50,000 IU weekly, for 1 month and then monthly for 1 year. With 25(OH)D replacement to levels >20 ng/ml, mean calcium and phosphate levels did not change. Calcium did not increase to >12 mg/dl during the study. PTH levels significantly decreased as early as 6 months (24%; *p* < 0.01, at 6 months; 26%, *p* < 0.01 at 12 months). Of note, two patients did develop hypercalciuria.

103. *(1C)* **Fujita T** et al. Adult-onset vitamin D–resistant osteomalacia with the unresponsiveness to parathyroid hormone. J Clin Endocrinol Metab 1980;50:927–931.

    A case report of a 50-year-old man with vitamin D–resistant osteomalacia.

104. *(1C)* **Itoi E** et al. Adult-onset vitamin D–resistant osteomalacia: A case with seventeen-year follow-up. J Bone Joint Surg Am 1991;73:932–937.

    Case report of prolonged follow-up of a patient with adult-onset vitamin D–resistant osteomalacia.

105. *(1C)* **Nelson A** et al. Fibroblast growth factor 23: A new clinical marker for oncogenic osteomalacia. J Clin Endocrinol Metab 2003;88:4088–4094.

    This is a case report of a patient with oncogenic osteomalacia and of the correlation found between this disease and FGF 23. The causative tumor stained for the FGF 23 mRNA and protein, and this patient's serum concentration of FGF 23 was elevated before resection of the mass, subsequently normalizing after its resection.

106. *(1C)* **Jonsson K** et al. Fibroblast growth factor 23 in oncogenic osteomalacia and x-linked hypophosphatemia. N Engl J Med 2003;348:1656–1663.

    This observational study demonstrated increased concentrations of FGF 23 in patients with oncogenic osteomalacia, which returned to normal after removal of the tumor.

107. *(1C)* **Leicht E** et al. Tumor-induced osteomalacia: Pre- and postoperative biochemical findings. Hormone Metab Res 1990;22:640–643.

    A case report of a patient who was successfully treated with surgical resection of the tumor, calcitriol, and phosphorus.

108. *(1C)* **Shane E** et al. Tumor-induced osteomalacia: Clinical and basic studies. J Bone Miner Res 1997;12:1502–1511.

    Case report.

109. *(1C)* **Tebben P** et al. Whole-body ^{99m}Tc-sestamibi scintigraphy to localize tumors causing oncogenic osteomalacia: An abstract presented at the AACE Annual Session, 2005, Washington, D.C.

    This is a case report of three patients with oncogenic osteomalacia, in which whole-body ^{99m}Tc-sestamibi scans localized the causative tumors.

110. *(2A)* **Carpenter TO** et al. 24,25-Dihydroxyvitamin D supplementation corrects hyperparathyroidism and improves skeletal abnormalities in X-linked hypophosphatemic rickets: A clinical research center study. J Clin Endocrinol Metab 1996;81:2381–2388.

This prospective, 1-year placebo-controlled trial compared 24,25(OH)$_2$D$_3$ supplementation with standard treatment in 15 patients with X-linked hypophosphatemia. In nine patients, 24,25(OH)$_2$D$_3$ normalized PTH values [peak PTH was 46.5 ± 6.6 pmol/L at entry, 42.3 ± 5.9 pmol/L after placebo, and 23.3 ± 5.4 pmol/L after 24,25(OH)$_2$D$_3$]. Nephrogenous cyclic adenosine monophosphate decreased at night, coincident with the decrease in PTH, and serum phosphorus level was slightly higher with 24,25(OH)$_2$D$_3$. Radiographic features of rickets improved during 24,25(OH)$_2$D$_3$ supplementation in children, and osteoid surface decreased in adults.

111. *(2A)* **Seikaly MG** et al. The effect of recombinant human growth hormone in children with X-linked hypophosphatemia. Pediatrics 1997;100:879–884.

A randomized, double-blind, crossover study was performed throughout a 24-month period in five children with X-linked hypophosphatemia. Results indicated that growth hormone therapy improved the height SD score (Z score) from a baseline of -2.66 ± 0.21 to -2.02 ± 0.25 and to -1.46 ± 0.28, after 3 and 12 months, respectively. The growth-velocity SD score was -1.90 ± 0.40 in the placebo group and $+4.04 \pm 1.50$ in the treated group. An increase in serum phosphate from 0.88 ± 0.07 mmol/L to 1.17 ± 0.14 mmol/L and tubular maximum for phosphate reabsorption (TmP/GFR) from 2.12 ± 0.15 to 3.41 ± 0.25 mg/dl was observed after 3 months of rhGH therapy. However, both serum phosphate and TmP/GFR were unchanged from baseline after 6, 9, and 12 months of therapy.

112. *(1C+)* **Verge CF** et al. Effects of therapy in X-linked hypophosphatemic rickets. N Engl J Med 1991;325:1843–1848.

Twenty-four patients with X-linked hypophosphatemic rickets (nine boys and 15 girls), aged 1 to 16 years (median, 5.3 years), were observed for 0.3 to 11.8 years (median, 3.0 years). Patients treated for ≤2 years before the onset of puberty (n = 19) had a mean height SD score of -1.08, compared with -2.05 in the untreated historic controls. The 13 patients who were treated with calcitriol and phosphate for ≤2 years had an increase in the mean height SD score of 0.33 (CI, 0–0.67; p = 0.05). Nineteen of 24 patients (79%) had nephrocalcinosis on renal ultrasonography. The grade of nephrocalcinosis was significantly correlated with the mean phosphate dose (r = 0.60; p = 0.002) but not with the dosage of vitamin D or the duration of therapy.

113. *(1C)* **Weinstein RS, Whyte MP.** Heterogeneity of adult hypophosphatasia: Report of severe and mild cases. Arch Intern Med 1981;141:727–731.

Two cases with varying clinical presentations were presented.

114. *(1C)* **Deal C, Whyte M.** Adult hypophosphatasia treated with teriparatide. J Bone Miner Res 2005;20:S1–S10.

A case report of the use of teriparatide in adult hypophosphatasia.

115. *(1C)* **Camacho P** et al. Treatment of adult hypophosphatasia with teriparatide. In preparation.

A case report of the use of teriparatide in adult hypophosphatasia.

Reproductive Disorders

Steven Petak and Rhoda H. Cobin

AMENORRHEA

Definition

Amenorrhea is the absence of menstruation in a woman during her reproductive years. Primary amenorrhea is the absence of menstrual periods in a girl without developed breasts by age 14 or the absence of menses in a girl with breast development by age 16. Secondary amenorrhea is the absence of menses in a woman who has previously had established menstrual function. The length of time defining secondary amenorrhea is widely variable; authorities place it between 3 and 12 months.

Etiology

Considerable overlap exists between primary and secondary amenorrhea. Ovarian failure and müllerian defects, including uterine and outlet disorders, account for about 60% of patients with primary amenorrhea. Premature ovarian failure and hyperandrogenic disorders account for about 72% of patients with secondary amenorrhea. Pregnancy should always be considered as a diagnosis. Constitutional delay of puberty is often responsible for what would otherwise appear to be primary amenorrhea.

Epidemiology

The incidence of primary amenorrhea varies from 0.48% to 1.2%. That of secondary amenorrhea is about 4.9%.

Pathophysiology

The approach to amenorrhea depends on whether it is primary or secondary. In the former, defects may be present at any level of the reproductive system (i.e., hypothalamus, pituitary, ovaries, uterus, or vaginal outflow tract). In women who have had prior menses, it is clear that not only must the woman have had an anatomically normal uterus and outflow tract, but that prior normal stimulation with estrogen has occurred, implying ovarian function.

Pregnancy should always be excluded in any patient first seen with amenorrhea, particularly secondary amenorrhea or primary amenorrhea with normal development. Thyroid abnormalities are commonly associated with menstrual disorders and should be sought with an initial thyroid-stimulating hormone (TSH) level.

A history and physical examination will help to define the problem and suggest appropriate laboratory investigation.

Primary Amenorrhea

Vaginal, Uterine, and Ovarian Disorders

Imperforate hymen will be seen with normal growth and development, normal secondary sexual characteristics, and, often, premenstrual molimina and lower abdominal cramping at the time of expected menses. The diagnosis is made by physical examination, and the treatment is surgical hymenectomy.

Müllerian agenesis (Mayer–Rokitansky syndrome) occurs with normal growth and development of secondary sexual characteristics. A rudimentary vaginal canal may be present but with absent uterus and fallopian tubes. Associated abnormalities (including scoliosis, unilateral renal agenesis, and rarely cardiac defects) may be found [1]. Although the disorder is usually sporadic, various genetic etiologies have been proposed [2,3]. The diagnosis is made with sonography. Levels of estrogen and gonadotropins are normal. Treatment may include vaginal reconstructive procedures.

Failure of normal ovarian development may be due to Turner syndrome, which may be clinically suspected by the observation of undeveloped secondary sexual characteristics, short stature, and somatic abnormalities including widely spaced nipples, low-set hairline, and other skeletal abnormalities. The diagnosis of an ovarian etiology is confirmed with the finding of an elevated follicle-stimulating hormone (FSH; due to lack of ovarian inhibin production), and the genetic basis of the syndrome is confirmed with an abnormal karyotype. XO is the most frequent genetic abnormality, but other X chromosome abnormalities and mosaicism may be present. Variants with Y chromosomal material may have mild virilization. The presence of Y chromosome increases the risk of gonadoblastomas, and thus gonadectomy should be considered (4).

Primary ovarian dysgenesis with XX karyotype is a rare condition that may be inherited as an autosomal recessive trait and does not have the associated somatic features of Turner syndrome; it may be associated with tall stature. Failure of development of secondary sexual characteristics, ovarian dysgenesis, and normal uterine and vaginal structures are noted. FSH is elevated [5,6].

Rarely autoimmune oophoritis will be seen as primary amenorrhea, although it is more likely to occur as secondary amenorrhea with evidence of ovarian failure (i.e., elevated FSH). Anti-ovarian antibodies are sometimes detectable, and a strong association exists with other autoimmune diseases.

Androgen insensitivity syndrome results from mutations in the androgen receptor of varying types and severity with corresponding variation in clinical presentation, including phenotypic females with normal breast tissue, modest axillary and pubic hair, and absent müllerian structures. The incidence is higher in females with inguinal hernias [7,8]. The diagnosis is made with sonography and the finding of a male-range testosterone. The karyotype is XY.

Pituitary/Hypothalamic Disease

Hypogonadotrophic hypogonadism [low luteinizing hormone (LH) and FSH] may be seen as primary amenorrhea with or without anosmia (Kallmann syndrome). Various mutations in the KAL gene, which cause abnormal migration of gonadotropin-releasing hormone (GnRH)-producing cells to the hypothalamus have been described [9]. Other less common syndromes first seen as primary hypogonadotrophic hypogonadism include Prader–Willi syndrome and Laurence–Moon–Biedel syndrome.

Pituitary and hypothalamic tumors, especially craniopharyngioma, as well as infiltrative diseases occasionally are initially seen as primary amenorrhea with low gonadotropins, although they are rare in children and generally appear as secondary amenorrhea (vide infra).

Secondary Amenorrhea

Vaginal / Uterine Disorders

In patients with previously normal menses, secondary amenorrhea with normal hormonal function and abnormal uterine function may develop. A history of pelvic infection, dilation and curettage, or uterine instrumentation in a patient with secondary amenorrhea should suggest Asherman syndrome. Cyclic estrogen–progestin therapy can be administered to determine whether a functional endometrium is present. If no bleeding occurs, hysteroscopy or hysterosalpingography should be considered to establish the diagnosis.

Ovarian Failure

Autoimmune oophoritis will occur as secondary amenorrhea with evidence of ovarian failure (i.e., elevated FSH). Anti-ovarian antibodies are sometimes detectable, and a strong association with other autoimmune diseases is present. Premature ovarian failure may be familial and may be found with no evidence of autoimmune disease.

Pituitary and Hypothalamic Disease

Women with normal or low gonadotropins, normal pelvic structures, and normal androgens may be suspected of having hypothalamic or pituitary disease. Although the latter is often functional, it is imperative to image the pituitary to rule out pituitary tumors or other lesions in this area, which may affect normal hypothalamic–pituitary function. Usually this is seen as secondary amenorrhea, although occasionally the onset is early enough in life to appear as primary amenorrhea.

A high prolactin level may indicate either prolactin production from a pituitary adenoma or stalk compression, causing reduced dopaminergic negative regulation of pituitary prolactin production. Because the level of prolactin is usually proportionate to the size of the tumor in pure prolactin-secreting tumors, tumors disproportionately large compared with the serum prolactin level should be suspected of being non-prolactinomas, which are not amenable to therapy with dopaminergic agents and may be considered for surgery.

Hypothalamic amenorrhea is a very common cause of secondary amenorrhea and an occasional cause of primary amenorrhea. Laboratory studies reveal normal to low gonadotropins and estrogen, and normal androgens and prolactin levels. Anatomic pathology is absent. A thorough and sensitive history must be obtained, because emotional stress, excessive exercising, weight loss, dieting, and eating disorders such as anorexia and bulimia may be difficult to elicit on initial history. Once rapport is established, the patient may be more comfortable in discussing these important etiologic factors and their management.

Hyperandrogenism

Excessive androgen production is associated with both primary and secondary amenorrhea and may be due to either ovarian or adrenal sources.

The most common cause of primary amenorrhea with excess androgen production is adrenal hyperplasia, most frequently 21-hydroxylase deficiency. The frequency of this disorder is variable, depending on ethnic origin. Presentation may be at birth with ambiguous genitalia, or it may be delayed until later in life, particularly in the non–salt-wasting variety. In childhood, accelerated growth and bone maturation and signs of hyperandrogenism (hirsutism, acne, increased musculature, alopecia) appear. If untreated, amenorrhea and short final adult stature are found (because of early closure of the epiphyses secondary to androgenic stimulation). The diagnosis is made with the finding of elevated 17-OH progesterone, either in the basal state or with adrenocorticotropic hormone (ACTH) stimulation. Genetic testing will confirm the presence of a variety of mutations of the CYP21 gene on chromosome 6 [10]. Treatment consists of glucocorticoid replacement to suppress excess ACTH and hence adrenal androgen production, with care to avoid excess glucocorticoid, which can cause growth retardation, osteopenia, and iatrogenic Cushing disease [11,12].

Other less common enzyme defects causing adrenal hyperplasia include 11-hydroxylase deficiency, which occurs with amenorrhea, hyperandrogenism, hypertension, and hypokalemia; 3β-hydroxysteroid dehydrogenase deficiency, which causes hyperandrogenism, and 17-hydroxylase deficiency, which occurs with sexual infantilism.

Polycystic ovarian syndrome (PCOS) affects between 6% and 10% of women of reproductive age and typically occurs with oligomenorrhea dating from the onset of puberty, along with variable hyperandrogenism. PCOS is strongly associated with insulin resistance and carries a high risk of glucose intolerance, frank diabetes, hypertension, dyslipidemia, and an increased frequency of myocardial infarction and cerebrovascular disease in later life, making a diagnosis is critical [13].

Signs or symptoms of hyperandrogenism may include acne, hirsutism, and alopecia. More severe hyperandrogenism (virilization) including increased muscle mass, clitoromegaly, deepening of the voice, and male-pattern baldness is indicative of higher testosterone levels (vide infra), usually not seen with PCOS.

Diagnosis

Androgen concentrations including total and free testosterone, androstenedione, and dehydroepiandrosterone sulfate (DHEA-S) should be measured. A testosterone level between 40 and 200 mg/ml is consistent with diagnosis of PCOS or other forms of hyperandrogenemia. A testosterone level more than 200 mg/ml suggests an ovarian tumor, adrenal tumor, or hyperthecosis; therefore appropriate imaging studies are needed. An elevated DHEA-S level may indicate adrenal hyperandrogenism or an adrenal tumor.

17α-Hydroxyprogesterone elevation either in the basal state or after ACTH stimulation will make a diagnosis of 21-hydroxylase adrenal hyperplasia, the most common variety of acquired adrenal hyperplasia.

Treatment

Therapy for amenorrhea should be directed at the underlying cause. If outflow obstruction or Asherman syndrome is present, surgical consultation with a gynecologist is needed. For ovarian failure secondary to gonadal dysgenesis with a Y chromosome or fragment, surgical removal of the gonads at the time of diagnosis has been recommended because of the high risk of gonad-related malignancy. In androgen-insensitivity syndrome, removal of the gonads may be deferred until immediately after pubertal maturation because the risk of malignancy appears to be low until after puberty [14]. Psychological counseling is also needed in patients with gonadal dysgenesis and androgen insensitivity syndromes.

Management of Turner syndrome is complex and focuses on recognizing and monitoring the associated anomalies [15]. About 30% of patients with Turner syndrome have congenital heart defects (e.g., bicuspid aortic valve and coarctation of the aorta), and 30% have renal anomalies [15]. The risk of death from aortic aneurysm is high [relative risk (RR) of 63.23, with a 95% CI of 20.48–147.31] and an initial evaluation with periodic echocardiography and follow-up by a cardiologist are needed [15,16]. Thyroid disease may occur in up to 30% of affected patients; therefore TSH levels should be measured every 1 to 2 years or if symptoms suggestive of thyroid disease develop [15]. Short stature can be improved significantly with the early use of growth hormone, and consideration for use should be given if and when the height is less than the 5th percentile [11,17]. Estrogen use will cause fusion of the epiphyses and may therefore limit final adult height, depending on the total length of growth hormone therapy before starting estrogen [18]. However, starting growth hormone early may allow the use of estrogen at age 12 or 13 without compromising height gain [19]. Early use of estrogen may have some benefit on motor and nonverbal function in girls with Turner syndrome [20], although this must be reconciled with the goal of increasing height. Bone-density studies should be done in adults and periodically thereafter [15]. Patients with Turner syndrome, particularly those demonstrating symptoms of mosaicism and other forms of ovarian failure, have a possibility of pregnancy. The potential for pregnancy does not improve with medical interventions [21]. Cyclic hormone replacement therapy [11] is justified by recent studies that suggest a beneficial effect of estrogen therapy on bone density and fracture risk in such patients [22–27].

Pituitary tumors may require surgical therapy, whereas the majority of prolactin-secreting tumors may be managed with dopamine agonist therapy.

Treatment of adrenal hyperplasia consists of replacement glucocorticoid to suppress ACTH and hence adrenal androgen production while avoiding excessive steroid levels, which may cause growth retardation. Occasionally adrenalectomy may be required. Ovarian and adrenal tumors are treated surgically. PCOS therapy is discussed in the section on hirsutism.

Hypothalamic dysfunction should be treated by addressing the underlying cause wherever possible. Weight gain in patients with anorexia may help normalize reproductive function and bone density [28,29]. Hormone replacement therapy is often initiated to optimize bone development in the setting of hypothalamic dysfunction, but results have been inconsistent [30]. Nutritional counseling as well as psychological counseling may be necessary and modification of exercise regimens may be helpful.

Table 5.1 is a summary of amenorrhea.

HIRSUTISM

Hirsutism is defined as male-pattern excessive growth of terminal hair in women. It may result from elevated androgen levels, produced by increased secretion from the ovary or the adrenal, from exogenous sources of androgen, or from increased conversion of androgen precursors to the more active male hormone dihydrotestosterone at the level of the hair follicle. Hirsutism may occur without actual elevation in androgen levels if increased target organ sensitivity to androgen action exists.

Hirsutism should not be confused with hypertrichosis, which is defined as the growth of hair on any part of the body, in excess of the amount usually present in persons of the same age, race, and sex. Hypertrichosis may be caused by many medications and poisons and repeated skin irritation or chronic inflammation. It may be associated with systemic nonendocrine disease.

Because hair distribution is both ethnic and familial, "excessive" hair growth should be diagnosed only in those contexts.

Etiology

Any disorder that produces excess androgen or androgen sensitivity in a female may cause hirsutism. Although the severity of the hirsutism is often proportional to the amount of androgen, remarkable individual variation exists in the manifestations of androgen excess. In general, women with significant androgen elevations will be amenorrheic, or at least oligomenorrheic and anovulatory.

Severe hyperandrogenism causes virilization, in which hirsutism is accompanied by male-pattern baldness, deepening of the voice, increased muscle development, and clitoromegaly. The presence of true virilization usually points to a serious underlying disorder, such as virilizing tumors of the ovary or adrenal gland or hyperthecosis ovarii [31].

PCOS is the most frequent cause of hirsutism. Insulin resistance may be closely associated with PCOS. Other causes of hirsutism include hyperprolactinemia (Table 5.2), congenital adrenal hyperplasia (CAH), insulin-resistance syndromes, ovarian tumors, and adrenal tumors. Medications such as danazol, phenytoin, levonorgestrel, nonprescription DHEA, and abuse of androgenic substances can result in hirsutism.

Epidemiology

The distribution and growth of body hair are variable among various ethnic groups, with populations from the Mediterranean basin in general having more body hair in

Table 5.1. Amenorrhea Summary

	Uterus	FSH	Prolactin	Testosterone	Karyotype	Special Considerations
Primary amenorrhea						
Turner syndrome	Yes	N	N	45,X; mosaic variants	Counseling; HRT consideration and discussion if appropriate	HRT?
Immune ovarian failure	Yes	N	N	46,XX	CV evaluation; thyroid tests; GH?	
Gonadal dysgenesis	Yes	N	N	46,XX; 46,XY	Glucocorticoids; remove gonads if Y or part of Y present	
17α-hydroxylase deficiency	Yes	N	N	46,XX	Glucocorticoids	
17α-hydroxylase deficiency	No	N	N	46,XY	Remove gonads	
Androgen insensitivity	No	N	N	46,XY	Remove gonads at maturity	
Müllerian agenesis/outlet	No	N	N	N	Surgical consideration; evaluate for urinary tract anomalies	
Kallmann syndrome	Yes	N	N	N	hMG/GnRH for fertility	
Hypothalamic dysfunction	Yes	N	N	N	hMG/GnRH for fertility if primary disease not treatable	
Prolactinoma	Yes	N	N		Dopamine agonists, surgery; hMG if hypopituitary for fertility	
Other pituitary tumor	Yes	N	N	N	Surgery, irradiation; hMG if hypopituitary for fertility	
Infiltrative disorders	Yes	N	N	N	Treat disease; hMG/GnRH if hypopituitary for fertility	

	Uterus	FSH	Prolactin	Testosterone	Karyotype	Special Considerations
Secondary amenorrhea						
Premature ovarian failure	Yes	N	N		46,XX	
Iatrogenic: radiotherapy, chemotherapy	Yes	N	N			
Low body weight/exercise						Weight gain as appropriate
Hypothalamic dysfunction	Yes	N	N	N		hMG/GnRH if cannot treat underlying disease for fertility
Sheehan syndrome	Yes	N	N	N		hMG/GnRH if cannot treat underlying disease for fertility
Prolactinoma	Yes	N	N			Dopamine agonists, surgery; hMG if hypopituitary for fertility
Hyperprolactinemia	Yes	N	N			Change of medications possible? Treat underlying medication problem
Other pituitary tumor	Yes	N	N	N		Surgery, irradiation; hMG if hypopituitary for fertility
Infiltrative disorders	Yes	N	N	N		Treat disease; hMG/GnRH if hypopituitary for fertility
PCOS	Yes	N	N			Weight control; see section on hirsutism
Asherman syndrome	Yes	N	N	N		Surgery if appropriate

GH, growth hormone; GnRH, gonadotropin-releasing hormone; hMG, human menopausal gonadotropin; HRT, hormone replacement therapy; N, normal; PCOS, polycystic ovarian syndrome.

Table 5.2.   Medications That Can Cause Hyperprolactinemia

Dopamine receptor blockers
Catecholamine or dopamine depletors
Phenothiazines and other neuroleptics
Antidepressants
Antihypertensives
Estrogens
Opiates

normal individuals than do those from other parts of the world. Because of these population differences, it is difficult to determine the prevalence of hirsutism in the general population. In a prospective study of the prevalence of PCOS in the Southeastern United States, between 2% to 8% of whites and blacks had hirsutism, and the prevalence of PCOS was 3.5% to 11.2% [32].

Diagnosis
The purposes of making a conclusive diagnosis are as follows:

1. To exclude serious, though rare disorders, including androgen-secreting tumors of the ovary and adrenal gland as well as Cushing syndrome.
2. To establish a diagnosis of PCOS, which is strongly associated with insulin resistance, and therefore carries a high likelihood of serious metabolic and cardiovascular risk. Patients with this disorder require not only therapy for hyperandrogenism, but also life-long follow-up to prevent, detect, and treat glucose intolerance, hypertension, obesity, and other cardiovascular risks [33].
3. To establish a diagnosis of adrenal hyperplasia, which may benefit by the use of low-dose (suppressive) glucocorticoid replacement.

Using appropriate ranges, most patients with clinical hyperandrogenism will have testosterone levels greater than 40 ng/dl [34], because normal women generally have testosterone levels below this [35].

Free testosterone levels may be useful in compensating for either elevated or decreased sex hormone–binding globulin and may give a more accurate representation of biologically active hormone. Although no studies are available, a level greater than 150 ng/dl is often used to indicate the possible presence of an androgen-secreting tumor, requiring further evaluation. Sex hormone–binding globulin (SHBG) may be combined with total testosterone to compute a free-androgen index. Free testosterone levels are highly assay dependent but may be useful in obesity in which the SHBG is low. DHEA-S is a marker of adrenal androgen production and may indicate the presence of partial 21-hydroxylase deficiency. This disorder is diagnosed by the finding of an elevated 17α-hydroxyprogesterone concentration (the immediate substrate of the 21-hydroxylase enzyme) either in the basal state or after stimulation with ACTH. The study should be done in the morning in the follicular phase of the menstrual cycle in women with menses. A very high DHEA-S, generally over 600, may suggest an adrenal tumor.

Treatment
Treatment is directed at the underlying cause of the hirsutism, when possible. Nonpharmacologic therapy includes hair removal by shaving, depilatories, bleaching, and wax. Medical therapy often takes 6 months or more to show a response. The choice of therapy options also depends on whether the patient is planning pregnancy, because most medications used for hirsutism are contraindicated in pregnancy. No long-term studies of safety or efficacy beyond 1 to 2 years have been done. For PCOS and the insulin-resistance syndrome, life-style changes are recommended to encourage weight loss if the patient is overweight. Appropriate diet and exercise programs should be

instituted in such patients and can be effective in controlling these disorders, including the associated hirsutism [36].

Oral contraceptives (OCPs) are generally considered first-line agents for the treatment of hirsutism, although studies with OCPs have generally been on a small scale. OCPs with antiandrogenic progestogens, particularly drosperinone in the United States (and cyproterone in Europe) should be used in this population [37].

The use of OCPs may exacerbate insulin resistance in susceptible individuals, and care should be taken, particularly in patients with PCOS, who are usually insulin resistant as part of the syndrome. Care should be taken to test this group periodically for impaired glucose tolerance and/or overt diabetes [38].

Spironolactone is an antiandrogen that inhibits testosterone binding at the receptor level. It is rated as pregnancy category C by the U.S. Food and Drug Administration (FDA). In a review of six small, randomized, controlled trials, a significant benefit was noted after 6 months taking spironolactone, 100 mg/day, compared with placebo [39]. The effects of spironolactone on hirsutism are at least comparable with those of flutamide and finasteride [40]. Spironolactone is often combined with an OCP to help prevent pregnancy, to maintain regular menstrual cycles, and to augment therapeutic efficacy. Cyproterone acetate is a progestin that acts as an antiandrogen and is frequently used worldwide for hirsutism, but it is not available in the United States. Other antiandrogens and some OCPs have been demonstrated to be as effective as cyproterone acetate in most studies [41]. Flutamide is an antiandrogen that inhibits testosterone binding at the receptor level. It is FDA category D for pregnancy. It is as effective as spironolactone and finasteride in treatment of hirsutism [39–42]. Use of this agent in hirsutism should be limited to investigational studies because of the lack of improved efficacy, the potential for hepatic toxicity, the high cost, and its potential for fetal harm.

Finasteride inhibits 5α-reductase, which controls the conversion of testosterone to dihydrotestosterone. Although it is specific for the enzyme type found in the prostate, it has clinical effects on decreasing hair growth as well. It is FDA category X for pregnancy, showing fetal risk, and is therefore contraindicated in pregnancy and in women at risk for pregnancy. For hirsutism, it is slightly less effective in most studies compared with spironolactone and flutamide, although it may provide additional improvement in combination with some antiandrogenic OCPs [39,42]. Because of the significant risk of fetal harm, high cost, and lack of greater efficacy than other agents, use of finasteride for hirsutism should be limited to investigational studies.

Gonadotropin-releasing hormone (GnRH) agonists are expensive and produce hypogonadism. Their use should be limited to investigational studies [42].

Metformin is an oral biguanide approved for the treatment of type 2 diabetes. Its effects on hirsutism have been modest [43], but further studies are needed in view of the beneficial effects on insulin resistance syndrome and associated hyperandrogenism. Dopamine agonists may improve hyperandrogenism in patients with hyperprolactinemia [44]. Eflornithine is a topical ornithine decarboxylase inhibitor that is FDA approved for hirsutism on the face and chin. Long-term prospective trials are not available.

In patients with PCOS with insulin resistance, a role may exist for insulin sensitization with thiazolidinediones, either in conjunction with OCPs and/or metformin [45,46].

PRECOCIOUS PUBERTY

Definition

Precocious puberty is defined as the premature development of secondary sex characteristics. In girls, this generally constitutes breast budding (thelarche) or development of pubic hair (pubarche) before age 7 in whites and age 6 in blacks. In boys, testicular enlargement before age 9 would indicate precocious puberty [47].

In contrast, premature adrenarche refers to inappropriately early development of axillary and pubic hair, whereas premature thelarche refers to early breast development. Either or both may be associated with true precocious puberty, which is associated with progressive development, accelerated growth velocity, and ultimately menses in girls. Whereas precocious puberty leads to premature closure of the epiphyses and short adult final stature, the former two conditions are not progressive and do not carry this risk. They are generally static, and children enter full puberty at a normal age.

Pathophysiology
Central precocious puberty (CPP) is defined as early activation of pulsatile GnRH activity in an otherwise normal hypothalamopituitary–gonadal axis. Pseudopuberty occurs when true central activation is absent.

Etiology and Diagnosis
Premature adrenarche and thelarche are characterized by prepubertal luteinizing hormone (LH), FSH, testosterone, and estradiol levels, and bone age demonstrates that no progression is occurring. In premature adrenarche, a significantly elevated DHEA-S level requires further evaluation for CAH or adrenal tumor would be needed. Girls with premature adrenarche may be at risk for PCOS and insulin resistance. Periodic monitoring for both conditions is indicated to ensure they do not progress.

In girls, CPP is overwhelmingly idiopathic but may result from a hypothalamic hamartoma that secretes pulses of GnRH. Bone-age testing should be undertaken to assess the effect on growth rate and to gauge progression and response to therapy. MRI of the brain/pituitary is needed in all cases of CPP to exclude disease affecting the central nervous system.

In boys, CPP is nearly always secondary to a tumor, irradiation, or septooptic dysplasia with premature activation of GnRH secretion. Discontinuation after exposure to exogenous sex steroids may also result in activation of the central axis, resulting in acquired CPP. MRI of the brain and hypothalamopituitary region should be done, as well as a bone-age test. Pseudopuberty in girls is associated with prepubertal levels of LH and FSH, LH unresponsive to GnRH stimulation, and sex hormones in the pubertal range or higher. Causes in girls include ovarian follicular cysts, McCune–Albright syndrome (associated with café-au-lait spots and polyostotic fibrous dysplasia), and stromal cell tumors of the ovary. A pelvic ultrasound should be done to look for cysts or masses in the ovary. Thyroid studies should be done to evaluate for hypothyroidism.

In boys, autonomous testicular function may be present secondary to a Leydig cell tumor, human chorionic gonadotropin (hCG)-secreting tumor, McCune–Albright syndrome (activated G protein), or familial male precocious puberty (abnormal activated LH receptor). LH and FSH levels will be in the prepubertal range, with pubertal range or higher testosterone levels. With a Leydig cell tumor, a testicular mass may be noted on examination or ultrasound. An hCG level should be checked in boys with precocious puberty, because tumors that secrete hCG can stimulate testicular testosterone production. These tumors may occur in the gonads, pineal, liver, posterior mediastinum, or retroperitoneum.

Other causes of pseudopuberty include abuse of exogenous androgens, congenital adrenal hyperplasia, and a pituitary gonadotroph-secreting adenoma. Thyroid studies (TSH, FT4) should be done to evaluate for hypothyroidism.

Treatment
For all patients with precocious puberty, it is important to provide the child and family with professional counseling services, although no formal studies have been reported with clinical outcomes. Patients with isolated premature thelarche or premature adrenarche should be examined periodically to ensure that precocious puberty is not developing. Girls with premature adrenarche should be monitored especially for development of the PCOS and the insulin-resistance syndrome. Treatment of pseudoprecocious puberty must be directed at the underlying disease. Surgery, irradiation, and chemotherapy options exist for tumors causing precocious puberty. Aromatase inhibitors may be used for gonadotropin-independent precocious puberty [48,49].

Treatment of boys with familial male-limited precocious puberty with spironolactone and testolactone helps controls symptoms of acne, erectile function, and aggression, but without a significant improvement of predicated final adult height [50]. Activation of the central axis with development of CPP in response to circulating sex hormones limits the usefulness of this combination alone. Combination of spironolactone and testolactone with triptorelin/jargone (GnRHa) to prevent the activation of the central axis is more effective, with an improvement in final predicated adult height [51]. Further long-term studies are needed to document the efficacy and safety of this combination therapy. In a small study, resistant cases may respond to ketoconazole [52].

No unanimity exists about treatment of CPP. Treatment goals include the preservation of the potential for normal adult height, prevention of premature sexual activity, improvement of psychosocial problems related to the disorder, and prevention of early menarche [53]. Proposed criteria for therapy with GnRH agonists are as follows: patients that clearly meet the definition for precocious puberty with documentation of an active GnRH axis by GnRH stimulation testing or sleep studies and sex hormone levels in the pubertal range with limited predicted adult height (<5th percentile) or significant psychosocial problems from menses or early development [54]. Generally, therapy is initiated in very young children to prevent sexual development and in older children when bone-maturation acceleration outpaces linear growth velocity, resulting in premature closure of the epiphyses and diminished final adult height. No studies document the benefits of GnRH therapy on ultimate psychosocial well-being in children with this disorder. Quality-of-life issues should enter into therapy considerations but must be individualized and have not been well studied. Long-term safety issues pertaining to the use of GnRH agonists are largely unknown. A review of earlier trials of GnRHa use suggests that therapy should be started before age 8 years to have a significant impact [53]. Therapy with GnRHa generally produces a height increase of 3 to 8 cm over that in untreated patients, but typically 1 to 7 cm below the normal predicted adult height [53]. Newer studies suggest that a final adult height appropriate for midparental height prediction is achieved by 85% to 90% of patients. Some studies suggest that weight gain may be associated with therapy with GnRH analogues [55,56].

Addition of growth hormone in small studies has generally shown significantly improved heights in girls [57–59] but has not been clearly shown to have value in boys [53], although sample sizes in the studies have been small. Larger, more recent studies suggest a therapeutic benefit with a gain between pretreatment predicted adult height (PAH) and final height of 8.2 ± 4.8 cm according to tables for accelerated girls and 12.7 ± 4.8 cm according to tables for average girls in patients treated with GH plus GnRHa. In patients treated with GnRH alone, the gain calculated between pretreatment PAH for accelerated girls was just 2.3 ± 2.9 cm and 7.1 ± 2.7 cm greater than pretreatment PAH for average girls. The difference between the gain obtained in the two groups (~6 cm) remained the same, however the PAH was calculated [60]. The most powerful predictors of a good response are early age of disease, early age at therapy, rapidity of bone advancement, and initial predicted height to target height deficit [61].

MALE HYPOGONADISM

Definition
Hypogonadism is inadequate gonadal function, as manifested by deficiencies in sperm production and/or the secretion of sex steroids. Hypogonadism may manifest with testosterone deficiency, infertility, or both conditions.

Etiology and Diagnosis
Disorders of male hypogonadism are generally divided into those that produce hypogonadotropic hypogonadism and those that produce hypergonadotropic hypogonadism. Hypogonadotropic disorders are associated with inappropriately normal or low FSH and LH levels and may be idiopathic or secondary to pituitary tumors or infiltrative disorders of the hypothalamus or pituitary. The initial hormonal evaluation of hypogonadism should include FSH, LH, testosterone, and prolactin levels (Table 5.3). MRI

Table 5.3. Male Hypogonadism Disorders: Evaluation and Therapy Considerations

Testicular Size[a]	FSH	LH	Testosterone[b]	Semen Analysis	Diagnosis	Evaluation of Treatment
Not palpable	↑	↑	↓	Azoospermia	Anorchism	Surgical exploration
Not palpable	↑	↑	N[b]/↓	Azoospermia	Bilateral cryptorchidism	Surgical exploration
<5 ml	↓	↓	↓	Azoospermia, oligospermia	Kallmann's syndrome, hypogonadotropic hypogonadism	T to virilize; hCG, hMG (or FSH) or GnRH for spermatogenesis
<5 ml	↑	↑	N[b]/↓	Azoospermia	Klinefelter's syndrome; other hypergonadotropic syndromes	Karyotype to confirm; T to virilize
8–15 ml	↑	N	N	Azoospermia, oligospermia	Germinal damage; toxins, idiopathic	Fertility: IVF with ICSI(?)
10–20 ml	↓	↓	↓	Oligospermia	Adult acquired hypogonadotropic hypogonadism	Pituitary MRI; prolactin. Treat pituitary disorder if present; otherwise treat as Kallmann's syndrome
10–20 ml	N/↑ (variable)	N[b]/↑ (variable)	N/↓	Variable	Senescence	T if symptomatic with low TB
15–20 ml	N/↑	N	N	Oligospermia	Varicocele, drugs, idiopathic	Fertility; varicocele repair if significant varicocele present. Optimize wife; IVF with ICSI
Variable phenotype	↑ (variable)	↑ (variable)	↑	Variable	T receptor defects, Reifenstein's syndrome	Variable (depending on degree); medical or surgical therapy

[a] Normal testicular size is 20–30 ml. Testicular size is used here as a clinical finding to help narrow the differential diagnosis. Some variation beyond the listed ranges may exist for a specific condition. Use of this variable is optional; the diagnosis should be based on the total clinical picture.

[b] Because of changes in SHBG levels, total testosterone may be in the normal range in the setting of low testosterone production. An SHBG level or free testosterone should be used in this setting to determine whether treatment options should be considered.

FSH = follicle-stimulating hormone; GnRH = gonadotropin releasing hormone; hCG = human chorionic gonadotropin; hMG = human menopausal gonadotropin; ICSI = intracytoplasmic sperm injection; IUI = intrauterine insemination; IVF = in vitro fertilization; LH = luteinizing hormone; MRI = magnetic resonance imaging; N = normal; SHBG = sex hormone-binding globulin; T = testosterone

Adapted from American Association of Clinical Endocrinologists. Medecal Guidelines for clinical practice for the evaluation and treatment of hypogonadism in adult male patients—2002 update. Endocr Tract 2002;8:440–456.

of the brain and pituitary may be needed to evaluate further for secondary causes in men with a testosterone less than 150 ng/dl if gonadotropins are not elevated.

Congenital Male Hypogonadism

Congenital male hypogonadism is seen with failure of sexual development. Hypogonadotrophic disorders have absent or abnormal GnRH secretion and may occur in the setting of anosmia (Kallmann syndrome). Other syndromes include Prader–Willi syndrome and Lawrence–Moon–Biedel syndrome. Gonadotropin levels (LH/FSH) are low in these disorders.

Congenital causes of hypergonadotropic hypogonadism (high LH and FSH) include Klinefelter syndrome (47,XXY) and other chromosomal abnormalities.

Acquired Male Hypogonadism

Acquired hypogonadotrophic disorders include prolactinomas and other pituitary tumors, infiltrative disorders such as sarcoidosis, histiocytosis or hemochromatosis, infection, pituitary apoplexy, injury, severe illness, glucocorticoids, pituitary surgery, and irradiation.

Hypergonadotropic disorders are associated with high FSH and LH levels. Acquired testicular failure with compensatory hypergonadotropin secretion may result from muscular dystrophy, cryptorchidism, varicocele, mumps orchitis, HIV, testicular trauma, torsion, chemotherapy, chronic diseases, or irradiation. Many cases are idiopathic.

Testosterone deficiency associated with aging (andropause) may be associated with loss of energy, decreased libido, erectile dysfunction, mood disturbances, loss of muscle mass, increased fat mass, decreased strength, and loss of bone density. Approximately 30% of men 60 to 70 years old and 70% of men from 70 to 80 years have low bioavailable or free testosterone levels. Symptoms and findings of testosterone deficiency may be difficult to differentiate from aging and/or depression. They include loss of energy, depressed mood, decreased libido, erectile dysfunction, decreased muscle mass and strength, increased fat mass, frailty, osteopenia, and osteoporosis [62]. Several small clinical trials indicate that testosterone replacement therapy can improve many of these findings; however, the studies have not been powered to assess potential risks, including exacerbation of benign prostatic hyperplasia, development of a clinical prostate cancer, or cardiovascular events. Criteria for the treatment of older men are still being evaluated. It has been suggested that older men with symptoms and testosterone levels below 200 to 300 ng/dl should be considered for replacement therapy if not otherwise contraindicated [63,64], although no long-term studies document efficacy and safety. Studies substituting testosterone in elderly men with low serum testosterone have shown that men with clinical symptoms identical to the symptoms of classic hypogonadism will benefit most from such therapy. Therefore it is the general consensus to treat men with age-related hypogonadism only when clinical symptoms are present that can be potentially corrected by testosterone administration [65].

Treatment

Treatment should be directed first at any underlying disorders. The goal of therapy is to relieve symptoms of hypogonadism and preserve bone density. Testosterone is contraindicated if a testosterone-dependent neoplasm (e.g., prostate cancer), hyperviscosity, or sleep apnea is present. In adult men with hypergonadotropic hypogonadism and in men with hypogonadotropic hypogonadism not desiring fertility, testosterone therapy should be considered as first-line therapy. In hypogonadal men, testosterone therapy improves bone density, lean body mass, hemoglobin, energy levels, and sexual function with increases in prostate volume [66]. No improvement may be found in underlying depression [67]. HIV-positive hypogonadal men may have significant improvements in libido, energy levels, depression, and muscle mass [68]. In boys who have not gone through puberty, low doses of testosterone should be used with gradual increases, because aggressive behavior may occur [69].

Preparations of testosterone include testosterone enanthate or cypionate by intramuscular injection, transdermal testosterone by scrotal patch, transdermal testosterone through normal skin, and testosterone gel. Oral testosterone preparations should not be used because of poor potency and risk of hepatic injury. Intramuscular preparations of testosterone should be given every 7 to 14 days. Intramuscular injection of testosterone undecanoate is an attractive new therapy that can be administered quarterly. Monitoring of testosterone levels with the gel or patches can be done randomly, and dosing adjusted to keep the level in the normal range. For injections, the midpoint between-injections dose should be in the midnormal range. Improvement in clinical parameters should also be monitored, such as muscle mass, bone density, well-being, erectile function, and libido. Prostate size and prostate-specific antigen (PSA) should be monitored at least annually. If the PSA is above 4 ng/ml at outset or if it increases, referral of the patient to a urologist for possible ultrasound and biopsy is needed. For selected men, serial measurement of bone mineral density during androgen therapy might be helpful to confirm end-organ effects. Hematocrit should be monitored to detect polycythemia [70].

Treatment of male infertility in men with hypogonadotropic hypogonadism is covered in the section on infertility.

INFERTILITY

Definition

A couple is considered infertile if they are unable to conceive after 12 months or more of unprotected intercourse in the absence of surgical sterility or contraception. Primary infertility refers to couples that have never had a pregnancy. Secondary infertility refers to couples having had a prior pregnancy.

Etiology and Diagnosis

In a study of 708 couples with infertility in England, the common causes of infertility were noted to be idiopathic (28% of cases), male factor (24%), ovulatory dysfunction (21%), tubal disease (14%), endometriosis (6%), sexual dysfunction (6%), or cervical defects or mucus problems (3%) [71]. About 15% to 20% of infertile couples have both male and female factors reducing fertility. Therefore the initial evaluation should include a thorough history and physical examination to evaluate both male and female factors. A normal semen analysis will exclude a male factor, whereas an abnormal study should prompt further investigation.

A sperm count exceeding 48 million/ml with more than 63% motility is considered fertile; a count between 13.5 and 48 million/ml with motility of 32% to 63% is considered indeterminate; and a count less than 13.5 million/ml with less than 32% motility is considered subfertile [72]. Genetic studies to assess for Y-chromosome abnormalities may be considered if the couple is considering intracytoplasmic sperm injection (ICSI).

Ovulatory function can be assessed by the menstrual history, BBT charts, midcycle measurement of urinary gonadotropins ovulation kits [73], a midluteal progesterone level, or endometrial biopsy.

When ovulatory failure is diagnosed, an etiology should be determined. Studies should include an early follicular phase FSH to determine whether ovarian failure is present, a prolactin test to evaluate for hyperprolactinemia, and measurement of testosterone and DHEA-S levels to test for hyperandrogenism. Female infertility with ovulatory sufficiency should prompt an investigation of anatomic disease (e.g., tubal obstruction, uterine abnormalities, or endometriosis) assessed by ultrasound, hysterosalpingography, laparoscopy, and hysteroscopy, as clinically indicated.

The cervical factor can be assessed by a midcycle postcoital test wherein the presence and motility of sperm is assessed in a cervical swab after intercourse. If sperm are inactivated by the cervical mucus and they are motile without contact, a "cervical factor" may be operative.

Epidemiology

According to the National Center for Health Statistics, the estimated number of women aged 15 to 44 with infertility was 6.1 million, and the number seeking fertility services was 9.3 million in 1995.

Treatment

Treatment of male infertility should be directed at the underlying disorder. If a large varicocele is present, surgery may improve sperm counts and fertility rates [74]. Men with hypogonadotropic hypogonadism may respond to therapy with gonadotropin or GnRH therapy. Men with acquired disease may respond to hCG injections alone at 1,500 to 2,000 IU, 3 times a week. Intramuscular and subcutaneous preparations are available. Response to therapy, as measured on semen analysis, may take 6 to 12 months. Human menopausal gonadotropin can be added if no response is noted to hCG alone at doses of 37.5 to 75 IU, 3 times a week. It may take 12 months or more for a response. Pulsatile GnRH subcutaneously or intravenously has been success-fully used in the treatment of hypogonadotropic hypogonadism in men. Testosterone therapy with the hopes of rebound improvement in sperm counts and pregnancy rate is ineffective and does not improve pregnancy rates or semen parameters [75]. Antie-strogen therapy with clomiphene citrate or tamoxifen can improve testosterone levels in men but has no significant effect on pregnancy rate [76]. In men with low sperm counts, intrauterine insemination (IUI) can significantly improve the chances for pregnancy over timed intercourse with natural cycles and with controlled ovarian hy-perstimulation cycles [77]. ICSI with in vitro fertilization (IVF) is associated with sig-nificantly higher oocyte fertilization rates than is IVF alone in men with male factor infertility [78]. In unexplained infertility, pregnancy rates with IVF are not signifi-cantly different than those from IUI with and without controlled hyperstimulation [79]. IVF is indicated if infertility from tubal disease is present that cannot be cor-rected or in male factor, especially when combined with ICSI. In the treatment of women with unexplained infertility, clomiphene citrate has been found to be effective, based on randomized prospective trials with an odds ratio (OR) of 2.5 (95% CI, 1.35–4.62) [80]. In women with ovulatory dysfunction, clomiphene citrate is even more effective, with an OR of 3.41 (95% CI, 4.23–9.48) [81]. Risk of ovarian cancer, however, may be increased in women with infertility, although it is has not been di-rectly linked with fertility medications [82]. For unexplained infertility, IUI combined with superovulation is more effective than IUI or intracervical insemination (ICI) with superovulation and in turn more effective than ICI alone [83].

As a final note, it is critical to discuss issues of age-related decrease in reproductive function in older women contemplating future pregnancy. The infertility rate is about 6% at age 20 to 24 years, about 9% at 25 to 29 years, about 15% at 30 to 34 years, about 30% at 35 to 39 years, and about 64% at 40 to 44 years. Assessment of repro-ductive potential can be done by using the clomiphene challenge test [84].

MENOPAUSE

Definition

Menopause (adult-onset ovarian failure) occurs after the last menstrual period, al-though symptoms may start much earlier. After 1 year of amenorrhea, menopause is likely and can be confirmed by an elevated FSH if needed. The average age of menopause is 51 years.

Diagnosis

Diagnosis can be confirmed by an elevated FSH level. If cycles are still present, peri-menopausally, the early follicular phase FSH will be increased.

Treatment

The primary purpose of therapy is to relieve any significant menopausal symptoms. The decision to treat must be individualized in light of the potential benefits and risks of hormone replacement therapy. Clear evidence exists that vasomotor symptoms are significantly relieved by hormone replacement therapy (HRT) compared with placebo [85,86]. Vaginal dryness and urogenital atrophy are significantly improved by estrogen [86,87]. Urinary tract infections have improved in some studies [87,88], but no benefit on urinary tract infection was noted in the Heart and Estrogen/Progestin Replacement Study (HERS) study [89]. Depression in postmenopausal women may respond significantly to estrogen therapy, even in the absence of vasomotor symptoms [90,91], although only women with vasomotor symptoms improved in the HERS study [92]. Other potential benefits include prevention of bone loss and osteoporosis-related fracture and reduced risk of colorectal cancer. The issue of dementia prevention is still controversial, because some studies suggest benefit, whereas no benefit and increased risk of cognitive impairment were found in the Women's Heath Initiative study [93,94].

HRT does not appear to protect against heart disease in recent primary and secondary prevention trials such as HERS and the Women's Health Initiative [95,96]. Other risks include an increased risk of thromboembolism and biliary tract disease [97]. The risk of breast cancer appears increased after 5 or more years of use [98]. The use of estrogen for 10 years or more may be associated with an increased risk of ovarian cancer [99]. Other risks of HRT include an increased incidence of endometrial cancer (with unopposed estrogen use), bronchospasm, dry-eye syndrome, and an increased incidence of lupus.

At present, recommendations are to use as low a dose of HRT as possible for treatment of significant vasomotor symptoms or vaginal dryness and for as brief a period as required. Alternatives for protection against osteoporosis and heart disease should be discussed. Small trials have been done showing some benefit for treatment of vasomotor symptoms with selective serotonin reuptake inhibitors, clonidine, megestrol, and gabapentin, but no comparison trials with estrogen have been conducted.

REFERENCES

Amenorrhea

1. (*2C*) **Pittock ST** et al. Mayer-Rokitansky-Kuster-Hauser anomaly and its associated malformations. Am J Med Genet A 2005;135:314–316.

   Retrospective chart review of 25 patients between 1975 and 2002 found 20% scoliosis, 28% unilateral renal agenesis, 16% nonvertebral skeletal anomalies, and 44% vertebral anomalies; two had unilateral ovarian agenesis. Cardiac anomalies occurred in 16%, including truncus arteriosus, PDA, patent foramen ovale, and mitral valve disease.

2. (*2C*) **Zenteno JC** et al. Molecular analysis of the anti-müllerian hormone, the anti-müllerian hormone receptor, and galactose-1-phosphate uridyl transferase genes in patients with the Mayer-Rokitansky-Kuster-Hauser syndrome. Arch Gynecol Obstet 2004;269:270–273. Epub 2002 Dec 19.

   Fifteen patients with müllerian agenesis underwent molecular analysis of antimüllerian hormone and its receptor genes. No deleterious mutations were found. Although new polymorphisms were identified, they were not different between subjects and controls, making this an unlikely genetic cause of the syndrome.

3. (*2C*) **Biason-Lauber A** et al. A WNT4 mutation associated with müllerian-duct regression and virilization in a 46,XX woman. N Engl J Med 2004;351:792–798.

   A single case report of a loss-of-function mutation in the WNT4 gene, which codes for a protein that suppresses male sexual differentiation and represses biosynthesis of gonadal androgens in females, was found in an 18-year-old with primary amenorrhea and absent müllerian-derived structures. This suggests that WNT4 is important in maintenance of the female phenotype.

4. (*1C*) **Patsalis PC**. Detection and incidence of cryptic Y chromosome sequences in Turner syndrome patients. Clin Genet 1998;53:249–257.

   The presence of Y chromosome sequences in Turner syndrome (TS) patients may predispose them to gonadoblastoma formation with an estimated risk of 15%–25%. Fifty Turner syndrome patients were screened for the presence of Y chromosome material by using a combination of polymerase chain reaction (PCR) and nested PCR followed by Southern blot analysis of three genes: the sex-determining region Y (SRY), testis-specific protein Y encoded (TSPY), and RNA-binding motif protein (RBM) (previously designated as YRRM), and nine additional STSs spanning all seven intervals of the Y chromosome. Karyotypes were divided in four groups: five (23.8%) of the 21 TS patients that have the 45,X karyotype (group A) also have cryptic Y sequences; none of the seven patients who have karyotypes with anomalies on one of the X chromosomes have Y mosaicism (group B); one (6.3%) of the 16 patients with a mosaic karyotype has Y material (group C); and six (100%) six patients with a supernumerary marker chromosome (SMC) have Y chromosome sequences (group D).

5. **Meyers CM**. Gonadal dysgenesis in 46 XX individuals: Frequency of the autosomal recessive form. Am J Med Genet 1996;63518–63524.

Gonadal (ovarian) dysgenesis with normal chromosomes (46,XX) clearly is a heterogeneous condition. In some forms, the defect is restricted to the gonads, whereas other affected females show neurosensory hearing loss (Perrault syndrome). Nongenetic causes exist as well. To elucidate the proportion of XX gonadal (ovarian) dysgenesis due to autosomal recessive genes, the authors used segregation analysis of 17 published and 18 unpublished families having at least two female offspring. Analysis was restricted to cases in whom ovarian failure was documented by the presence of streak ovaries (published cases) or elevated gonadotropins (unpublished cases). The segregation ratio estimate was 0.16, suggesting that many 46,XX females with gonadal (ovarian) dysgenesis represent a disorder segregating as an autosomal recessive trait, placing sisters of these cases at a 25% risk for this disorder.

6. (*1C*) **Ogata T**. Short stature homeobox-containing gene duplication on the der(X) chromosome in a female with 45X/46,X,der(X), gonadal dysgenesis and tall stature J Clin Endocrinol Metab 2000;85:2927–2930.

Chromosomal analysis of the X chromosome of a Japanese female with 45,X[40]/46,X, der(X)[60], primary amenorrhea, and tall stature was performed. Fluorescence in situ hybridization analysis for 10 loci/regions on the X-chromosome together with the whole X-chromosome and the Xp-specific and Xq-specific paintings showed that the der(X) chromosome was associated with duplication of roughly distal half of Xp, including SHOX (short stature homeobox-containing gene), and deletion of most of Xq. The authors suggest that the tall stature of this female is caused by the combined effects of SHOX duplication on the der(X) chromosome and gonadal estrogen deficiency. They note that the similarity in the growth pattern between this female and patients with estrogen resistance or aromatase deficiency implies that the association of an extra copy of SHOX with gonadal estrogen deficiency may represent another clinical entity presenting as tall stature resulting from continued growth in late teens or into adulthood.

7. (*1C+*) **Sarpel U** et al. The incidence of complete androgen insensitivity in girls with inguinal hernias and assessment of screening by vaginal length measurement. J Pediatr Surg 2005;40:133–136.

A prospective study of prepubertal girls with inguinal hernias revealed an incidence of complete androgen insensitivity syndrome of 1.1% in these girls, with short vaginal length being a marker for suspicion of the syndrome.

8. (*1C+*) **Ledig S** et al. Novel and recurrent mutations in patients with androgen insensitivity syndromes. Horm Res 2005;63:263–269. Epub 2005 May 26.

Twenty-four patients with AIS were studied by sequencing androgen-receptor gene. Nineteen of the investigated patients were affected by complete androgen insensitivity syndrome (CAIS), and five had partial androgen insensitivity syndrome (PAIS). Twelve unreported mutations were found, as well as nine recurrent mutations (three recurrent mutations were detected twice) in exons 2–8 of the androgen-receptor gene. Apart from truncating mutations, a reliable genotype/phenotype correlation cannot be established. Therefore modifying factors must be effective.

9. (*1C+*) **Quinton R** et al. Idiopathic gonadotropin deficiency: Genetic questions addressed through phenotypic characterization. Clin Endocrinol 2001;55:163–174.

A clinical study of 170 male and 45 female IHH patients. Eighty percent of data were obtained from case records, and 20% were collected prospectively. Parameters assessed included olfaction, testicular volume, family history of hypogonadism, anosmia or pubertal delay, and history or presence of testicular maldescent or neurologic, renal, or craniofacial anomalies. Olfactory acuity was bimodally distributed. Testicular volume, a marker of integrated gonadotropin secretion, did not differ significantly between anosmic and normosmic patients. The prevalence of cryptorchidism was nearly 3 times greater in anosmic (70.3%, of which 75.0% are bilateral) than in normosmic (23.2%, of which 43.8% are bilateral) patients. Disorders of eye movement and hearing occurred only in association with KS. The findings revealed a clear phenotypic separation between KS and nIHH. Pedigree studies suggest that autosomal KS is a heterogeneous condition, with incomplete phenotypic penetrance within pedigrees, and that some cases of autosomal KS, nIHH, and isolated anosmia may have a common genetic basis. Most sporadic KS cases are presumed to have an autosomal basis.

10. (*1C+*) **Dolzan V** et al. Mutational spectrum of steroid 21-hydroxylase and the genotype-phenotype association in Middle European patients with congenital adrenal hyperplasia. Eur J Endocrinol 2005;153:99–106.

The molecular genetic basis of 21-hydroxylase deficiency is clearly demonstrated in this large-scale study in a European registry. By genotyping for the most common point mutations, CYP21 gene deletion/conversion and the 8-bp deletion in exon 3, it was possible to identify the mutation in 94% to 99% of the diseased alleles in this population. Steroid 21-hydroxylase (CYP21) and the genotype–phenotype correlation were assessed in 432 patients with congenital adrenal hyperplasia (CAH) and 298 family members of middle European ancestry. CYP21 gene deletion and In2 and Ile172Asn mutation accounted for 72.7% of the affected alleles in the whole study group. A good genotype–phenotype correlation was observed, with the exception of Ile172Asn and Pro30Leu mutations. In 37% of patients, low-resolution genotyping could not identify the causative mutation or distinguish homozygosity from hemizygosity. With high-resolution genotyping, the causative mutations could be identified in 341 of 348 analyzed patients. A novel mutation Gln315Stop was found in one simple virilizing CAH (SV-CAH) patient. In the remaining seven patients, polymorphisms were identified as the leading sequence alteration. In patients with a mild form of the disease and no detectable mutation, CYP21 gene polymorphisms should be considered as a plausible disease-causing mutation. The presence of elevated basal and ACTH-stimulated 17-hydroxyprogesterone, premature pubarche, advanced bone age, and clitoral hypertrophy directly implicated Asn493Ser polymorphism in the manifestation of nonclassic (NC)- and SV-CAH.

11. (*1C+*) **King JA** et al. Long term corticosteroid replacement and bone mineral density in adult women with classical congenital adrenal hyperplasia. J Clin Endocrinol Metab 2005; Epub ahead of print.

The risk of overtreatment of adrenal hyperplasia was demonstrated in this observational study of 11 women with salt-losing (SL) CAH and 15 with the simple virilizing (SV) 21 hydroxylase deficiency who underwent DEXA measurement of spine and whole-body bone density and compared with nine unaffected sisters as controls. Osteopenia was noted in 45% of SL, 13% of SV, and 11% of controls. Lumbar spine and whole-body BMDs of CAH subjects were lower than those of controls. CAH patients with osteopenia had lower levels of DHEA-S and DHEA compared with similar patients with normal bone density. Adrenal androgen levels were particularly suppressed among postmenopausal women receiving glucocorticoid replacement. Oversuppression of adrenal androgens is associated with increased risk for bone loss in this population.

12. (*1C*) **Rivkees SA, Crawford JD.** Dexamethasone treatment of virilizing congenital adrenal hyperplasia: The ability to achieve normal growth. Pediatrics 2000;106:767–773.

Long-acting steroid suppression with dexamethasone resulted in favorable growth patterns and appropriate timing of puberty. The use of dexamethasone at a dose of 0.27 ± 0.01 mg/m^2/d in 17 boys and nine girls with simple virilizing CAH over approximately 7 years resulted in a final adult height comparable to estimated midparental height in nine boys and six girls. The seven children who were started on therapy with more advanced bone age had shorted predicted/final heights, although these improved during the course of therapy. During treatment, 17-ketosteroid excretion rates were normal for age, and 17-hydroxyprogesterone values were 69.6 ± 18 ng/dl. Testicular enlargement was first detected at 10.7 ± 0.8 years.

13. **Cobin RH** et al. Writing Committee, American Association of Clinical Endocrinologists Position Statement on Metabolic and Cardiovascular Consequences of Polycystic Ovary Syndrome, 2005, Endocrine Practice, 11(2):125–134.

14. (*1C*) **Manuel M** et al. The age of occurrence of gonadal tumors in intersex patients with a Y chromosome. Am J Obstet Gynecol 1976;124:293–300.

A retrospective study of 320 cases of gonadal dysgenesis, asymmetric gonadal differentiation, and male hermaphrodites demonstrated a significant increase in gonadal tumors shortly after puberty. Testicular feminization patients had a lower risk of 3.6% up to age 25. In testicular feminization, it may be acceptable to wait until after puberty, although gonads should be removed on diagnosis in Y chromosome–containing disorders.

15. **Saenger P** et al. Recommendations for the diagnosis and management of Turner syndrome: Fifth International Symposium on Turner Syndrome. J Clin Endocrinol Metab 2001;86:3061–3069.

Comprehensive recommendations on the diagnosis of Turner syndrome and the care of affected patients were published in 1994. In the light of recent advances in diagnosis and treatment of Turner syndrome, an international multidisciplinary workshop was convened in March 2000 to update these recommendations. This article details the outcome of this workshop, describing the genetics and diagnosis of the syndrome, and presenting practical treatment guidelines.

16. (*1C*) **Swerdlow AJ** et al. Mortality and cancer incidence in persons with numerical sex chromosome abnormalities: A cohort study. Ann Hum Genet 2001;65:177–188.

This cohort observational study included 400 patients with Turner syndrome and 8,609 person-years of follow-up. The RR of death was high at 4.1, with deaths from aortic aneurysm having a RR of 63.2. Other congenital abnormalities were also noted.

17. (*1B*) **Sas TC** et al. Normalization of height in girls with Turner syndrome after long-term growth hormone treatment: Results of a randomized dose-response trial. J Clin Endocrinol Metab 1999;84:4607–4712.

This was a randomized trial of 68 girls aged 2 to 11 with Turner syndrome randomly assigned to one of three doses of GH. Estradiol was added at the age of 12, and follow-up was continued until final height occurred. A normal range of adult height was achieved in 85%, with an estimated gain of about 4 in the higher dose groups after an average of about 7 years of GH use.

18. (*2B*) **Chernausek SD** et al. Growth hormone therapy of Turner syndrome: the impact of age of estrogen replacement on final height: Genentech, Inc, Collaborative Study Group. J Clin Endocrinol Metab 2000;85:2439–1245.

This was a randomized controlled trial of estrogen plus GH in girls with Turner syndrome. At entry, the girls were all younger than 11 years, with a mean age of 9.5 years. Estrogen was either added at age 12 or at age 15. The height gain in girls begun on estrogen at age 15 was 8.4 6 4.3 cm and the height gain in girls started on estrogen at age 12 was only 5.1 6 3.6 cm ($p < 0.01$). Final height was most dependent on number of years of GH therapy before starting estrogen.

19. (*1C*) **Reiter EO** et al. Early initiation of growth hormone treatment allows age-appropriate estrogen use in Turner's syndrome. J Clin Endocrinol Metab 2001;86:1936–1941.

A population of 344 girls with Turner syndrome followed up in the National Cooperative Growth Hormone Study database was assessed for GH and estrogen therapy in relation to final height. In girls started on GH early, greater gains in height were shown despite estradiol therapy. If estrogen is needed because of behavioral issues, then early treatment with GH can help preserve final height.

20. *(2B)* **Ross JL** et al. Effects of estrogen on nonverbal processing speed and motor function in girls with Turner's syndrome. J Clin Endocrinol Metab 1998;83:3198–3204.

This was a double-blind randomized control trial demonstrating that motor skills in 10- to 12-year-old girls with Turner syndrome were significantly improved with estrogen therapy.

21. *(2B)* **van Kasteren YM** et al. Premature ovarian failure: A systematic review on therapeutic interventions to restore ovarian function and achieve pregnancy. Hum Reprod Update 1999;5: 483–492.

Meta-analysis of seven controlled trials with a total of 194 women with premature ovarian failure assessed for ovulatory status and pregnancy in response to various interventions. Interventions included gonadotropins (e.g., human menopausal gonadotropin), estrogen, growth hormone, GnRH agonists and antagonists, danazol, clomiphene, birth control pills, and glucocorticoids. None of the treatments increased the rate of ovulation or pregnancy with an expected basal pregnancy rate of 5% to 10%.

22. *(1C)* **Hogler W** et al. Importance of estrogen on bone health in Turner syndrome: A cross-sectional and longitudinal study using dual-energy X-ray absorptiometry. J Clin Endocrinol Metab 2004;89:193–199.

Eighty-three patients with Turner syndrome age 4 to 24 were followed longitudinally with DEXA. In subjects who remained prepuberal, bone density decreased, whereas it increased in subjects entering puberty with hormonal therapy.

23. *(1C)* **Bakalov VK** et al. Bone mineral density and fractures in Turner syndrome. Am J Med 2003;115:259–264.

Areal bone density corrected for skeletal size in 40 women with estrogen-treated Turner syndrome was compared with that in 40 age-matched healthy women. Structured personal interviews were used for the determination of fracture and estrogen use. Bone density was measured in subjects and control. The prevalence of osteoporosis and fractures was similar in both groups. Women shorter than 150 cm are more likely to be misdiagnosed with osteoporosis when areal bone density is measured unless adjusted for height. This study indicates that the historical observation of osteoporosis and fractures in untreated Turner syndrome can be compared with a favorable prognosis with the use of estrogen.

24. *(1C)* **Hanton L** et al. The importance of estrogen replacement in young women with Turner syndrome. J Womens Health (Larchmt) 2003;12:971–977.

Structured personal interview was used to determine estrogen use, and spine BMD was measured by DEXA and QCT in 30 women with Turner, ages 30 to 59 years. Thirty-four subjects had received HRT according to guidelines, whereas the rest had not. The untreated group had a reduced spine QCT by 20%, with six of 16 with osteoporosis and three of 16 having vertebral fractures as compared with none of 34 in the treated group.

25. *(2C)* **Gravholt CH** et al. Increased fracture rates in Turner's syndrome: A nationwide questionnaire survey. Clin Endocrinol (Oxf) 2003;59:89–96.

A previous registry study of Turner syndrome patients revealed an increased risk of osteoporosis and fractures. In this study, 322 patients in Denmark were compared with 1,888 controls matched for age and geographic region by questionnaire. Of the patients with Turner syndrome, 71% had taken HRT beginning at a mean of 16 years of age, and 16% had used growth hormone. The hazard risk for fracture in the Turner group was 1.35 (CI 1.04–1.75; $p < 0.03$) with time to first fracture age 53 in TS vs. 63 years in controls. This study did not correlate the use of HRT/GH with fractures among the subgroups with Turner.

26. *(1C+)* **Costa AM** et al. Bone mineralization in Turner syndrome: A transverse study of the determinant factors in 58 patients. J Bone Miner Metab 2002;20:294–297.

Fifty-eight patients with Turner syndrome were studied with DEXA; 86% had z scores less than -1 SD, and 46% had z scores less than -2.5 SD. BMD was negatively correlated with age and height and positively correlated with weight and BMD. A higher BMD was observed in those who used hormone replacement for a longer period.

27. *(1C+)* **Benetti-Pinto CL** et al. Factors associated with the reduction of bone density in patients with gonadal dysgenesis. Fertil Steril 2002;77:571–575.

Thirty-eight women, aged 16 to 35 years (mean, 24.6 years) with Turner syndrome or pure gonadal dysgenesis were studied with DEXA, and variables associated with BMD were evaluated by multiple linear regression analysis: 90% had osteopenia or osteoporosis of the spine, and 55% in the femoral neck. The length of estrogen therapy and the BMI showed a positive association with BMD at the lumbar spine and femoral neck.

28. *(2B)* **Grinspoon S** et al. Prevalence and predictive factors for regional osteopenia in women with anorexia nervosa. Ann Intern Med 2000;21:33:790–794.

DEXA of the spine and femoral neck was measured in 130 women with anorexia nervosa. Bone mineral density (BMD) was reduced by at least 1.0 SD at one or more skeletal sites in 92% of patients and by at least 2.5 SD in 38% of patients. Weight was the most consistent predictor of BMD at all skeletal sites.

Twenty-three percent of patients were current estrogen users, and 58% were previous estrogen users. BMD did not differ by history of estrogen use at any site. Weight, but not estrogen use, is a significant predictor of BMD in this population at all skeletal sites.

29. (*1C+*) **Miller KK** et al. Preservation of neuroendocrine control of reproductive function despite severe undernutrition. J Clin Endocrinol Metab 2004;89:4434–4438.

In total, 116 women were studied: 42 low-weight women who fulfilled all DSM4 diagnostic criteria for AN, except for amenorrhea; and 74 women with AN and amenorrhea for at least 3 months. The two groups were similar in body mass index, percentage ideal body weight, duration of eating disorder, age of menarche, and exercise. Eumenorrheic patients had a higher mean estradiol level than did amenorrheic subjects. Mean percentage body fat, total body fat mass, and truncal fat were higher in eumenorrheic than amenorrheic patients. The mean leptin level and IGF-1 levels were higher in the eumenorrheic than in the amenorrheic group. Only minor differences in severity of eating disorder symptoms were seen, as measured by the Eating Disorders Inventory, and where differences were observed, eumenorrheic subjects manifested more severe symptoms than did amenorrheic subjects. Mean BMDs at the spine were low in both groups, but were higher in patients with eumenorrhea than in those with amenorrhea, but menstrual function was not protective at the hip. It was concluded that fat mass may be important for preservation of normal menstrual function in severely undernourished women, and this may be in part mediated through leptin secretion, and that nutritional intake and normal hormonal function may be independent contributors to maintenance of trabecular bone mass in low-weight women.

30. (*1A*) **Grinspoon S** et al. Effects of recombinant human IGF-I and oral contraceptive administration on bone density in anorexia nervosa. J Clin Endocrinol Metab 2002;87:2883–2891.

In a blinded, placebo-controlled study, 60 osteopenic women with anorexia nervosa, ages 18 to 38 years, body mass index (17.8 ± 0.3 kg/m^2), spinal bone mineral density T score ($-2.1 ± 0.1$ SD), were randomized to receive either recombinant IGF-I and OCP, OCP alone, IGF-I alone, or no therapy for 9 months. All subjects received calcium, 1,500 mg/d, and a standard multivitamin containing 400 IU of vitamin D. The rhIGF-I was titrated to maintain IGF-I levels within the age-adjusted normal range for each patient. Spine BMD increased significantly in response to rhIGF-I and all rhIGF-I groups vs. all placebo treated, by analysis of covariance. OCP alone did not improve BMD over placebo, but increased to the greatest extent in the combined treatment group compared with placebo-treated patients. The data indicate that osteopenic women with anorexia nervosa treated with rhIGF-I showed more beneficial changes in bone density, compared with patients not treated with rhIGF-I. OCP therapy alone is not sufficient to improve bone density in undernourished patients, but may augment the effects of rhIGF-I in a combined treatment strategy.

31. **Cobin RH**. The case of the Elusive Androgen, 2002, Endocrine Practice, 8(6):433-438.

A case report and review of the literature indicating that more serious disorders such as adrenal and ovarian tumors and hyperthecosis ovarii are usually associated with more severe elevations of androgen levels and correspondingly worse clinical hirsutism and virilization.

Hirsutism

32. (*2C*) **Knochenhauer ES** et al. Prevalence of the polycystic ovary syndrome in unselected black and white women of the southeastern United States: A prospective study. J Clin Endocrinol Metab 1998;3:3078–3082.

In a prospective study of 369 women, hirsutism was present in 2% to 8%, and PCOS, in 3.5% to 11.2%.

33. (*1C+*) **Ehrmann DA** et al. Prevalence and predictors of the metabolic syndrome in women with polycystic ovary syndrome (PCOS). J Clin Endocrinol Metab 2005; Epub ahead of print.

In 394 PCOS women, clinical, hormonal, and OGTT results were evaluated; components of the metabolic (insulin-resistance) syndrome were measured, including waist circumference, fasting glucose, HDL cholesterol and triglyceride concentrations, and blood pressure. Twenty-six (6.6%) subjects had diabetes. Among the 368 nondiabetics, the prevalence for individual components composing the metabolic syndrome were waist circumference, >88 cm in 80%; HDL cholesterol,<50 mg/dl in 66%; triglycerides, ≥150 mg/dl in 32%; blood pressure, ≥130/85 mm Hg in 21%; and fasting glucose concentrations, ≥110 mg/dl in 5%. Three or more of these individual criteria were present in 123 (33.4%) subjects overall. The prevalence of the metabolic syndrome did not differ significantly between racial/ethnic groups. The prevalence of the metabolic syndrome from lowest to highest quartile of free testosterone concentration was 19.8%, 31.3%, 46.9%, and 35.0% respectively ($p = 0.056$, adjusted for BMI). None of the 52 women with a BMI < 27.0 kg/m^2 had the metabolic syndrome; those in the top BMI quartile were 13.7 times more likely (95% CI, 5.7–33.0) to have the metabolic syndrome compared with those in the lowest quartile; 38% of those with the metabolic syndrome had impaired glucose tolerance compared with 19% without the metabolic syndrome.

34. (*1C+*) **Steinberger E** et al. Utilization of commercial laboratory results in management of hyperandrogenism in women. Endocr Pract 1998;4:1–10.

A review of testosterone levels from 17 studies of 649 total normal women demonstrated a mean testosterone level of 32.0 6 2.7 ng/dl with a 95% CI of 22.1 to 33. The average weighted mean testosterone level in women with symptoms of hyperandrogenism in 14 studies of 996 patients was 62.1 ± 3.2 ng/dl (95% CI, 55.5–68.7). With a typical upper limit of testosterone of 90 to 95 ng/dl in commercial laboratories, most patients with hyperandrogenism are not diagnosed with elevated testosterone levels. An upper limit of 40 ng/dl is recommended.

35. (*1C+*) **Ayala C** et al. Serum testosterone levels and reference ranges in reproductive-age women. Endocr Pract 1999;5:322–329.

The authors performed a cross-sectional retrospective study of 271 reproductive-age women encountered at an endocrinology clinic for complaints of potential thyroid problems. They had no clinical signs of hyperandrogenism and had not used oral contraceptives or glucocorticoids. The serum testosterone level in women with no acne, hirsutism, or menstrual dysfunction was 14.1 ± 0.9 ng/dl (mean $\pm$ standard error of the mean) (95% CI, 12.4–15.8). This group was considered our study reference population. In women with menstrual dysfunction but no acne or hirsutism, the mean testosterone level was significantly higher (17.9 $\pm$ 1.1 ng/dl; 95% CI, 15.7–20.0; $p < 0.002$); with mild hirsutism, it further increased (38.4 $\pm$ 5.1 ng/dl; 95% CI, 27.4–49.4; $p < 0.005$); and with moderate to severe hirsutism, it was still higher (49.0 $\pm$ 2.3 ng/dl; 95% CI, 44.4–53.6; $p < 0.003$). Serum DHEAS levels showed similar patterns. The upper limit (mean $\pm$ 2 standard deviations) of testosterone in our study reference population was 28 ng/dl, a level that provided a sensitivity of 84% for detecting hyperandrogenemia. The authors comment that detection of hyperandrogenemia is essentially impossible when the upper limit of the reference range for testosterone from commercial laboratories (95 ng/dl) is used and suggest a reassessment of the normal range in reference laboratories.

36. (*1C*) **Pasquali R** et al. Clinical and hormonal characteristics of obese amenorrheic hyperandrogenic women before and after weight loss J Clin Endocrinol Metab 1989;68:173–179.

Prospective study of 20 women with obesity and amenorrhea observed the weight-reducing diets. The mean body weight and testosterone levels significantly decreased from 63.8 ng/dl to 40.7 ng/dl ($p < 0.001$). The normal reference range for testosterone used was 26.2 6 7.8 ng/dl. The hirsutism score average before therapy was 16.0 and decreased to 13.6, a reduction of 55% ($p < 0.01$).

37. (*1B*) **Ibanez L, De Zegher F**. Flutamide-metformin plus an oral contraceptive (OC) for young women with polycystic ovary syndrome: Switch from third- to fourth-generation OC reduces body adiposity. Hum Reprod 2004;19:1725–1727. Epub 2004 June.

In this small randomized trial, the antiandrogenic progestogen was compared with standard progestational agent in OCP in lean PCOS women already receiving the antiandrogen flutamide in a study group that had already demonstrated the usefulness of flutamide itself and with OCP. Twenty-nine lean 20-year-old PCOS women who had been taking a combination of flutamide (62.5 mg/day), metformin (850 mg/day), and ethinylestradiol-gestodene for 8 to 15 months were enrolled in an open-label study and were randomized for replacement of the gestodene OC by a drospirenone OC. Assessments were made at randomization and after 6 months of therapy. The switch to drospirenone OC was accompanied by a reduction of total and abdominal fat (mean, −0.8 and −0.5 kg) and by an increment of lean body mass (+0.6 kg; all $p < 0.01$), so that body adiposity was strikingly reduced without changing body weight.

38. (*2B*) **Cagnacci A** et al. Glucose metabolism and insulin resistance in women with polycystic ovary syndrome during therapy with oral contraceptives containing cyproterone acetate or desogestrel. J Clin Endocrinol Metab 2003;88:3621–3625.

Oral contraceptives decrease insulin sensitivity. To determine whether OCPs exacerbate insulin resistance in polycystic ovary syndrome (PCOS), two different OCPs with different progestogens were used. In a 6-month study, lean women with PCOS received either biphasic 40/30 µg ethinyl estradiol (EE) and 25/125 µg desogestrel (DSG; $n = 10$) or monophasic 35 µg EE and 2 mg cyproterone acetate (CPA; $n = 10$). Glucose and C-peptide response to oral glucose were measured, and the minimal model method applied to frequently sampled intravenous GTT was used to calculate glucose utilization. EE/DSG increased the response of C-peptide to OGTT area under the curve and the C-peptide/insulin ratio, implying increased insulin resistance. It impaired insulin-mediated glucose utilization. EE/CPA did not modify responses to OGTT of glucose, insulin, C-peptide, or C-peptide/insulin ratio. It improved insulin sensitivity. The clinical implications of these findings should be studied in larger, more long-term studies.

39. (*1B*) **Farquhar C** et al. Spironolactone versus placebo or in combination with steroids for hirsutism and/or acne (Cochrane Review). In: The Cochrane Library Issue 3, 2002. Oxford, Update Software.

All known randomized controlled trials of spironolactone compared with placebo were identified. After study evaluation, six small trials were further reviewed. Spironolactone at 100 mg daily resulted in statistically significant decreases in hair growth and lower Ferriman–Gallwey scores after 6 months. No clear effect on acne was noted.

40. (*2B*) **Moghetti P** et al. Comparison of spironolactone, flutamide, and finasteride efficacy in the treatment of hirsutism: A randomized, double-blind, placebo-controlled trial. J Clin Endocrinol Metab 2000;85:89–94.

This trial observed 40 hirsute women with a mean age of 20.4 years for 6 months taking placebo, spironolactone (100 mg), flutamide (250 mg), or finasteride (5 mg). After 6 months, the patients receiving active medications all demonstrated significant improvement with no significant difference between the treatment groups. About a 30% reduction in hirsutism score was observed compared with placebo ($p < 0.01$).

41. (*2B*) **Pazos F** et al. Prospective randomized study comparing the long-acting gonadotropin-releasing hormone agonist triptorelin, flutamide, and cyproterone acetate, used in combination with an oral contraceptive, in the treatment of hirsutism. Fertil Steril 1999;71:122–128.

This prospective randomized trial of 39 hirsute women compared GnRHa, cyproterone acetate, and flutamide in combination with a birth control pill over a 9-month period. Although all drugs were effective, the Ferriman–Gallwey scores demonstrated the most rapid response at 3 months with flutamide and cyproterone acetate. The most reduction was seen in the flutamide group by 9 months.

42. *(2B)* **Muderris I** et al. A prospective, randomized trial comparing flutamide (250 mg/d) and finasteride (5 mg/d) in the treatment of hirsutism. Fertil Steril 2000;73:984–987.

This is a randomized prospective study of 70 hirsute women observed for 1 year randomized to either flutamide, 250 mg daily, or finasteride, 5 mg daily. The hirsutism score for flutamide went from 17.8 at baseline to 4.8 at 12 months, a 71% reduction ($p < 0.001$). For finasteride, the hirsutism score went from 19.1 at baseline to 11.3 at 12 months, a 41% reduction ($p < 0.001$). Flutamide was more effective and had fewer side effects than finasteride in this study.

43. *(2B)* **Kelly CJ, Gordon D.** The effect of metformin on hirsutism in polycystic ovary syndrome. Eur J Endocrinol 2002;147:217–221.

This was a randomized, double-blind, placebo-controlled, crossover study of 10 hirsute women over 14 months. The hirsutism score on metformin was 15.8 and 17.5 with placebo ($p = 0.025$). Cycle frequency ($p = 0.008$) also improved, and weight was reduced with metformin ($p = 0.009$).

44. *(2B)* **Hagag P** et al. Androgen suppression and clinical improvement with dopamine agonists in hyperandrogenic-hyperprolactinemic women. J Reprod Med 2001;46:678–684.

Eighty hirsute women with hyperprolactinemia secondary to medications, prolactinomas, and some idiopathic findings. Dopamine agonists were given for about 11 months. The hirsutism scores, prolactin, free testosterone, DHEA-S, and androstenedione levels were significantly improved by therapy.

45. *(1C)* **Lemay A** et al. Rosiglitazone and ethinyl estradiol/cyproterone acetate as single and combined treatment of overweight women with polycystic ovary syndrome and insulin resistance. Hum Reprod 2005; Epub ahead of print.

Twenty-eight obese women with PCOS and elevated insulin levels not improved with diet were treated with either OCP containing ethinyl estradiol and the antiandrogen cyproterone acetate or the thiazolidinedione rosiglitazone for 6 months. After this, both groups received a combination of both agents. In the first group, androgen levels and hirsutism were improved, but an increase in triglycerides and LDL cholesterol was found with no improvement in insulin sensitivity. In the second group, insulin sensitivity improved, with little effect on lipids, androgens, or hirsutism. In combination, improvement occurred in all parameters without a difference in side effects.

46. *(1A)* **Baillargeon JP** et al. Effects of metformin and rosiglitazone, alone and in combination, in nonobese women with polycystic ovary syndrome and normal indices of insulin sensitivity. Fertil Steril 2004;82:893–902.

One hundred lean PCOS subjects were randomized to receive either metformin, 850 mg, rosiglitazone, 4 mg, placebo, or both. Frequencies of ovulation were higher after treatment with an insulin-sensitizing drug (ovulations per subject in 6 months: metformin, 3.3; rosiglitazone, 2.4; and combination, 3.4) than with placebo (0.4). Ovulatory frequencies increased significantly more with metformin than with rosiglitazone, and the combination was not more potent. After treatment, serum free-T levels were comparable among all active treatment groups (metformin, 2.34 pg/ml; rosiglitazone, 3.06 pg/ml; and combination, 2.39 pg/ml) and were significantly lower than in the placebo group (7.26 pg/ml). Compared with placebo, fasting insulin levels, area under the insulin curve during OGTT, the homeostatic model assessment of insulin sensitivity, and OGTT-derived insulin sensitivity index improved significantly after metformin or combination therapies but not after rosiglitazone alone.

Precocious Puberty

47. *(1C+)* **Kaplowitz PB, Oberfield SE,** for the Lawson Wilkins Pediatric Endocrine Society: Reexamination of the age limit for defining when puberty is precocious in girls in the United States: Implications for evaluation and treatment. Pediatrics 1999;104:936–941.

Recommendations based on the Pediatrics Research in Office Settings Network cross-sectional study of 17,077 girls between the ages 3 and 12 years. Breast development occurred earlier than in earlier studies at about age 9.96 years in whites and 8.87 in blacks. With 2.5 to 3 SDs below normal mean, white girls younger than age 7 and black girls younger than age 6 would be considered precocious.

48. *(2B)* **Feuillan PP** et al. Long-term testolactone therapy for precocious puberty in girls with the McCune-Albright syndrome. J Clin Endocrinol Metab 1993;7:647–651.

This was a prospective study of 12 girls at the National Institute of Child Health and Human Development using the aromatase inhibitor testolactone in the treatment of precocious puberty secondary to the McCune–Albright syndrome. The response to treatment was variable and had no impact on final predicated adult height because of the development of CPP triggered by early exposure to sex hormones.

49. *(2C)* **Roth C** et al. Effective aromatase inhibition by anastrozole in a patient with gonadotropin-independent precocious puberty in McCune-Albright syndrome. J Pediatr Endocrinol Metab 2002;15(suppl 3):945–948.

A patient with McCune–Albright syndrome [café-au-lait spots; thelarche at age 2–6/12 yr; menarche at 5–5/12 yr; accelerated bone age (BA, 10 yr)] was treated with the highly selective aromatase inhibitor anastrozole (1 mg once per day). Estradiol levels were normal; anastrozole treatment and accelerated BA progressed only 6 months during 2.5 years of treatment. The potent estrogen-suppressive action and simple dosage regimen of anastrozole suggest it may be advantageous compared with other aromatase inhibitors such as testolactone or antiestrogens.

50. (2B) **Laue L** et al. Treatment of familial male precocious puberty with spironolactone and testolactone. N Engl J Med 1989;320:496–502.

This was a small study of nine boys between ages 3.3 and 7.0 with familial male precocious puberty. After the failure of single-agent therapy, spironolactone and testolactone were combined for a period of 6 to 12 months. This combination controlled symptoms of acne, erectile function, and aggression in all boys. Mean predicted height before and after therapy were not significantly different. With therapy, six of nine boys had development of CPP, which limited overall benefit.

51. (2B) **Leschek EW** et al. Six-year results of spironolactone and testolactone treatment of familial male-limited precocious puberty with addition of deslorelin after central puberty onset. J Clin Endocrinol Metab 1999;84:175–178.

Combined treatment with spironolactone, testolactone, and GnRHa (to help prevent central activation) was studied in 10 boys with familial male-limited precocious puberty. GnRHa was added an average of 2.6 years after starting the earlier therapies. The growth rate normalized by 1 year and remained normal for the remaining 5-year treatment ($p < 0.001$).

52. (2B) **Holland FJ** et al. Ketoconazole in the management of precocious puberty not responsive to LHRH-analogue therapy. N Engl J Med 1985;312:1023–1028.

This was a 1-year study of 3 boys aged 3.3 to 3.9 years old with precocious puberty unresponsive to GnRHa treated with ketoconazole. The testosterone level decreased by 2 days and normalized in two boys and reduced significantly in the third boy, with clinical improvement in behavior and growth velocity.

53. (1C) **Partsch CJ** et al. Management and outcome of central precocious puberty. Clin Endocrinol 2002;56:129–148.

GnRH testing is needed for diagnosis of CPP. Earlier GnRHa trials demonstrate preserved height potential with treatment, although no randomized trials exist on final height in CPP. GnRHa therapy does not improve final height if given past age 8 years in girls.

54. (1C) **Rosenfield RL.** Selection of children with precocious puberty for treatment with gonadotropin-releasing hormone analogs. J Pediatr 1994;124:989–991.

Review of the literature and recommendations for GnRH analogues in CPP based on the literature. Because few prospective data are available, these recommendations remain to be tested in long-term prospective studies.

55. (1C+) **Paterson WF** et al. Auxological outcome and time to menarche following long-acting goserelin therapy in girls with central precocious or early puberty. Clin Endocrinol (Oxf) 2004;61:626–634.

In a study of 46 girls treated with GnRH analogue, 11 had reached their final height of 159.7 cm (-0.63 SD) compared with the mean parental target height of 160.9 cm. Nine of the 11 girls (82%) attained final heights within or above their target range. This subset of girls gained a statistically insignificant excess of weight, but returned to pretreatment BMI at their final heights.

56. (1C+) **Tanaka T** et al. Results of long-term follow-up after treatment of central precocious puberty with leuprorelin acetate: Evaluation of effectiveness of treatment and recovery of gonadal function: The TAP-144-SR Japanese Study Group on Central Precocious Puberty. J Clin Endocrinol Metab 2005;90:1371–1376. Epub 2004 Dec 14.

The effect of leuprorelin treatment on adult height (AH) and recovery of reproductive function was observed in 63 girls and 13 boys with central precocious puberty (CPP). Mean treatment durations were 3.8 ± 2.0 and 4.1 ± 2.5 years, and post-treatment follow-up durations were 3.5 ± 1.3 and 2.6 ± 1.1 yr for girls and boys, respectively. AH was 154.5 ± 5.7 cm for girls, and 89.5% of girls reached AH within their target height range. For boys, AH was 163.2 ± 13.0 cm, and 90.9% reached target height range.

57. (2B) **Walvoord EC, Pescovitz OH.** Combined use of growth hormone and gonadotropin-releasing hormone analogues in precocious puberty: Theoretic and practical considerations. Pediatrics 1999;104:1010–1014.

Review of earlier trials with GnRHa only reveal final adult heights that are 1 to 7 cm below that of the predicted height, although measurements improved 3 to 8 cm over those in patients who were not treated. The studies using combinations of GH with GnRHa have been small and inconsistent but tend to indicate benefit.

58. (2B) **Pasquino AM** et al. Adult height in girls with central precocious puberty treated with gonadotropin-releasing hormone analogues and growth hormone. J Clin Endocrinol Metab 1999;84:449–452.

This was a small prospective study of 10 girls with CPP treated with depot GnRHa plus GH compared with 10 girls with CPP treated with GnRHa alone. Final adult height gain with GnRHa with GH group was 7.9 cm compared with 1.6 cm with GnRHa alone ($p = 0.001$).

59. (2B) **Pasquino AM** et al. Combined treatment with gonadotropin-releasing hormone analog and growth hormone in central precocious puberty. J Clin Endocrinol Metab 1996;81:948–951.

Ten girls and four boys with idiopathic CPP with low predicted height were studied with GnRHa plus growth hormone and compared with findings in 10 girls and four boys who received only GnRHa. After 3 years, the predicted adult height was increased significantly at 13.6 cm in the girls receiving combined therapy. No significant height difference was found in the boys.

60. (*2B*) **Pucarelli I** et al. Effects of combined gonadotropin-releasing hormone agonist and growth hormone therapy on adult height in precocious puberty: A further contribution. J Pediatr Endocrinol Metab 2003;16:1005–1010.

     This study compared 18 girls with idiopathic central precocious puberty treated with a combination of GnRH analogue and growth hormone with 17 subjects who declined growth hormone therapy. Treatment lasted 2 to 4 years. The GnRH agonist–alone group did not achieve an increase of final adult height above predicted adult height calculated for girls with accelerated growth, whereas it was higher than that calculated for average girls. The group treated with combination therapy achieved a final adult height significantly greater than predicted with either method. The second group gained an additional 6 cm of adult height compared with the first. The study demonstrates safety but still with a limited number of subjects.

61. (*2B*) **Heger S** et al. Long-term outcome after depot gonadotropin-releasing hormone agonist treatment of central precocious puberty: Final height, body proportions, bone mineral density, and reproductive function. J Clin Endocrinol Metab 1999;84:4583–4590.

     This was a prospective multicenter trial of 50 women with CPP treated with depot GnRHa for a mean of 4.4 years with therapy ending at a mean age of 11.0 years. About 80% of the women reached a final height within the target height range, whereas before treatment, only 56% of the women had a predicted adult height within the target range.

Male Hypogonadism

62. **Hijazi RA, Cunningham GR.** Andropause: Is androgen replacement therapy indicated for the aging male? Annu Rev Med 2005;56:117—137.

     This review article describes the demographics of androgen deficiency in the aging male as well as the potential risks and benefits of therapeutic intervention.

63. (*2B*) **Sih R** et al. Testosterone replacement in older hypogonadal men: A 12-month randomized controlled trial. J Clin Endocrinol Metab 1997;82:1661–1667.

     This small randomized trial of 15 hypogonadal men (mean age, 68 years) observed over a 1-year period demonstrated improved grip strength and increased hemoglobin levels but no change in memory.

64. (*2C*) **Basaria S, Dobs AS.** Hypogonadism and androgen replacement in elderly men. Am J Med 2001;110:563–572.

     Based on earlier studies, this article recommends treatment of older men with testosterone levels that measure less than 300 ng/dl.

65. **Jockenhovel F.** Testosterone therapy–what, when and to whom? Aging Male 2004;7:319–324.

     This review article outlines the indications for therapy in men with primary or secondary hypogonadism as well as age-related androgen deficiency. Various testosterone preparations are reviewed.

66. (*2C*) **Snyder PJ** et al. Effects of testosterone replacement in hypogonadal men. J Clin Endocrinol Metab 2000;85:2670–2677.

     Prospective study of 14 hypogonadal men taking transdermal testosterone followed up for 3 years showed increased spine and hip bone mineral density and improved energy level and sexual function. Knee-flexion strength was unchanged. Fat-free mass decreased, and lipid levels did not change.

67. (*2B*) **Seidman SN** et al. Testosterone replacement therapy for hypogonadal men with major depressive disorder: A randomized, placebo-controlled clinical trial. J Clin Psychiatry 2001;62: 406–412.

     Thirty-two men with hypogonadism and depression were randomized to placebo or testosterone and observed during a 6-week follow-up. No difference was found between placebo and testosterone groups in depression, although the testosterone-treated group had improved sexual function.

68. (*2B*) **Rabkin JG** et al. A double-blind, placebo-controlled trial of testosterone therapy for HIV-positive men with hypogonadal symptoms. Arch Gen Psychiatry 2000;57:141–147.

     This double-blind, placebo-controlled 3-month trial of testosterone therapy in 74 patients demonstrated significant improvements in muscle mass, libido, energy levels, and depression.

69. (*2B*) **Finkelstein JW** et al. Estrogen or testosterone increases self-reported aggressive behaviors in hypogonadal adolescents. J Clin Endocrinol Metab 1997;82:2423–2438.

     This randomized, double-blind, placebo-controlled, crossover study included 35 hypogonadal boys starting depotestosterone who demonstrated increased physical aggression.

70. **Darby E, Anawalt BD.** Male hypogonadism: An update on diagnosis and treatment. Treat Endocrinol 2005;4:593–309.

     A review article outlining the differential diagnosis of male hypogonadism, appropriate laboratory studies, and therapeutic options.

Infertility

71. (*2C*) **Hull MG** et al. Population study of causes, treatment, and outcome of infertility. Br Med J 1985;291:1693–1697.

     Specialist infertility practice was studied in a group of 708 couples within a population of residents of a single health district in England. At least one in six couples needed specialist help at some time in their lives because of an average infertility of 2.5 years, 71% of whom were trying for their first baby. Those seen at gynecology clinics comprised 10% of new and 22% of all patient visits. Failure of ovulation (amenorrhea or oligomenorrhea) occurred in 21% of cases and was successfully treated (2-year conception rates of 96% and 78%, respectively). Tubal damage (14%) had a poor outlook (19%) despite surgery. Endometriosis accounted for infertility in 6%, although seldom because of tubal damage, cervical mucus defects, or dysfunction in 3%, and coital failure in up to 6%. Sperm defects or dysfunction were the most common defined cause of infertility (24%) and led to a poor chance of pregnancy (0–27%) without donor insemination. Obstructive azoospermia or primary spermatogenic failure was uncommon (2%), and hormonal causes of male infertility were rare. Infertility was unexplained in 28%, and the chance of pregnancy (overall, 72%) was mainly determined by duration of infertility. IVF could benefit 80% of cases of tubal damage and 25% of unexplained infertility (that is, 18% of all cases, representing up to 216 new cases each year per million of the total population).

72. (*1C*) **Guzick DS** et al. Sperm morphology, motility and concentration in fertile and infertile men. N Engl J Med 2001;345:1388–1393.

Two semen specimens from each of the male partners in 765 infertile couples and 696 fertile couples at nine sites were evaluated. Classification and regression-tree analysis were used to estimate threshold values for subfertility and fertility with respect to the sperm's concentration, motility, and morphology. Receiver-operating-characteristic curves were used to assess the relative value of these sperm measurements in discriminating between fertile and infertile men. The subfertile ranges were a sperm concentration less than 13.5×10^6/ml, less than 32% of sperm with motility, and less than 9% with normal morphologic features. The fertile ranges were a concentration of more than 48.0×10^6/ml, more than 63% motility, and more than 12% normal morphologic features. Values between these ranges indicated indeterminate fertility. Extensive overlap was noted between the fertile and the infertile men within both the subfertile and the fertile ranges for all three measurements. Although each of the sperm measurements helped to distinguish between fertile and infertile men, none was a powerful discriminator. The percentage of sperm with normal morphologic features had the greatest discriminatory power. Threshold values for sperm concentration, motility, and morphology can be used to classify men as subfertile, of indeterminate fertility, or fertile. None of the measures, however, is diagnostic for infertility.

73. (*1C*) **Nielsen MS** et al. Comparison of several one-step home urinary luteinizing hormone detection test kits to OvuQuick. Fertil Steril 2001;76:384–387.

This prospective cohort study examined the accuracy and ease of use of one-step home urinary LH-detection kits in 81 cycles in women undergoing artificial insemination. Three different kits detected an LH surge within 12 hours, all with similar accuracy, making the detection of ovulation for fertility management easy and accurate.

74. (*2B*) **Madgar I** et al. A controlled trial of high spermatic vein ligation for varicocele in infertile men. Fertil Steril 1995;63:120–124.

In this randomized, controlled study of high-ligation treatment of varicocele, a significant increase in pregnancy was seen in the first year after surgery compared with findings in a group that waited 1 year before having surgery, with 44.4% pregnancies in the first year compared with 10% in the nonoperated-on group. The group that waited also had a significant increase in pregnancies in the year after surgery, at 60% over a 1-year period.

75. (*2C*) **Vandekerckhove P** et al. Androgens versus placebo or no treatment for idiopathic oligo/asthenospermia (Cochrane Review). In: The Cochrane Library, Issue 3, 2002. Oxford, Update Software.

The 11 trials of 930 men determined whether androgen suppression followed by rebound would improve fertility. No significant benefit was found, with an OR of 1.10 (95% CI, 0.75–1.61). No difference was seen in semen parameters.

76. (*2B*) **Vandekerckhove P** et al. Clomiphene or tamoxifen for idiopathic oligo/asthenospermia (Cochrane Review). In: The Cochrane Library, Issue 3, 2002. Oxford, Update Software.

Five prospective, randomized studies involving 738 men demonstrated a beneficial effect of antiestrogens on testosterone levels, but no difference in the pregnancy rate was found with an OR of 1.26 (95% CI, 0.99–1.56). The overall pregnancy rate was 15.4% in the treated groups compared with 12.5% in the control groups.

77. (*1C*) **Cohlen BJ** et al. Timed intercourse versus intra-uterine insemination with or without ovarian hyperstimulation for subfertility in men (Cochrane Review). In: The Cochrane Library, Issue 3, 2002. Oxford, Update Software.

Seventeen trials comprising 3,662 completed cycles were studied and demonstrated improved pregnancy rates with natural cycle IUI compared with timed intercourse. The OR was 2.43 (95% CI, 1.54–3.83). When combined with controlled ovarian hyperstimulation, IUI improved pregnancy rates compared with timed intercourse with an OR of 2.14 (95% CI, 1.30–3.51).

78. (*1C*) **van Rumste MME** et al. Intra-cytoplasmic sperm injection versus partial zona dissection, subzonal insemination and conventional techniques for oocyte insemination during in vitro fertilization (Cochrane Review). In: The Cochrane Library, Issue 3, 2002. Oxford: Update Software.

A review of 10 studies, eight of which compared ICSI with conventional IVF. In men with normal semen on analysis, no difference in pregnancy rates occurred with ICSI compared with conventional IVF. With a borderline result on semen analysis, ICSI was significantly better than conventional IVF with an OR of 3.79 (95% CI, 2.97–4.85) for fertilization rate per oocyte, although no data on pregnancy rate were compiled.

79. (*1C*) **Pandian Z** et al. In vitro fertilisation for unexplained subfertility (Cochrane Review). In: The Cochrane Library, Issue 3, 2002. Oxford: Update Software.

Four randomized, controlled trials of IVF were studied in unexplained infertility. No difference was noted in pregnancy rates between IVF and IUI with and without hyperstimulation, with an OR of 0.51 (95% CI, 0.23–1.1) in nonstimulated IUI cycles and with an OR of 0.87 (95% CI, 0.42–1.8) in IUI cycles with ovarian stimulation.

80. (*1B*) **Hughes E** et al. Clomiphene citrate for unexplained subfertility in women (Cochrane Review). In: The Cochrane Library, Issue 3, 2002. Oxford, Update Software.

In six studies, clomiphene citrate demonstrated improved pregnancy rates compared with placebo, with an OR of 2.5 (95% CI, 1.35–4.62). It was noted that the risk of ovarian cancer may be increased in women who had 12 cycles of clomiphene or more, although it is not clear whether the infertility is the cause of this finding or whether the medication was responsible.

81. (*1B*) **Hughes E** et al. Clomiphene citrate for ovulation induction in women with oligo-amenorrhea (Cochrane Review). In: The Cochrane Library, Issue 3, 2002. Oxford: Update Software.

Four crossover studies are reviewed. Clomiphene treatment increased pregnancy rate, with an OR of 3.41 (95% CI, 4.23–9.48).

82. (*2C*) **Bristow RE, Karlan BY**. Ovulation induction, infertility, and ovarian cancer risk. Fertil Steril 1996;66:499–507.

This review of four earlier case–control studies, three retrospective cohort studies, and a meta-analysis of three case–control studies and three retrospective cohort studies, as well as a large meta-analysis of three additional case–control studies, indicates that infertility is an independent risk factor for ovarian cancer, and the increased risk is not likely related to fertility medications.

83. (*1B*) **Guzick DS** et al. Efficacy of superovulation and intrauterine insemination in the treatment of infertility. N Engl J Med 1999;340:177–183.

This was a randomized controlled clinical trial of 932 couples with unexplained infertility comparing treatment with ICI, IUI, IUI with superovulation, and ICI with superovulation. IUI with superovulation produced a pregnancy rate of 33%, which was significantly increased over ICI and IUI alone, compared with 18% in the IUI-alone group, 19% in the superovulation with ICI group, and 10% with the ICI-alone study subjects. IUI-alone and ICI with superovulation outcomes were significantly improved over ICI alone.

84. (*1C*) **Klein J, Sauer MV**. Assessing fertility in women of advanced age. Am J Obstet Gynecol 2001;185:758–770.

If the basal FSH is normal, further assessment should be obtained by administering clomiphene, 100 mg, days 5 to 9, with a repeated FSH on day 10. If the pretreatment day 3 FSH or day 10 posttreatment FSH is elevated, then the patient has diminished ovarian reserve and is less likely to become pregnant.

Menopause

85. (*1B*) **MacLennan A** et al. Oral oestrogen replacement therapy versus placebo for hot flushes (Cochrane Review). In: The Cochrane Library, Issue 3, 2002. Oxford, Update Software.

This is an analysis of 21 double-blind, randomized, placebo-controlled trials of oral HRT therapy involved 21 a total of 2,511 women observed from 3 months to 3 years. HRT decreased hot flashes by 77% (95% CI, 58.2–87.5) compared with findings in placebo.

86. (*1B*) **Notelovitz M, Mattox JH**. Suppression of vasomotor and vulvovaginal symptoms with continuous oral 17-beta-estradiol. Menopause 2000;7:310–317.

Oral 17β-estradiol was studied in a randomized, double-blind, multicenter, parallel-group study of 145 postmenopausal women. Hot flashes were significantly reduced by 83% ($p < 0.001$) in the estrogen-treated group. Vaginal dryness was reduced 86.1% with estrogen.

87. (*1B*) **Eriksen B**. A randomized, open, parallel-group study on the preventive effect of an estradiol-releasing vaginal ring (Estring) on recurrent urinary tract infections in postmenopausal women. Am J Obstet Gynecol 1999;180:1072–1079.

This was a randomized prospective study of 53 women treated with a vaginal estrogen ring compared with 55 untreated women. Incidence of urinary tract infection was significantly higher in the untreated women ($p = 0.008$).

88. (*1B*) **Cardozo L** et al. Meta-analysis of estrogen therapy in the management of urogenital atrophy in postmenopausal women: Second report of the Hormones and Urogenital Therapy Committee. Obstet Gynecol 1998;92:722–727.

This meta-analysis of nine randomized controlled studies demonstrated a significant benefit of estrogen, regardless of route of administration, on urogenital atrophy.

89. (*1B*) **Brown JS** et al. Urinary tract infections in postmenopausal women: Effect of hormone therapy and risk factors. Obstet Gynecol 2001;98:1045–1052.

HERS was a randomized, blinded secondary prevention trial of HRT [conjugated equine estrogen/medroxyprogesterone acetate (CEE/MPA)] and heart disease in 2,763 postmenopausal women (aged 44–79 years).

Urinary tract infection frequency was not improved in the HRT group, with an OR of 1.16 (95% CI, 0.99–1.37).

90. (*2B*) **Soares CN** et al. Efficacy of estradiol for the treatment of depressive disorders in perimenopausal women: A double-blind, randomized, placebo-controlled trial. Arch Gen Psychiatry 2001;58:529–534.

This was a randomized, double-blind, placebo-controlled trial of estrogen in 50 postmenopausal women with depressive disorders. Depression significantly decreased in 68% of women treated with 17β-estradiol compared with 20% of placebo-treated patients (*p* = 0.001).

91. (*1B*) **Zweifel JE, O'Brien WH**. A meta-analysis of the effect of HRT upon depressed mood. Psychoneuroendocrinology 1997;22:189–212.

This was a meta-analysis of 14 randomized controlled trials and 12 cohort studies of estrogen and depression in postmenopausal women, demonstrating significant improvement on estrogen.

92. (*1B*) **Hlatky MA** et al., for the Heart and Estrogen/Progestin Replacement Study (HERS) Research Group. Quality-of-life and depressive symptoms in postmenopausal women after receiving hormone therapy: Results from the Heart and Estrogen/Progestin Replacement Study (HERS) trial. JAMA 2002;287:591–597.

This was a randomized clinical trial of HRT therapy in older postmenopausal women with preexisting coronary heart disease. Most women did not have vasomotor symptoms and did not improve with HRT. In women with vasomotor symptoms, depression was improved by HRT.

93. (*1B*) **Espeland MA** et al. Women's Health Initiative Memory Study: Conjugated equine estrogens and global cognitive function in postmenopausal women: Women's Health Initiative Memory Study. JAMA 2004;23:2959–2968.

In this randomized double-blind placebo-controlled trial, 2,808 (ages 65–79) women enrolled in the WHI and "free of probable dementia" were assessed for global cognitive function with a Modified Mini-Mental State Examination (3MSE) yearly for a mean of 5.4 years. The 1,387 subjects receiving 0.625 mg of conjugated estrogen were compared with 1,421 placebo-treated matched controls. The estrogen-treated group had a lower score (and estrogen plus progesterone in another arm of the trial also yielded lower results; *p* < 0.04 for estrogen alone, and *p* < 0.006 for estrogen plus medroxyprogesterone acetate). The risk of having a 10-unit decrease in the 3MSE score was 1.47 (CI, 1.04–2.07) for estrogen versus placebo. It was noted that having a lower cognition at baseline worsened the outlook, but removing women with stroke, dementia, and mild cognitive impairment from the analysis lessened the difference.

94. **Maki PM**. A systematic review of clinical trials of hormone therapy on cognitive function: Effects of age at initiation and progestin use. Ann N Y Acad Sci 2005;1052:182–197.

This literature review suggested that a potential benefit of postmenopausal estrogen use may exist in selected cognitive domains, especially in newly menopausal and symptomatic women and little evidence for benefit at ages older than 65.

95. (*1B*) Writing Group for the Women's Health Initiative Investigators. Risks and benefits of estrogen plus progestin in healthy postmenopausal women. JAMA 2002;288:321–333.

The CEE/MPA arm of the study was a randomized, placebo-controlled primary prevention trial of 16,608 women between 50 and 79 years of age without hysterectomy. This portion of the study was stopped on May 31, 2002, after an average of 5.2 years because of an increased risk of invasive breast cancer, although it was not statistically significant, and lack of cardiovascular benefit exceeding the safety parameters set previously. The absolute risks (per 10,000) and hazard ratios (HRs) with 95% CI noted seven more coronary heart disease sequelae (HR, 1.29; CI, 1.02–1.63), eight more strokes (HR, 1.41; CI, 1.07–1.85), eight more pulmonary emboli (HR, 2.13; CI, 1.39–3.25), and eight additional invasive breast cancers (HR 1.26; CI, 1.00–1.59). The rate of all-case mortality was not affected. It was also noted that there were six fewer colon cancers per 10,000 (HR, 0.63; CI, 0.43–0.92) and five fewer hip fractures (HR, 0.66; CI, 0.45–0.98). These results may be dependent on the use of progestin or a specific progestin and may not apply to other estrogen/progestin combinations and different routes of administration. The CEE-only arm of the study is continuing.

96. (*1B*) **Grady D** et al. Cardiovascular disease outcomes during 6.8 years of hormone therapy: Heart and Estrogen/Progestin Replacement Study follow-up (HERS II). JAMA 2002;288:49–57.

The cohort of 2,321 women observed during follow-up after HERS I, a randomized, double-blind, placebo-controlled secondary prevention trial for cardiovascular disease, for a total of 6.8 years on CEE/MPA. No reduction in cardiovascular events was found in the HRT treatment group. The unadjusted RR was 0.99 (CI, 0.81–1.22) in HERS I and 1.00 (CI, 0.77–1.29) in HERS II.

97. (*1B*) **Hylley S** et al. Noncardiovascular disease outcomes during 6.8 years of hormone therapy (HERS II). JAMA 2002;288:58–66.

The RR for venous thromboembolism in HERS II was 2.08 overall over a 6.8-year period (CI, 1.28–3.40). The RR for biliary surgery was 1.48 (CI, 1.12–1.95), but no difference was found in overall mortality rates.

98. (*1B*) Collaborative Group on Hormonal Factors in Breast Cancer. Breast cancer and hormone replacement therapy: Collaborative reanalysis of data from 51 epidemiological studies of 52,705 women with breast cancer and 108,411 women without breast cancer. Lancet 1997;350:1047–1059.

Meta-analysis of 51 studies and 52,705 women. For patients who had had estrogen replacement therapy for 5 years or longer, the RR of breast cancer was 1.35 (CI, 1.21–1.49) with little effect of estrogen preparation or dose, but limited information was gathered on long-term use of specific preparations.

99. (*1C*) **Lacey JF** et al. Menopausal hormone replacement therapy and risk of ovarian cancer. JAMA 2002;288:334–341.

This is a prospective cohort study of 44,241 women who were studied over a mean of 13.4 years. The "ever" use of estrogen had a RR of 1.6 (CI, 1.2–2.0) and was related to the duration of therapy. For women receiving HRT for between 10 and 19 years, the RR was 1.8 (CI, 1.1–3.0), and for longer than 20 years, the RR was 3.2 (1.7–5.7).

Diabetes Mellitus

Haitham S. Abu-Lebdeh

TYPE 1 DIABETES MELLITUS

Definition

Type 1 diabetes mellitus (DM) is a chronic metabolic disorder of glucose homeostasis that manifests secondary to absolute lack of insulin.

Etiology

It is thought that, in humans, environmental factors such as diet, severe stress, and possibly viral infections, among other unknown factors, may trigger a T-cell–mediated autoimmune destruction of pancreatic beta cells in a susceptible host, which leads to onset of type 1 DM. Family studies failed to identify a specific mendelian pattern of inheritance for this disease [1,2]. However, multiple genetic loci are strongly linked to the development of this polygenic disorder, especially human leukocyte antigen (HLA)-DR and HLA-DQ alleles of the histocompatibility complex. Having a specific genotype that is associated with type 1 DM does not necessarily result in development of this disease; in more than half of monozygotic twins of diabetic patients, type 1 DM will not develop, which suggests an important role for environmental factors in the etiology of this disease. Furthermore, most patients (85%) lack a family history of a similar disorder.

Genetics

Major Histocompatibility Complex Genes

Major histocompatibility complex class II molecules attach to exogenous peptides and then present these peptides on the cell surface for T-cell (CD4) recognition. In humans, class II loci (HLA-DR, -DP, -DQ) of the MHC are located on chromosome six. The findings that type 1 DM develops in 30% to 50% of monozygotic twins, whereas it occurs in only 15% of HLA-identical sibs indicates that other genes must be involved in the etiology of this disease.

Insulin-Dependent Diabetes Mellitus Genes

Multiple other genes are suspected in the development of type 1 DM. These genes are termed insulin-dependent DM (IDDM) genes. IDDM 2 is a nonhistocompatibility gene located on chromosome 11, and it is related to the insulin gene, such that 90% of people with type 1 diabetes are homozygous for this gene compared with 60% of the general population. Other loci such as IDDM 4 (on chromosome 11), IDDM 5 (on chromosome 6), IDDM 8 (on chromosome 6), and IDDM 12 (on chromosome 2) may also play an important role [3].

Epidemiology

Based on National American Health Service surveys, the prevalence of diabetes among people younger than 20 years is around two per 1,000 in the United States. Worldwide incidence and prevalence rates vary significantly, depending on the population, ethnicity, and geography, which suggests an important role for environmental factors. In the United States, the overall incidence of type 1 DM is around 20 per 100,000 per year (Rochester, MN, data 1970–1979). Incidence of type 1 DM is 2 to 3 times more common in whites than in other ethnic groups in the United States.

Type 1 DM also develops in adults; the incidence is estimated around 8.2 per 100,000 annually [4].

Pathophysiology

The development of type 1 DM starts with an unknown precipitating event in a genetically susceptible host (stage 1) that triggers a T-cell–mediated autoimmune destruction of beta cells (stage 2). Over time, generally months to years, progressive loss of insulin is noted and can be detected by using intravenous glucose tolerance tests (stage 3). Subsequently, blood glucose starts to increase, indicating significant beta cell damage (stage 4); this stage may last for several months in children or a longer period in adults and is characterized by clinical diabetes in the presence of normal or low C-peptide levels. Finally, in stage 5, insulin and C-peptide production ceases, and the subject becomes dependent on exogenous insulin for survival.

Diagnosis

Screening

Diabetes develops in 2% to 5% of relatives of patients with type 1 DM. Numerous antibodies directed against islet cell antigens have been identified, but few are of value as research screening tools [5]. In the research setting, autoantibodies are commonly used to predict type 1 DM in studies involving relatives of diabetic patients [6]. Using low titers as diagnostic values predicts future development of type 1 diabetes in a highly sensitive manner, but this, of course, is associated with a significant number of false-positive results. Therefore researchers use combination autoantibodies with the intravenous glucose tolerance test to increase the specificity and yield of these tests.

Islet Cell Cytoplasm Antibodies

The presence of serum islet cell cytoplasmic antibodies (ICAs) is a highly predictive marker for future development of type 1 DM in relatives of family members with that disease. The sensitivity is higher than 80%, and the specificity is higher than 90%. However, these values change significantly depending on the cut-off titers used. The exact antigenic molecules responsible for ICAs are not fully identified, but glutamic acid decarboxylase (GAD) and ICA 512 are thought to contribute significantly to ICA reactivity, and specific assays are available for detection of these autoantibodies [7]. The sensitivity of GAD antibodies and ICA 512 is between 65% and 70% and is highly specific (typically >90%).

Insulin Autoantibodies

Insulin autoantibodies (IAAs) are less sensitive markers than ICAs (25% sensitivity); however, IAAs correlate well with the short duration to development of disease as well as young-age onset of disease. Risk for diabetes increases with higher titers of ICA and the presence of multiple autoantibodies. Autoantibodies may be of value to screen the high-risk population, but lack of an effective intervention is the main barrier against recommendation of such a practice.

First-Phase Insulin Release

Measuring first-phase insulin release during an intravenous glucose tolerance test increases the predicted value of screening with autoantibodies [8]. First-phase insulin release is consistent with progress of diabetes from stage 2 to stage 3. A finding of insulin release that is below the first percentile confers a 90% risk of type 1 diabetes in 3 years in patients with positive ICAs and positive IAAs.

Clinical Manifestations

The most common presenting symptoms are polydipsia and polyuria. Other symptoms frequently encountered in children and adolescents are fatigue, weight loss, and abdominal pain, as well as enuresis. Diabetic ketoacidosis (DKA) is a presenting symptom in 10% to 40% of cases. Frequency of this presentation varies significantly between different countries and may depend on public education, incidence of diabetes in that region, and presence of other people with diabetes in the family, resulting in early detection before development of DKA. These symptoms are not specific for type 1 diabetes and can occur in patients with type 2 diabetes, including DKA.

Most patients with type 1 diabetes are diagnosed at a young age (typically, 30 years); furthermore, in recent years, an increasing number of adolescents have been diagnosed with type 2 DM, especially those who are obese.

Laboratory Findings

The laboratory glucose values used for diagnosis type 1 DM are fasting plasma glucose of 126 mg/dl (7 mmol/L) on more than two occasions, or 2-hour glucose value of 200 mg/dl (11.1 mmol/L) or higher during oral glucose tolerance testing.

Prevention

Prevention of type 1 DM is still in early research stages [9,10]. Currently, no effective preventive strategies exist. Immunomodulating drugs (e.g., azathioprine and cyclosporine) and nicotinamide prevented further beta cell destruction in small studies for a short time. The short-term benefits were not sufficient to indicate long-term use of these potentially toxic medications. The Diabetes Prevention Trial (DPT-1) demonstrated that **using injectable insulin does not prevent diabetes in relatives of diabetic patients.**

Treatment

Insulin

Only insulin is used to control blood glucose in type 1 diabetes. Animal-derived insulins have long been passed over in favor of genetically engineered so-called human insulins. The goal of treatment is to achieve normal plasma glucose around the clock. Intensive therapy delays the onset and progression of microvascular complications of diabetes but may not affect macrovascular mortality [11,12]. The main disadvantages of intensive therapy are the increased frequency of hypoglycemia, ketoacidosis, and weight gain [13]. Ideally, reducing the hemoglobin A_{1c} to less than 7% (ADA) or less than 6.5% (American Association of Clinical Endocrinologists) is the goal in type 1 DM patients [14], but clinicians must also consider the risk of hypoglycemia and train patients to recognize it.

Insulin Regimens

Conventional Therapy. The regimen of twice-daily injections with basal insulin (typically intermediate-acting insulin) and a bolus insulin (regular or rapid-acting analogues)—known as conventional therapy—is associated with variable and inferior glycemic control in comparison with intensive insulin therapy regimens and therefore has been abandoned in favor of other insulin regimens. Evidence supports intensive glycemic control by using multiple daily injections or insulin pump rather than two-injection conventional therapy [15]. A twice-daily split insulin regimen (conventional therapy) and once-daily injections are not recommended because of difficulty in achieving the goal and the inability to adjust insulin doses appropriately to prevent hyperglycemia in type 1 DM. These two modalities of treatment, however, are frequently used by general practitioners at the onset of disease until the patient is transferred to the care of a specialist.

Intensive Insulin Therapy. Insulin Pump: Portable, external insulin infusion pumps have undergone significant improvement in the past two decades [16]. Insulin is delivered continuously at a set basal rate (~60% of total daily insulin). Pumps can be programmed to increase the basal insulin at night to counteract morning hyperglycemia. At mealtime, bolus doses of insulin are provided to cover meal glucose excursions. Use of such a pump requires frequent monitoring of blood glucose and predisposes to site infections and diabetic ketoacidosis, but usually results in better glycemic control.

Multiple Daily Injections: Multiple daily injections (MDIs) refers to three or more injections with very rapid acting analogues before meals. In addition, basal insulin is provided at dinner (glargine or detemir) or at bedtime (NPH or glargine or detemir) for background coverage over a 24-hour period. Frequently, if NPH or detemir is used, a second dose is provided before breakfast. In type 1 DM, intensive insulin therapy (pumps or MDIs) provides lower hemoglobin A_{1c} and significantly reduces the risk of microvascular complications. These data are derived primarily from the results of the Diabetes Control and Complications Trial (DCCT/EDIC) cohort, which also involved a comprehensive patient-support program of diet, exercise, and close supervision with instructions.

Types of Insulin

- *Inhaled insulin.* Available as exubera (1 or 3 mg) blisters of homogenized powder formulation. The powder is inhaled via a special inhaler. This form of therapy is contraindicated in patients who smoke or are diagnosed with chronic obstructive pulmonary disease (COPD) or asthma. A 1-mg blister provides an effect almost equivalent to 3 units of regular insulin, and a 3-mg blister is almost equivalent to 8 units of regular insulin.
- *Very rapid acting insulin analogues.* The available agents, insulin aspart (NovaLog), insulin glulisine (Apidra) or insulin lispro (Humalog), are engineered so that after injection, the insulin dissociates quickly from the aggregate. Therefore these insulins have rapid onset of action and short duration of activity (Table 6.1). These agents are used specifically to lower glucose after a meal and to correct postprandial hyperglycemia, and therefore are called "meal" insulins. These insulins are at least as effective as regular insulin [15,17–19]. Furthermore, their use can reduce the frequency of hypoglycemia and can be safely used in patients with unpredictable eating patterns.
- *Regular insulin.* The main disadvantage for use of regular insulin is the need to inject it 30 to 45 minutes before meals, which may be inconvenient or may be associated with hypoglycemia if the meal is delayed or not eaten at all.
- *Intermediate-acting insulin.* NPH and Lente insulin have a longer duration of action than regular insulin and are used mainly to provide basal insulin coverage [20]. These insulins are not used to control postprandial glucose levels but, when given appropriately, are effective in reducing fasting plasma glucose.

Table 6.1.   Insulin Types and Timeframe of Action

Insulin	Onset (hr)	Peak (hr)	Duration (hr)
Regular	0.5	2–4	6–8
Aspart, Glulisne, Lispro	0.2	1–2	2–4
Inhaled	0.1	1	6
NPH, Lente	2	6–10	12–18
Glargine	2	Peakless	24–30
Detemir	2	Peakless	6–24

- *Long-acting insulin analogues.* Glargine (Lantus) and detemir (Levemir) are long-acting synthetic preparations that are relatively peakless, with a lower incidence of hypoglycemia and a prolonged duration of action. The main disadvantage is that they cannot be mixed with other insulins. Detemir insulin has significantly shorter duration of action than glargine and may be more similar to NPH in clinical practice. However, it is associated with less nocturnal hypoglycemia than NPH.
- *Premixed insulins.* Mixtures of two kinds of insulin do not allow for flexibility and require more skill in adjustment of insulin to achieve a therapeutic end, and thus such a combination should not be the drug of choice.
- *Pramlintide*: Pramlintide (15–60 μg) is a synthetic analogue of human amylin that slows gastric emptying and improves A_{1c} concentrations mainly by reducing postprandial glucose excursions. In patients with type 1 diabetes, it is used only with meal insulins. It is recommended to reduce the insulin dose by 50% when pramlintide is started.

Diet

Dietary-management regimens improve glycemic control, but insufficient evidence is available to recommend a specific diet plan over another. Dietary knowledge is essential for carbohydrate counting if used in patients using MDIs or insulin pumps. Eating disorders are more common in type 1 DM, especially in adolescents [21], and this adversely influences glycemic control. Therefore regular psychological assessment and instruction regarding healthy eating habits are recommended [22].

Exercise

Aerobic exercise is recommended. In addition, persistent training with light weights and high repetitions could be useful [23]. Of note, exercise during a state of insulin deficiency as manifested by higher blood glucose before the activity, may be associated with hyperglycemia subsequent to exercise, and therefore blood glucose monitoring is helpful, especially in cases of unanticipated exercise [24]. Insulin should not be injected into the exercising limb because continuous muscle movement results in increased insulin release. The abdomen is the preferred site for insulin injection.

High-intensity exercise may result in increased albuminuria and may in theory be associated with adverse effects. However, no evidence supports clinical progression of retinopathy or kidney disease with high-intensity exercise. The risk of myocardial infarction (MI) is higher in people with type 1 DM, and thus the American Diabetes Association recommends cardiac-stress exercise testing for patients who are older than 35 years, who have been diagnosed with type 1 diabetes for longer than 15 years (especially those who have evidence of clinical autonomic neuropathy, peripheral vascular disease, or microvascular disease), or who have a significant cardiovascular risk profile. The evidence to support such recommendations is inadequate.

Blood Glucose Monitoring

Learning blood glucose self-monitoring skills is essential for type 1 DM. It is important for diabetic patients to monitor for hypoglycemia and significant hyperglycemia to avoid complications. Little evidence indicates that frequent blood glucose self-monitoring translates to better glucose control by using standard glucometers. This might be secondary to lack of adjustment or intervention by physicians or patients. Continuous-monitoring real-time glucose sensors are gaining acceptance among patients. Glucose measurements using these devices correlate very well with standard glucometer readings and are considered accurate within 95%. Such devices in patients with type 1 or type 2 DM were superior to standard meters in reducing duration of hyperglycemia and hypoglycemia.

Transplantation

Pancreas transplantation is considered in patients planning to have a kidney transplant for treatment of end-stage renal disease, given that pancreas transplantation may improve the survival of the transplanted kidney, may improve hypoglycemia, and may partially reverse neuropathy. Pancreas transplantation alone may be considered in patients with severe complications of diabetes. Islet cell transplantation has a significant advantage over whole-pancreas transplantation but requires special experience that is not available in many centers.

TYPE 2 DIABETES MELLITUS

Definition
Type 2 DM is a chronic disorder of glucose homeostasis characterized by hyperglycemia and impaired insulin action, with abnormal pancreatic insulin secretion as well as increased rates of hepatic glucose production. Unlike type 1 DM, no absolute physiologic lack of insulin is present.

Etiology
The concordance rate of type 2 DM in identical twins is 70% to 90%, with a strong familial clustering of type 2 DM, suggesting a genetic etiology. No specific gene has been identified as the cause of type 2 DM, and multiple genetic abnormalities may be involved. Insulin resistance alone does not explain diabetes; another defect superimposed on insulin resistance may be responsible for impaired insulin secretion. This defect may be environmental (associated with obesity, nutrition, or reduced activity) or genetic.

Risk Factors
1. Obesity. Risk for type 2 DM increases with obesity as measured by the body mass index in both men and women [25]. Central fat (so-called apple distribution) increases the risk of type 2 DM in addition to body mass index measurements. Weight gain in adulthood of more than 10 kg in men or more than 8 kg in women is associated with increased risks of DM regardless of the body mass index.
2. Ethnicity. The reasons behind ethnic variation are unclear, but general themes were observed among minorities at increased risk for diabetes. These include abandoning traditional lifestyle behaviors and adopting new behaviors that include reduced physical activity and increased caloric intake.
3. Family history of type 2 DM.
4. Subjects with elevated fasting glucose measurements or with high postprandial measurements are at increased risk for overt diabetes development.
5. Lack of exercise. This is an independent factor from the body mass index. Reduced activities are associated with the development of type 2 DM.
6. Diet. Consuming foods that are low in fiber and high in glycemic loads is associated with increased risk of DM.
7. Hypertension is associated with DM.

Epidemiology
Based on U.S. national health surveys, it is estimated that 6.2% of the U.S. population has diabetes. It is also estimated that for each 11 subjects diagnosed with diabetes, six others would meet the criteria for diagnosis of type 2 diabetes but have not been diagnosed. The prevalence of diabetes increases with age, and 20% of subjects older than 65 have diabetes. Worldwide, the prevalence of diabetes differs significantly between one region and another (Micronesian Naurans rates ~40%).

Diabetes is the sixth leading cause of death in the United States, and most deaths are attributed to heart disease. The American Diabetes Association estimates health care costs that are specifically due to diabetes (direct medical costs) at $44 billion in 1997, plus another $54 billion in indirect costs of disability, work loss, and premature mortality.

Pathophysiology
Type 2 diabetes is usually the result of three processes: insulin resistance, excess glucose production by liver, and impaired insulin secretion.

Early in diabetes, plasma glucose levels remain normal despite insulin resistance because beta cells compensate by increasing the insulin output. Eventually, beta cells are unable to sustain production, and impaired glucose tolerance develops. This is marked by postprandial glucose elevation.

Insulin resistance and impaired insulin secretion result in failure to suppress gluconeogenesis, thus causing fasting hyperglycemia and then overt diabetes. This also causes an inhibition of glucose storage after a meal, causing postprandial hyperglycemia. Other hormones may play a role in increasing hepatic glucose production, independent of insulin.

Diagnosis

Clinical Manifestations

Unlike patients with type 1 DM, most patients with type 2 diabetes do not show the classic symptoms of hyperglycemia, as mentioned previously. More than half of patients in the United States are not diagnosed. The most common classic symptoms in type 2 DM are excessive thirst followed by easy fatigability, neurologic symptoms, and blurred vision.

Laboratory Findings

Plasma glucose levels that are thought to be, in the long term, associated with retinopathy and proteinuria are used to diagnose diabetes. Several diagnostic modalities have been proposed to separate those patients with hyperglycemia who are at increased risk for development of microvascular complications from those who are at low risk but who do have hyperglycemia. Currently, two main diagnostic criteria are used: the American Diabetes Association criteria, which use fasting plasma glucose, and the World Health Organization criteria, which depend on oral glucose tolerance test results. Various populations were followed up prospectively by using a 2-hour glucose test after a 75-g glucose load for the development of microvascular complications. A postchallenge plasma glucose level of 200 mg/dl (11.1 mmol/L) seemed to differentiate reliably subjects who experience microvascular complications from those who do not. These studies are the basis of the World Health Organization diagnostic system.

In 1997, the American Diabetes Association Expert Committee recommended another set of criteria, which are more widely accepted and currently widely used in clinical practice. Based on studies that indicate a fasting plasma glucose level of 126 mg/dl (7 mmol/L) predicts a postchallenge plasma glucose level of 200 mg/dl (11.1 mmol/L), the American Diabetes Association recommends the use of a fasting glucose level of 126 mg/dl (7 mmol/L) as the cut-off point for diagnosis. Therefore fasting plasma glucose testing in the morning before 9 a.m. is the method routinely used in practice in the United States. Hyperglycemia that is below the cut-off point of 126 mg/dl (7 mmol/L) is termed impaired fasting glucose.

Screening

Identifying patients with asymptomatic diabetes is an effective strategy because of the availability of effective treatments that reduce the morbidity and the progression of disease. Screening adults 45 years or older every 3 years is the consensus. Screening adults younger than 45 years old with risk factors may also be a cost-effective strategy. Risk factors include family history of diabetes, overweight defined as body mass index of 25 kg/m^2 or higher, habitual physical inactivity, being a member of a high-risk ethnic or racial group, previously identified impaired fasting glucose or impaired glucose tolerance, hypertension, dyslipidemia, history of gestational DM or delivery of a baby weighing more than 9 lb (4 kg) [26], and polycystic ovary syndrome.

Prevention

The risk of type 2 DM in people with impaired glucose tolerance may be altered with metformin and lifestyle changes, as observed in the Diabetes prevention program, as well as Acarbose, as observed in the STOP-NIDDM study, and orlistat, as observed in the XENDOS study. Angiotensin-converting enzyme (ACE) inhibitors and angiotensin blockers have been observed (CAPPP, HOPE, ALLHAT, LIFE, SCOPE, and VALUE studies) to be associated with reduced rates of development of DM; however, this was not evaluated prospectively as a primary point. Results from ongoing prospective studies should confirm or refute this observation.

Treatment

Weight Reduction and Dietary Restrictions

The effect of diet on glucose control is observed early, before any demonstrable weight loss. Weight loss itself is also associated with significant improvement in glycemic control, whether it is through diet and exercise, behavioral modification, weight-loss medications, or bariatric surgery [27]. Programs that are associated with 5% to 10% weight loss in 3 to 4 months result in significantly improved glycemic control. Larger weight-loss percentage may result in normalization of fasting glucose in newly diagnosed diabetic patients. In the U.K. Prospective Diabetes Study (UKPDS), diabetic patients with mild fasting hyperglycemia were more likely to normalize glucose measurements than were patients with higher fasting glucose measurements [28]. Using a very-low-calorie diet (800 kcal/day) produces greater initial improvement in glycemic control than low-calorie diets (1,000–1,200 kcal/day), but no measurable difference exists between these diets in the long term at 6 to 12 months. Using Orlistat (120 mg TID) in patients with type 2 DM is associated with modest weight loss, but also with a reduced need for insulin or oral diabetes medicines and improved A_{1c} (0.5% over placebo). Other weight-loss medications are currently being developed and may provide additional forms of treatment for patients with type 2 DM. For example, rimonabant is the first in a new class of drugs that selectively block the cannabinoid-1 (CB1) receptor. This receptor system is involved in weight and appetite regulation. In the RIO-DIABETES trial, patients with type 2 diabetes received either 5 mg or 20 mg of rimonabant once daily or placebo. Patients receiving 20-mg rimonabant lost weight, and in addition, A_{1c} levels were reduced by 0.6% from baseline.

Exercise

Exercise in combination with diet results in maintenance of weight loss and therefore is recommended for patients with type 2 DM [29].

Drug Therapy

Biguanides

Metformin (500–2,550 mg/day) is available in immediate-release and also extended-release forms. In the UKPDS, overweight patients assigned to metformin had fewer diabetes-related complications and lower mortality rates than did those using insulin [30]. Compared with the conventionally treated group (using diet), patients using metformin had a 32% risk reduction for diabetes complications, a 42% risk reduction for diabetes-related death, and a 36% reduction for all-cause mortality. Therefore metformin is recommended as the first-line oral agent to be used in patients with type 2 DM [31]. Metformin reduces plasma glucose mainly by altering hepatic gluconeogenesis and thereby reducing hepatic glucose release. Furthermore, insulin-stimulated glucose uptake in the muscle is also enhanced by the use of metformin. Metformin does not increase insulin release, and therefore it is not associated with hypoglycemia and does not cause weight gain. Typically, metformin reduces hemoglobin A_{1c} by 1% to 2%. The most common side effects are gastrointestinal (diarrhea and indigestion), but lactacidosis, a very rare side effect, is the most serious adverse event and could be fatal, especially if metformin is used in patients with renal impairment, cardiac or pulmonary failure, or sepsis.

Sulfonylureas

Second-generation sulfonylureas are used mainly in the United States and have replaced the first-generation agents tolbutamide and chlorpropamide. All agents, however, reduce glucose levels effectively and are comparable in efficacy (lowering hemoglobin A_{1c} by 1%–2%). All sulfonylureas function by stimulating insulin release. Patients who fail to respond to sulfonylureas are typically thin and have low insulin levels [32]. The most common side effects are weight gain of 2 to 3 kg and hypoglycemia (1%–2%) especially in the elderly. The results of the UKPDS show that the use of sulfonylureas does not increase cardiovascular events or cardiovascular motility in comparison with findings in patients who are treated with diet alone [33]. Sulfonylureas are used in combination therapy with other oral agents, as well as insulin, with variable successful results [34–38].

α-Glucosidase Inhibitors
Acarbose (75–300 mg/day) and miglitol (75–300 mg/day) inhibit α-glucosidase activity in the luminal intestinal brush border, leading to delay in absorption of carbohydrates and therefore producing a reduction in postprandial glucose concentrations [39,40]. These agents are frequently associated with bloating, flatulence, and diarrhea, and therefore are not commonly prescribed. Typically, hemoglobin A_{1c} decreases by 0.5% to 1.8% without significant weight gain or hypoglycemia.

Meglitinides
Repaglinide (0.5–16 mg/day) and nateglinide (60–360 mg/day) stimulate insulin release through a mechanism different from that of sulfonylureas [41]. These medications have a short duration of action and therefore should be used before meals. Meglitinides effectively reduce hemoglobin A_{1c} by 1% to 2%. Side effects include hypoglycemia and weight gain.

Thiazolidinediones
Rosiglitazone (2–8 mg/day) and pioglitazone (15–45 mg/day) mediate their effect by binding to nuclear receptor peroxisome proliferator-activated receptor-γ and enhance tissue (muscle) sensitivity to insulin [42]. The most common side effects are weight gain and fluid retention (edema), so these medications should be avoided in patients with congestive heart failure, especially NYHA class III and IV. The original thiazolidinedione medication, troglitazone, was withdrawn from the market because of fatal hepatic disease. In clinical trials, rosiglitazone and pioglitazone did not show evidence of hepatotoxicity. These agents are effective as monotherapeutic agents or in combination therapy and reduce hemoglobin A_{1c} by 1.0% to 1.5%. They can be used in patients with renal impairments and have been used effectively in combination treatments and with insulin. Thiazolidinediones use is safe in relation to coronary disease or stroke, as observed in "PROactive" study.

Insulin
See the section on type 1 DM regarding types of insulins. Insulin therapy should not be delayed in patients with type 2 DM, especially if glycemic control is suboptimal with the use of oral agents [43,44]. The primary adverse effects are weight gain (4 kg) and hypoglycemia. No significant evidence indicates that exogenous insulin use is associated with cardiovascular events. In the UKPDS, the use of insulin or sulfonylureas was not associated with increased cardiovascular disease, in comparison with findings in patients treated with diet alone.

Once-daily injection regimen: Either intermediate- or long-acting insulin is used in this regimen. This regimen is associated with fewer hypoglycemic episodes but usually results in variable suboptimal glucose levels.

Twice-daily injection: Prebreakfast and predinner twice-daily NPH or Lente (so-called split regimen) is frequently used in type 2 DM patients. If prelunch or bedtime glucose are elevated, then very rapid acting insulin is added (i.e., split mixed regimen) with effective results. In some patients, this regimen can be substituted with premixed insulin, but this has the disadvantage of not allowing proper adjustments of insulin doses.

Intensive insulin therapy: Similar to type 1 DM, the MDI regimen is sometimes used in type 2 DM but is associated with weight gain.

Pramlintide
See section on type I DM. Pramlintide (60–120 μg) has been used in type 2 DM patients in combination with insulin, sulfonylureas, and metformin.

Exenatide (5–10 μg BID injections) is a long-acting glucagon-like peptide-1 (GLP-1) receptor agonist. The gut peptide GLP-1 is secreted in response to nutrients and stimulates glucose-dependent insulin secretion, promotes beta cell proliferation, and inhibits apoptosis. GLP-1 also inhibits gastric emptying, food intake, and glucagon secretion. Furthermore, GLP-1 potently stimulates insulin secretion and reduces blood glucose in human subjects with type 2 DM. Dipeptidyl peptidase-4 (DPP-4) degrades GLP in the plasma quickly. Exenatide is more resistant to DPP-4 than is natural GLP-1. Using exenatide is associated with mild to moderate gastrointestinal side effects but no weight gain. Other agents that use the GLP-1 system are currently being developed for the treatment of type 2 diabetes (DPP-4 inhibitors).

Combination Therapy
Several combination regimens of sulfonylureas, metformin, or thiazolidinediones with insulin have been investigated [45] and are successful in reducing hemoglobin A_{1c} as well as fasting plasma glucose measurements, but these combinations are more expensive than insulin alone.

Transplantation
Pancreatic transplantation is not recommended for patients with type 2 DM.

DIABETIC KETOACIDOSIS

Definition
DKA is an acute, life-threatening complication of diabetes characterized by hyperglycemia, ketonemia, and a wide anion-gap metabolic acidosis. DKA occurs mainly in patients with type 1 DM and may occur in other types of diabetes [46].

Etiology
Its etiology is absolute or relative insulin deficiency in the presence of excessive counter-regulatory hormones, leading to numerous metabolic abnormalities, diuresis, and ketoacid accumulation. The process could be triggered by various precipitating factors (e.g., pneumonia, urinary tract infections, and other infections; 25%) [47] or stress associated with severe or acute illness, including coronary disease, gastrointestinal hemorrhage, and trauma (10%–20%). It can also be the first presentation of diabetes in a previously undiagnosed patient (10%–30%). In insulin-requiring diabetic patients, omission of insulin or nonadherence to therapy or suboptimal dosing preoperatively or postoperatively may precipitate DKA (30%). In patients using insulin pumps, DKA occurs because of catheters that are dislodged or obstructed [13]. Finally, medications, especially those that increase insulin resistance (e.g., glucocorticoids, β-agonists, and sympathomimetics), can precipitate DKA.

Epidemiology
The incidence of DKA seems to be increasing. In the United States, the incidence of hospital admission increased from four per 1,000 to 12 per 1,000 from 1980 to 1989. Generally speaking, DKA occurs in patients with type 1 DM, but patients at high risk for DKA include those at extremes of age, those with poor prior glycemic control, and those who use insulin pumps [48,49].

Pathophysiology
Elevated levels of counter-regulatory hormones are necessary for the development of DKA in diabetic patients. Glycogenolysis is enhanced especially by glucagon, catecholamines, and low insulin levels. Furthermore, glucagon excess and insulin deficiency result in enzymatic changes in the liver that ultimately shift pyruvate away from glycolysis toward the glucose synthesis. Excessive counter-regulatory hormones in the absence of insulin lead to lipolysis and excess free fatty acid release from adi-

pose tissue, which is then converted to ketoacids in the liver. Ketoacids are buffered by bicarbonate, leading to its depletion.

Diagnosis

Laboratory Findings

No specific laboratory criteria exist for the diagnosis of DKA; however, the presence of wide anion gap $[(Na + K) - (Cl + HCO_3) > 16 \text{ mEq/L}]$ and ketonemia in a patient with diabetes is consistent with DKA. Most patients' glucose levels are high, exceeding 250 mg/dl (14 mmol/L), but occasionally glucose levels are normal, especially if the episode is preceded by long periods of fasting. Hematocrit and mean corpuscular volume increase in DKA. Glucose enters the red blood cell easily despite lack of insulin, which leads to osmotic swelling of the blood cell. Serum sodium levels vary significantly despite total body sodium deficit. Triglyceride levels are frequently elevated, mainly as a result of insulin deficiency and reduced clearance, but they typically return to normal with proper treatment of DKA. Initially, serum potassium levels are high or high normal secondary to the dehydration of acidosis, although total body potassium stores are depleted. Serum phosphate levels are also elevated initially, and both potassium and phosphate decrease quickly and significantly with treatment of DKA. Both amylase and lipase levels may be elevated in DKA without abdominal symptoms of pancreatitis or even hypertriglyceridemia; however, careful evaluation for possible pancreatitis should be pursued if lipase is elevated.

Clinical Manifestations

Symptoms develop rapidly in patients using pumps but may take several days in other diabetic patients. Ketonemia results in nausea and vomiting and the characteristic odor of acetone on the breath. Less frequently, abdominal pain is the presenting symptom. Hyperglycemia and diuresis produce symptoms of dehydration and may progress to hypovolemic shock. Metabolic acidosis causes rapid and deep respirations (Kussmaul sign). Impaired mentation is also seen in 10% of DKA patients and may quickly proceed to coma, especially if the serum osmolality exceeds 340 mOsm/kg.

Treatment

Fluid Replacement

Some controversy exists on how best to administer fluids in patients with DKA. In patients without renal impairment or shock, low-rate saline infusions of 500 ml/hr over 4 hours and then 250 ml/hr were more effective than more rapid rates of infusion. However, in the setting of hypotension, saline should be given more rapidly, and treatment should be guided by using central venous pressure measurements. Generally speaking, rates of 500 to 1000 ml/hr of normal saline for the first 1 to 2 hours have been used to expand circulatory volume, followed by 250 to 500 ml/hr of normal saline or half-normal saline. It is generally accepted that half the estimated fluid deficit should be corrected in the first 12 hours. Dextrose and water should be added after glucose levels decrease to 250 mg/dl (14 mmol/L).

Insulin

With equivalent doses, intravenous insulin was shown to be as effective as subcutaneous or intramuscular insulin in reducing length of hospital stay, but intravenous insulin led to a faster initial decline in glucose and had more predictable effects [50]. Intravenous insulin should be administered early to reduce hospital stay and to ensure faster recovery. Low-dose insulin (e.g., 0.1 unit/kg) is as effective as high-dose bolus therapy of 50 to 150 units but is associated with reduced instances of hypoglycemia and hypokalemia [51]. Therefore the recommendation is for low-dose insulin bolus intravenously followed by maintenance therapy.

Maintenance Insulin

Intravenous insulin at a rate of 0.1 to 0.2 units/kg/hr is maintained until acidosis is mostly corrected (pH > 7.3, bicarbonate > 18 mEq/L, or anion gap < 14 mEq/L).

Frequently, serum glucose decreases to less than 250 mg/dl (14 mmol/L) before acidosis is corrected. Insulin infusion should continue; however, a dextrose-and-water infusion should be started to prevent hypoglycemia. This practice of maintaining intravenous insulin is mainly to allow ketone clearance and correction of acidosis [52].

Bicarbonate
Controversy remains about the use of intravenous bicarbonate in DKA. No clear benefits were shown with intravenous bicarbonate administration with patients with pH that exceeds 6.9 [53,54], and it can be associated with adverse events of hypokalemia and cerebral edema in children [55]. Therefore bicarbonate use is not recommended. No studies have addressed the use of bicarbonate in patients with severe acidosis (pH < 6.9) or hypotension. In these patients, the practice has been to administer bicarbonate in doses of 44 to 133 mEq. No evidence supports or opposes such a practice.

Potassium
Potassium levels decrease quickly with management of acidosis because of intracellular compartment shift. Therefore if serum potassium levels are low or normal, intravenous potassium should be administered immediately. If potassium levels are elevated (>5.5 mEq/L), potassium administration could be delayed until levels decrease to less than 5.5 mEq/L and the patient can urinate. Potassium is administered in 20 to 40 mEq/L of fluid provided as potassium chloride.

Phosphate
Serum phosphate levels also decreased to normal levels with proper management of DKA. Potential risk is associated with moderate to severe hypophosphatemia, including rhabdomyolysis, hemolysis, and impaired cardiac function. However, these are rarely found clinically. In small studies, adding phosphate to intravenous fluid did not affect the rate of recovery and was associated with minimal and nonsignificant lower serum calcium levels [56]. Therefore phosphate treatment is not recommended unless evidence is found of significant hypophosphatemia.

Finally, in treating DKA, special attention should be directed to identifying as well as treating the triggering factors (e.g., urine culture, chest radiograph, and electrocardiogram).

Monitoring Therapy
Most patients with DKA experience hyperchloremic acidosis with therapy, especially in the first 8 hours. Therefore observing serum bicarbonate levels, anion gap, and pH is better than measuring any single parameter. Correction of two of the three parameters (bicarbonate >18, pH >7.3, and anion gap <14 mEq/L) is considered an adequate target of therapy. Assessing levels of urinary ketones as measured by standard assays measures only acetone and acetoacetate but not the primary ketone formed in DKA, which is β-hydroxybutyrate, and therefore management of urine ketones should not be a target of therapy. As DKA is treated, β-hydroxybutyrate is converted to acetoacetate as well as acetone, both of which are readily measured by urinalysis, and therefore excessive urine ketones can be seen, whereas serum levels of β-hydroxybutyrate have attained normal levels.

Prognosis
Mortality rates vary between 0.5% and 3.3%. Most patients at increased risk of death with DKA are elderly patients who have shock, altered mentation, acute respiratory distress syndrome, high osmolality, severe hyperglycemia, and acidemia. In children, cerebral edema carries a high risk of death or permanent damage [57–59]. In adults, clinically detectable cerebral edema is rare and usually asymptomatic, but minor elevation in cerebrospinal fluid pressures has been documented; however, it is usually transient.

HYPEROSMOLAR COMA

Definition
Hyperosmolar coma is defined as extreme hyperglycemia that is associated with hyperosmolality, dehydration, and altered mental status without overt ketosis.

Etiology
A serious infection or an acute illness usually precipitates hyperosmolar coma in diabetic patients. For many patients, hyperosmolar coma is the first manifestation of type 2 diabetes and may be related to severe dehydration and lack of access to drinking water [60]. Noncompliance with insulin treatment and surgical trauma are other important precipitating factors [61].

Pathophysiology
Reduced insulin sensitivity or relative insulin deficiency leads to hyperglycemia (discussed earlier in this chapter). Hyperglycemia causes osmotic diuresis and results in significant dehydration. Overt ketosis does not form because insulin is not lacking, and low levels of insulin prevent lipolysis.

Epidemiology
Hyperosmolar coma is an uncommon but potentially fatal complication of diabetes [62,63]. Some 4,500 hospitalizations in the United States resulted from hyperosmolar coma in 1990, most in women older than 60 years. Mortality rates are high, ranging from 15% to 60%. Mortality correlates with high osmolality, azotemia, and age [64].

Diagnosis

Clinical Manifestations
Polydipsia, polyuria, weakness, and fatigue are present in most patients and may precede hospitalization by weeks. These symptoms are usually followed by progressive mental-status impairment in 50% of patients. Seizures are not common, but symptoms may be similar to those of an acute stroke, and patients may be in a coma, especially if serum osmolality is very high. Fever, nausea, and vomiting are frequently present at diagnosis (40%–65%).

Laboratory Findings
Plasma glucose concentrations are usually significantly elevated—around 600 mg/dl (33 mmol/L) or higher. Serum osmolality is increased and usually more than 320 mOsm/L. Urea and sometimes creatinine are elevated because of dehydration. Minimal acidosis secondary to starvation and lactic acid accumulation as well as mild ketosis (i.e., starvation) may be present, but arterial pH is usually higher than 7.3.

Treatment
Treatment recommendations are derived from retrospective reports [65–68]. Very few studies have addressed treatment of hyperosmolar coma in diabetes [65]. Recommendations are derived from consensus statements and modified from treatment recommendations for ketoacidosis.

Fluids
The most essential part of such treatment is fluid management, preferably in the intensive care unit, with monitoring and under the guidance of central venous pressure measurements. Normal saline is infused at a rate of 1,000 ml/hr for 1 to 2 hours to normalize blood pressure. In cases of severe dehydration, hypernatremia usually is present, and therefore subsequent fluid infusions are managed with 0.45% saline or at rates of 250 to 500 ml/hr, or dextrose infusions can be used [65], especially if the glucose concentration decreases to 250 mg/dl (14 mmol/L) or lower. Typically, half the total body water deficit is corrected over a 12-hour period, and the remaining half is corrected over the next 1 or 2 days.

Insulin

Although evidence exists of insulin resistance in hyperosmolar conditions, high insulin doses are best avoided to reduce chances of hypoglycemia [52,67,68]. Insulin bolus of 0.05 to 0.1 unit/kg followed by infusion of 0.1 unit/kg/hr intravenously is frequently used. Insulin should be followed with dextrose-and-water fluid supplementation when plasma glucose is less than 250 mg/dl (14 mmol/L).

Electrolytes

In hyperosmolar coma, a state of total body potassium deficit is found. Serum potassium could decrease further with insulin treatment and dilution secondary to the effect of fluids. Potassium supplements should be provided as discussed in previous section.

Phosphate also is depleted, and monitoring phosphate levels is recommended. Providing phosphate in patients without moderate to severe hypophosphatemia remains controversial. Corrected serum sodium provides a better measure of sodium levels than does uncorrected sodium. Finally, tests to confirm an underlying etiology should be carried out (e.g., chest radiograph, urine and blood cultures, electrocardiogram, and others, as deemed necessary). After the episode has been treated and the etiology has been investigated, the patient is discharged, preferably while receiving insulin therapy.

HYPOGLYCEMIA

Definition

Hypoglycemia is defined as a plasma glucose level of 50 mg/dl (2.8 mmol/L) or less [69].

Classification

The term *asymptomatic hypoglycemia* describes the condition of patients whose laboratory glucose levels are low but who are not experiencing any symptoms. Mild hypoglycemia describes the condition in patients who experience adrenergic symptoms and respond quickly to an oral carbohydrate load. In moderate hypoglycemia, patients experience both adrenergic and neuroglycopenic symptoms but manage to treat themselves and initiate therapy. Severe hypoglycemia is a term limited to patients who need assistance to treat hypoglycemia and are unable to administer treatment by themselves. Severe hypoglycemia is a major factor preventing tight glucose control and is costly.

Etiology

This section focuses on the most common cause of hypoglycemia, which is exogenous insulin– or oral hypoglycemic agent–mediated hypoglycemia. Evidence supports the principle that glycemic goals and not the insulin regimen used determine the frequency of hypoglycemia [13]. Insulin treatment with rapid-acting agents is associated with a lower risk of hypoglycemia than is regular insulin [69], and the use of Glargine and Detemir insulin have been shown to be associated with less hypoglycemia than NPH insulin. Incidence of severe hypoglycemia is the same for animal-derived insulins and so-called human-engineered insulin treatments [70,71]. Most episodes of hypoglycemia are related to lifestyle factors, especially missing meals [72,73]. Other predictors of severe hypoglycemia are previous episodes of severe hypoglycemia [74], hemoglobin A_{1c} levels less than 7% [75], hypoglycemia unawareness [76], autonomic neuropathy [77], and long duration of diabetes.

Pathophysiology

When plasma glucose levels approach the hypoglycemic range, predictable physiologic changes occur. Pancreatic insulin release is suppressed at plasma glucose levels of 75 to 85 mg/dl (4.2–4.7 mmol/L). When glucose levels decrease to less than 70 mg/dl (3.9 mmol/L), counter-regulatory hormone (e.g., glucagon, epinephrine, and cortisol) and growth hormone secretion is enhanced, thus producing adrenergic symptoms. Finally, neuroglycopenic symptoms (impaired mental status) occur when glucose levels decrease to less than 45 to 50 mg/dl (2.5–2.8 mmol/L). These threshold numbers may vary with repeated recurrent hypoglycemia. For example, in patients with insulinoma or type 1 DM and frequent hypoglycemic episodes, the threshold for counter-regulatory hormone release and therefore the initial hyperadrenergic symptoms are possible with less-elevated findings. Hypoglycemia unawareness occurs when the threshold of adrenergic symptoms becomes lower than that of neuroglycopenic symptoms, so that patients may have impaired mental status as the first sign of hypoglycemia.

Epidemiology

Type 1 Diabetes Mellitus

In the DCCT [36,78,79], 65% of patients randomly assigned to the study's intensive insulin arm and 35% to the conventional arm experienced at least one episode of hypoglycemia that was considered severe over a period of 6.5 years. Most episodes of severe hypoglycemia occur at night, and adolescents are more prone than adults.

Type 2 Diabetes Mellitus

In the UKPDS during a 10-year period, 23% of patients treated with insulin experienced at least one episode of severe hypoglycemia compared with 4% treated with chlorpropamide and 6% with glibenclamide [36]. The difference between oral agents was not statistically significant. None of the patients using metformin experienced a major hypoglycemic episode in the UKPDS. Long-acting sulfonylureas (e.g., chlorpropamide and glibenclamide) can be associated with prolonged episodes [80]. Glimepiride may be associated with a lower incidence of hypoglycemia than glyburide [81]. α-Glucosidase inhibitors and thiazolidinediones should not induce hypoglycemia if used alone. Meglitinides use results in hypoglycemia probably similar to sulfonylureas' activity.

Diagnosis

The Whipple triad criteria may be used to diagnosis hypoglycemia: symptoms consistent with hypoglycemia, low plasma glucose concentrations, and relief of symptoms after a carbohydrate load. Visually interpreted Chemstrips or portable glucometers can be used to detect hypoglycemia reliably in patients with diabetes and then to initiate treatment.

Clinical Manifestations

Adrenergic symptoms frequently encountered include sweats, palpitations, anxiety, tremors, and sensations of hunger or nausea. Neuroglycopenic symptoms include confusion, impaired concentration, weakness, blurred vision, difficulty speaking, and drowsiness. Patients who are unable to recognize adrenergic symptoms (so-called hypoglycemia unawareness) may have serious neuroglycopenic symptoms of coma and seizures.

Treatment

Diabetic patients should consider glucose levels less than 70 mg/dl (4 mmol/L) as hypoglycemic and requiring treatment [82–84]. Hypoglycemia should be treated quickly. In most patients, an oral glucose load of 15 g is generally recommended. This would increase glucose levels by 40 mg/dl (2.1 mmol/L) within 20 minutes. Patients should typically check glucose at the onset of hypoglycemia and 20 minutes after starting treatment. If plasma glucose levels did not increase by 20 mg/dl (1 mmol/L) at 20 minutes after treatment, then retreatment with another 15 g of glucose is recommended. Glucose gel is significantly slower in increasing blood glucose, and buccal use should not be recommended because absorption is minimal.

In the unconscious patient, glucagon, 1 mg subcutaneously or intramuscularly, will increase plasma glucose measurements significantly after 10 to 15 minutes, and levels may peak an hour later. A trained spouse or a support person typically administers glucagon at home. In the hospital setting, intravenous glucose administration of 25 g over several minutes (e.g., 50 ml of D50) followed by dextrose 10% infusion is the standard effective treatment. For recurrent or unresponsive oral agent–induced hypoglycemia, oral or intravenous diazoxide or octreotide subcutaneously could be used.

Hypoglycemia Unawareness

It is postulated that with repeated episodes of hypoglycemia, the nervous system adapts to low glucose levels and maintains glucose uptake despite hypoglycemia without adrenergic effects, leading to unawareness of hypoglycemia. Hypoglycemia unawareness may produce serious adverse events in diabetic patients with tight glycemic control. Previous episodes of hypoglycemia are essential for the development of hypoglycemia unawareness. Therefore detection of episodes of hypoglycemia is important, especially nocturnal hypoglycemia, which is frequently not recognized.

Autonomic neuropathy leads to reduced epinephrine response to hypoglycemia and may contribute to development of severe hypoglycemia [77]. However, hypoglycemia unawareness may occur without autonomic neuropathy. Of note, glucagon response to hypoglycemia decreases with duration of diabetes.

Small studies showed that avoidance of hypoglycemia for days to months results in improvement of recognition of hypoglycemia or improved counter-regulatory response (epinephrine and glucagon) to hypoglycemia. Therefore aiming at higher glucose or hemoglobin A_{1c} goals and avoidance of hypoglycemia may improve hypoglycemia unawareness [85]. The use of caffeine or theophylline to stimulate the sympathetic–adrenal axis is of controversial clinical use.

Complications

In the DCCT, patients' neuropsychological tests did not distinguish between those treated with an intensive insulin regimen and those undergoing conventional therapy over the study's duration of 7 years, even in those patients who experienced episodes of coma or seizures. In small studies of children younger than 5 years, children with hypoglycemic seizures had poor results during neuropsychological testing [86], and therefore glucose goals should be relaxed to avoid severe hypoglycemia in children younger than 5 years. Furthermore, bedtime snacks are effective in reducing nocturnal hypoglycemia [87] and should be considered as part of the treatment protocol.

COMPLICATIONS OF DIABETES

Cardiovascular Disease

Epidemiology

Patients with diabetes are at more risk for developing cardiovascular disease than are patients without diabetes. Both men and women across all age groups with diabetes are at 2 to 4 times higher risk of death from cardiovascular disease. This increased risk is not, however, related solely to classic cardiac risk factors [88].

Etiology

Diabetes itself is an independent risk factor for development of cardiovascular disease, regardless of other risk factors. Plasma glucose levels predict development of cardiovascular disease in type 1 as well as type 2 DM. In the UKPDS, each 1% increase in hemoglobin A_{1c} was associated with 15% increase in the incidence of myocardial infarction [89]. Glucose elevations above the reference range also are associated with increased cardiovascular disease, even if they do not meet criteria for diagnosis of DM. This might be related to increased glycated end products and low-density lipoprotein (LDL) oxidation. Traditional risk factors such as age, smoking, gender, hypertension, hyperlipidemia, and obesity play an important role in the development of cardiovascular disease of diabetes. Microalbuminuria is associated with a significant increase in cardiovascular events and might be a marker of an underlying progressive subclinical atherosclerosis [90]. Visual complications of DM, such as proliferative retinopathy, are also associated with cardiovascular disease. Obviously, retinopathy and microalbuminuria are not causal factors but might be indicators of other causal factors. Insulin resistance, as measured by "clamp" techniques or mathematical homeostasis model assessment, may be associated with cardiovascular events, as shown in several studies. The association, however, is weaker than the other risk factors already mentioned. In the UKPDS, the use of exogenous insulin was not associated with increased cardiovascular disease.

Diagnosis

Patients with diabetes in whom cardiovascular diseases develops may not initially have classic symptoms.

No evidence exists that cardiac tests perform differently in diabetic patients than in nondiabetic patients, and therefore the diagnostic approach should be similar to that with other nondiabetic populations.

Prevention and Treatment

Glucose Control

In the UKPDS [36], treatment of overweight type 2 diabetes patients with metformin and intensively controlling glucose levels was associated with a 36% reduction in all-cause mortality. Therefore metformin should be used as the drug of choice for patients with type 2 DM who are overweight. However, in the main UKPDS study, achieving tight control with insulin or oral agents was associated with a trend for reduced cardiovascular events, which did not reach statistical significance. Other small trials examined the effect of glycemic control with variable results. Thiazolidinediones therapy is associated with reduced C-reactive protein and other markers of macrovascular disease, independent of glycemic control. Pioglitazone efficacy in reducing a composite of (all-cause mortality, nonfatal myocardial infarction, and stroke) in patients with DM and existing macrovascular disease in the "PROactive" study. The use of pioglitazone was associated with 16% reduction in that composite. However, these agents may precipitate congestive heart failure and can induce edema. Acarbose therapy in the STOP-NIDDM trial significantly reduced the risk of macrovascular disease and hypertension.

For type 1 DM, the DCCT demonstrated a nonsignificant reduction in cardiovascular disease events in patients treated with intensive insulin therapy. A meta-analysis of epidemiologic studies of type 1 DM also demonstrated a nonsignificant reduction in the first cardiovascular events but reported a significant reduction in the total number of cardiovascular subsequent events.

Blood Pressure Control

Reducing blood pressure significantly reduces cardiovascular disease in diabetic patients [91–93]. Evidence supports the use of ACE inhibitors and angiotensin-receptor blockers as first-line therapy in diabetic patients. However, β-blockers, calcium-channel blockers, and diuretics may be safely used in patients with type 2 DM to reduce cardiovascular risk. The use of α-blockers in diabetic patients to control blood pressure is controversial because of potentially increased numbers of cardiovascular events. Multiple studies addressed systolic blood pressure goals in epidemiologic studies: the lowest risk was seen in those with systolic blood pressure less than 120 mm Hg. The ADA consensus goal has been a systolic blood pressure less than 130 mm Hg. Diastolic blood pressure control to less than 80 mm Hg is desirable.

Aspirin

The use of aspirin has been shown in meta-analyses to reduce cardiovascular events similar to its effects in patients without diabetes, but use of aspirin should be gauged carefully to balance potential risk for bleeding. Doses of 75 to 325 mg/day have been effective.

Lipid Control

Specific trials addressing lipid control in DM also are lacking, but indirect evidence exists to support low-density lipoprotein (LDL) reduction by using a "statin" in preventing cardiovascular disease in primary and secondary intervention [94,95]. The recommended goal is LDL less than 100 mg/dl (2.6 mmol/L). Reducng triglycerides and increasing high-density lipoprotein (HDL) levels with a fibrate could also reduce cardiovascular disease events in subgroup analyses of major trials [96].

Thrombolysis

Thrombolytic therapy has been shown to reduce mortality after acute myocardial infarction (MI) in diabetic patients without increased risk of hemorrhage compared with findings in the general population. Thrombolytic therapy should not be withheld because of concern about retinal hemorrhage in patients with retinopathy. However, the same contraindications for the use of thrombolysis in the general population apply to the diabetic population.

Angioplasty for Acute Myocardial Infarction

Primary angioplasty was shown to be successful in patients with DM and may be superior to thrombolysis in patients with MI.

Postinfarction Insulin

The use of intensive insulin treatment after MI reduces mortality in type 2 DM by 29% [97]. Although post-MI insulin use reduces mortality, it does not prevent recurrent MI.

β-Blockers

The use of β-blockers in patients with DM after MI is not contraindicated, and β-blockers should be considered for all patients after MI, including diabetic patients.

ACE Inhibitors

Using an ACE inhibitor within the first 2 days after MI for at least 4 weeks reduces mortality, especially in patients who are at high risk, such as those with intercurrent congestive heart failure. For this reason, ACE inhibitors should be used in patients while serum potassium levels and renal status are being monitored.

Antiplatelet Therapy

Adding clopidogrel to aspirin reduces the risk of stroke and fatal as well as nonfatal MI by 20% in patients with symptoms of acute coronary syndromes. However, risk of bleeding should be balanced.

Coronary Bypass

Patients with DM are at increased risk of surgical complications, restenosis, and death after coronary bypass graft. This increased risk may be secondary to associated diffuse arthrosclerosis, diabetic cardiomyopathy, or renal disease. However, the Bypass Angioplasty Revascularization Investigation demonstrated that coronary bypass using the internal mammary artery was superior to angioplasty [98]. Therefore in patients with DM and multivessel disease, coronary artery bypass graft is recommended over angioplasty.

Stents

Patients with DM undergoing angioplasty should use stents and receive antiplatelet therapy. Use of stents improves outcome in comparison with angioplasty without stents.

Eye Disease

Etiology

Visual impairment in diabetic patients is mainly secondary to retinopathy and cataracts. The most important risk factor for the development of progressive retinopathy in type 1 or type 2 DM is glucose control, measured as glycated hemoglobin. Other factors include hypertension, duration of diabetes, elevated triglyceride levels, total cholesterol, low HDL cholesterol, and pregnancy. Smoking and alcohol use, however, are not considered risk factors for retinopathy.

Pathophysiology

Loss of vision in type 1 DM is most likely associated with proliferative retinopathy (80%), but in type 2 DM, it is most likely secondary to macular edema. Development of new vessels and glial proliferation in the retina may result in hemorrhage, macular distortion, and retinal detachment, leading to visual loss. Reduced capillary profusion and ischemia break the blood–retinal barrier with resultant fluid leakage, edema, endothelial proliferation, and formation of microaneurysms, thickening of the retinas, and neuronal necrosis.

Multiple types of retinal lesions develop in patients with DM secondary to the process mentioned.

Epidemiology

The prevalence of legal blindness in the diabetic population of southern Wisconsin was 3.6% in type 1 DM and 1.6% in type 2 DM. In type 1 DM patients, 20% had impaired vision 30 years after the diagnosis of diabetes, whereas 35% of type 2 DM patients had impaired vision 20 years after diagnosis. The estimated incidence of blindness is 3.3 per 100,000 annually.

Diagnosis

Screening by using direct ophthalmoscopy and retinal digital photography is effective at detecting unrecognized retinopathy. More than one third of patients with type 2 DM have retinopathy at diagnosis, and therefore annual screening examinations are recommended for all patients with type 2 DM, starting at the time of diagnosis. In type 1 DM, retinopathy develops after the onset of puberty, and therefore screening should start at age 12, or if the disease is diagnosed after puberty, then 3 years after diagnosis.

Prevention and Treatment

Glucose Control

The DCCT demonstrated that intensive management control of glucose prevents the development or progression of retinopathy in type 1 DM (76% primary prevention and 54% secondary prevention) compared with less-tight control [11]. Other studies provided similar results [36]. Several studies reported a transient deterioration of retinopathy with acute control, usually lasting several months. Therefore if severe retinal disease or visual loss exists, eye disease should be treated before rapid control of glucose. In type 2 DM, tight glucose control with insulin or oral agents resulted in reduced retinopathy by 20% to 25% as well as reduced surgical intervention. Early tight control is not associated with transient deterioration of retinopathy. Reducing hemoglobin A_{1c} to 7% or less is likely to reduce visual loss and eye disease.

Blood Pressure Control

Control of blood pressure to target reduces the rate of progression of retinopathy and progression to visual loss by 50% in people with type 1 DM [99] and by 30% in those with type 2 DM. The effect is noted earlier than effects of blood glucose control and is not related to the use of a special blood pressure agent. Both β-blockers and ACE inhibitors were similarly effective. These conclusions are also likely to be valid for patients with type 1 DM.

Antiplatelet Therapy

Use of aspirin with or without dipyridamole versus ticlopidine reduced microaneurysm formation in early retinopathy but did not prevent the development of high-risk proliferative retinopathy or cataract formation. Aspirin did not increase the risk of vitreous hemorrhage; therefore aspirin is not contraindicated in diabetic patients with retinopathy.

Aldose Reductase Inhibitors

Theoretically, the use of aldose reductase inhibitors may reduce tissue damage and oxidative stress as well as glycated end products. In clinical trials, however, these agents did not show an effect on slowing the progression of retinopathy.

Laser Photocoagulation

In diabetic proliferative retinopathies, scatter photocoagulation significantly reduced progression of disease and was associated with reduced new-vessel formation and reduced visual loss by 50%. The Early Treatment Diabetic Retinopathy Study (ETDRS) studied patients with proliferative diabetic retinopathy in at least one eye or severe nonproliferative diabetic retinopathy in both eyes and studied the photocoagulation effects [100–102]. ETDRS showed a significant reduction of sudden visual loss or vitrectomy; therefore scatter laser treatment is recommended for patients with proliferative diabetic retinopathy [103]. No clear-cut evidence indicates that patients with mild or moderate nonproliferative eye disease would benefit from photocoagulation. However, patients with type 2 DM or older patients with DM who are older than 40 years with severe nonproliferative diabetic retinopathy would benefit from photocoagulation [104].

Macular edema is treated with focal photocoagulation even before visual acuity is affected and regardless of the severity of nonproliferative diabetic retinopathy. This mode of therapy reduces future visual loss.

Vitrectomy
In type 1 DM, early vitrectomy results in reduction of visual loss by 10% in patients who have persistent vitreous hemorrhage when compared with delayed vitrectomy (1 year later) over a period of 4 years. This is not the case in patients with type 2 DM, in whom early and delayed vitrectomy have similar outcomes. In patients with tractional retinal detachment or severe fibrovascular proliferation and reduced visual acuity, early vitrectomy reduced sudden visual loss by 15.9% over a 4-year period.

Diabetic Neuropathy

Classification
The most common form of diabetic neuropathy is distal symmetric polyneuropathy. Another common form is mononeuropathy, such as carpal tunnel syndrome, ulnar neuropathy, peroneal neuropathy, or cranial nerve neuropathies. Less common are radiculopathies, such as diabetic lumbar plexopathy and intercostal (truncal) radiculopathy. Autonomic neuropathy usually involves multiple systems and may present with gastroparesis, hyperhidrosis, anhidrosis, or bladder dysfunction.

Pathophysiology
Several hypotheses explain the pathophysiology of diabetic neuropathy. Increased glycols influx in Schwann cells through the aldose reductase system leads to depletion of sodium/potassium adenosine triphosphatase and slowing of nerve-conduction velocities. Advanced glycation of essential nerve proteins also leads to several pathologic changes and is postulated to result in neuropathy. Ischemia secondary to microvascular damage results in multifocal loss of exons. Finally, it is thought that a deficiency of nerve growth factors and other trophic factors in diabetes increases neuropathy.

Epidemiology
Prevalence of neuropathy is estimated around 34% in type 1 and 26% in type 2 DM [105]. Neuropathy may occur early in the disease, especially with suboptimal glycemic control. In the DCCT, clinically detectable neuropathy developed in 10% after 5 years of enrollment. In type 2 DM, the incidence is around 6% per year.

Diagnosis

Clinical Manifestations
The history and physical examination—including sensory testing and evaluation of light touch, pinprick perception, thermal sensitivity, and vibration sensation by using a 128- or 256-Hz tuning fork—provide adequate information for diagnoses. The use of monofilament as a screening tool should not replace the neurologic examination, although it has been widely accepted as a reliable method.

Sensory loss, paresthesia, neuropathic pain, autonomic abnormalities, and motor weakness are prominent symptoms.

Laboratory Findings
Several tests are used for the diagnosis of diabetic neuropathy. In the Rochester Diabetic Study, the most sensitive tests were nerve-conduction studies and autonomic

testing by using heart-rate (i.e., R-R interval) change during the Valsalva maneuver [106]. Quantitative sensory threshold tests were less sensitive in diagnosing neuropathy, but combination thermal and vibration sensory thresholds provide high sensitivity and specificity.

Sural Biopsy
Small-nerve biopsy should not be a diagnostic tool because of the associated morbidity, pain, and invasiveness.

Treatment
Currently no pharmacologic therapeutic modalities reverse or cure diabetic neuropathy. Treatment is focused on pain control.

Glucose Control
With intensive therapy, clinically detectable neuropathy is reduced in patients with type 1 DM (DCCT findings) and type 2 DM.

Aldose Reductase Inhibitors
These agents reduce the accumulation of sorbitol in nerve cells. Meta-analysis demonstrated some benefits for motor neuropathy, but generally these are associated with adverse effects and no demonstrable efficacy with autonomic or sensory neuropathy [107].

Tricyclic Antidepressants
This class is considered a first-tier therapy [108]. Amitriptyline is useful in the treatment of painful polyneuropathy, but its use is limited because of the adverse-effect profile and sedation. Nortriptyline and desipramine may also be used for the same indication and are associated with lower levels of sedation. Tricyclic antidepressants are also useful for the treatment of pain secondary to lumbar plexopathy.

Duloxetine
This is another first-tier therapy. In two randomized studies, duloxetine was effective in reducing pain scores. A dose of 60 mg daily is safe and effective in reducing pain, even in patients older than 65 years. Side effects include constipation and somnolence.

Pregabalin
Pregabalin also is considered first-tier therapy. In randomized double-blind studies, this agent was effective in doses of 300 to 600 mg daily. Side effects include dizziness, somnolence, and edema.

Other Agents
Oxycodone, gabapentin, venlafaxine, lamotrigine, tramadol, carbamazepine, and capsaicin [108–110] are effective in controlling painful neuropathy by 25% to 50% compared with placebo.

Surgery
Surgical decompression reverses entrapment neuropathies such as carpal tunnel syndrome. Other entrapment neuropathies have less successful outcomes with surgery.

Renal Disease

Definition
Microalbuminuria is one of the earliest manifestations of diabetic renal disease, characterized by increased secretion of albumin greater than 30 mg/day. Diabetic nephropathy is an advanced stage of diabetic renal disease in which albumin excretion is more than 300 mg/day.

Etiology
Glycation end products and sorbitol interaction with growth factors and structural proteins lead in the presence of altered hemodynamic process to glomerular lesions that progress in a predictable pattern, leading to impaired renal function.

Pathophysiology

Early in the course of DM, increased glomerular volume and glomerular capillary pressure lead to increased glomerular filtration rate and kidney size. With progression of diabetes, the basement membranes of the glomerulus, tubules, and the Bowman capsule thickens. This is followed by mesangial expansion and accelerated damage of arterioles as well as reduced filtration rates. This process progresses to diffuse glomerular sclerosis. Kimmelstiel–Wilson nodular lesions are present in 20% of renal biopsies of diabetic patients.

Epidemiology

The cumulative incidence rate of diabetic nephropathy is 30% at 30 years of duration of diabetes. In types 1 and 2 DM, the prevalence of microalbuminuria is variable and depends on multiple factors such as duration of diabetes, hypertension, smoking, and hyperlipidemia. The average time for progression from microalbuminuria to diabetic nephropathy in type 1 DM is around 8 years [111]. Overall incidence of developing end-stage renal disease in patients with type 1 DM regardless of albuminuria is 14% over a period of 10 years. It is estimated that up to 50% of type 1 DM patients with diabetic nephropathy will develop end-stage renal disease after 10 years.

In type 2 DM, the cumulative incidence is estimated at around 25% at 20 years of duration of diabetes. However, a significant proportion (8%) may have microalbuminuria at diagnosis. In fewer than 0.5% of patients with type 2 DM without proteinuria, end-stage renal disease develops within 10 years, but in 8% to 10% with baseline proteinuria, end-stage renal disease develops during the same period.

Diagnosis

The standard urine dipstick is not sensitive to measure albumin less than 300 mg/24 hr. The best test is radioimmunoassay measurement of microalbumin in a 24-hour urine sample. However, 4-hour, 12-hour, and overnight collections achieve similar results (95% correlation). Albumin concentration measurements from spot urine are also a useful diagnostic test, especially if coupled with creatinine as the albumin-to-creatinine ratio. Special microalbumin dipsticks are of variable sensitivity and specificity and therefore, depending on the amount of urine dilution, these tests would provide variable results and are not as reliable as the standard tests. The use of the albumin/creatinine ratio compensates for urine dilution with a high sensitivity and specificity.

In type 1 DM, minor elevations in blood pressure precede diabetic nephropathy by years. No role exists for kidney biopsy in diagnosing diabetic nephropathy in patients with elevated urine microalbumin and a typical history as well as diabetic retinopathy. Nearly all (>98%) biopsies performed in patients with type 1 DM indicate diabetic nephropathy, especially if the patient has prolonged duration of diabetes (>5 years) in the absence of a clinically apparent secondary cause.

In type 2 DM, hypertension precedes diabetic nephropathy by years. Frequently proteinuria is present at diagnosis. Approximately 12% to 20% of all renal biopsies performed on patients with proteinuria in patients with type 2 DM are due to nondiabetic etiology. Biopsy could be considered if the duration of diabetes is short in the absence of retinopathy.

Prevention and Treatment

Glucose Control

In the DCCT, patients who achieve tight glycemic control reduce the risk of development of microalbuminuria by 39% and the progression of albuminuria by 54%, although the conventionally treated group reported 6.5% increase in albumin excretion per year. In the UKPDS, tight control leads to a 33% relative risk reduction for the development of microalbuminuria; therefore tight glucose control is recommended in type 1 and type 2 DM patients to reduce the development of renal disease and progression of existing microalbuminuria.

Blood Pressure Control

Meta-analysis of several studies on the effect of blood pressure control on proteinuria demonstrated that a 10-mm Hg decrease in blood pressure by using ACE inhibitors was adequate to show a significant reduction of proteinuria. In the UKPDS, intensive blood pressure control to less than 144/82 was compared with conventional control to less than 154/87, which led to 8% absolute risk reduction of microalbuminuria over a 6-year period [112,113].

In type 1 DM, patients with nephropathy whose main arterial pressure was 6 mm higher than the treated group tripled their urine microalbumin excretion over a 2-year period. Therefore blood pressure control is important in controlling albuminuria and nephropathy.

ACE Inhibitors

ACE inhibitors function by reducing blood pressure as well as glomerular pressure and appear to be effective in delaying the progression of proteinuria in both type 1 [114,115] and type 2 [116] DM. ACE inhibitors decrease microalbuminuria and are effective in reducing diabetic nephropathy and delaying the progression toward end-stage renal disease.

Angiotensin-Receptor Blockers

Evidence supports the use of these agents in patients with type 2 DM. Combining angiotensin receptor blockers with maximal doses of ACE inhibitors may further reduce blood pressure and albuminuria.

Aldosterone Inhibitors

A small dose of spironolactone, 25 mg/day, or eplerenone added to an ACE inhibitor reduced albuminuria significantly (40%).

Protein Restriction

A high-protein diet leads to hyperfiltration, and therefore it is not advised in patients with DM. Protein restriction was also shown to reduce the decline in glomerular filtration rate in a meta-analysis of smaller studies [117].

INTENSIVE GLYCEMIC MANAGEMENT

Definition

Intensive glycemic management indicates tight control of blood glucose, aiming at near normal blood glucose measurements. In patients with type 1 DM, this is achieved with multiple daily insulin injections or insulin pumps (continuous subcutaneous insulin infusions) and is also known as intensive insulin therapy or flexible insulin therapy. In patients with type 2 DM, tighter control may be achieved with oral agents (at least for the short term), or combination oral agents and insulin or with multiple daily insulin injections.

Etiology/Rationale

The significant long-term benefits noted with large studies, the DCCT (type 1 DM) and UKPDS (type 2 DM) were associated with tighter glucose control. This is the basis for recommending intensive glycemic management.

In the fasting state, the human pancreas secretes insulin continuously, which prevents lipolysis and other catabolic activities; this is referred to as basal insulin. During eating, insulin levels increase immediately and stay elevated for 1 to 4 hours. This meal-related insulin production is proportional to the amount of the carbohydrate in the meal and constitutes approximately 50% of the total daily insulin release. Intensive insulin therapy means providing a continuous supply of insulin to mimic natural pancreatic basal secretion and also providing meal insulin in doses according to the size of the meal to mimic natural pancreatic insulin secretion. Because meal timing (and therefore insulin) is variable and flexible, this regimen is also referred to as flexible insulin therapy.

Outpatient Setting
Refer to previous sections on type 1 and type 2 for additional discussion.

Type 1 DM
The DCCT and other studies showed that intensive glycemic control can be achieved by MDI by providing short-acting insulin to cover meals; however, short-term insulin use was accompanied by hypoglycemia [118] and also by postprandial hyperglycemia. The very rapid acting insulin analogues increase rapidly after injection and may better control postprandial hyperglycemia [119,120]. These agents have a short duration of action and therefore better mimic natural insulin meal release. Therefore very rapid acting insulin analogues are used frequently as meal insulins. Insulin preparations used in the DCCT/MDI regimen to cover basal insulin were either intermediate-acting or long-acting Ultralente. Their peak activity was also associated with nocturnal hypoglycemia. Glargine, which does not exhibit peaks or troughs, is widely used in practice now to provide basal insulin around the clock and is used frequently as basal insulin in the MDI program [121,122]. The evidence obtained from the DCCT and other studies [123] supports the use of intensive insulin therapy to achieve near-normal A_{1C} percentage through MDI or insulin infusions. The use of pramlintide as an adjunctive agent may provide an additional (but small) improvement to glycemic control [124].

Type 2 DM
The UKPDS showed that adequate glucose control can be achieved by using oral agents; however, this is dependent on beta cell function, which declines over a short period, resulting in adding a second oral agent and insulin. Evidence supports the use of dual agents to achieve adequate glucose control, but a significant number of patients (40%) would require insulin over a period of several years. Combining insulin and oral agents is also effective and safe. The evidence from the UKPDS supports the use of antidiabetic agents to achieve a near-normal A_{1C} percentage with metformin, sulfonylureas, insulin, or combination therapy. The use of pramlintide as adjunctive therapy adds little to the degree of control, and it is not indicated to be used as a stand-alone agent [125]. Exanetide, conversely, may provide an additional (but small) improvement in glycemic control [126]. Acarbose could be used and may have an additional benefit of reducing the risk of hypertension and cardiovascular events, but patients frequently discontinue using this agent because of side effects [127].

The Inpatient Setting
Epidemiology
People with DM are frequently (25% annual rate) admitted to the hospital and on average stay longer than those without DM. Hospital mortality rates are higher for patients with hyperglycemia, even if they are not diagnosed with DM [128].

Pathophysiology
During hospitalization, glycemic control in patients with DM becomes a significant problem because of anorexia, frequent episodes of fasting for tests, reduced activity, newly prescribed medications (especially corticosteroids), intravenous glucose infusions, parenteral nutrition, inappropriate timing of meals, and most important, stress of illness or surgery. These factors may lead to excessive hyperglycemia or serious hypoglycemia if antidiabetic therapy is not adjusted. Furthermore, in patients without DM, high glucose values may develop secondary to acute illness.

Hospitalized patients are at increased risk for severe hypoglycemia, which may result in coronary events, arrhythmias, and seizures, and are also at increased risk from severe hyperglycemia including dehydration, ketoacidosis, hyperosmolar coma, increased infection rates, impaired immune function [129], and increased mortality [130–132]. Evidence supports avoidance of excessive hyperglycemia in hospitalized patients at risk for infection [133], critical illness, and during myocardial infarction.

Myocardial Infarction

The use of insulin in acute MI in nondiabetic patients reduces hospital mortality by 4.9% (absolute risk reduction) [134]. It is recommended to use an insulin infusion to normalize glucose levels, even in patients without prior diagnosis of DM, especially in those with a complicated course.

Critical Illness

The use of insulin infusion to target glucose value of 80 to 110 mg/dl (4.4–6.1 mmol/L) reduced ICU mortality by 42 % [135]. Evidence supports the use of insulin infusion in ICU patients aiming at tight control [136]

Hospitalized Patients in Other Circumstances

Lacking adequate data, the general recommendations are based on epidemiologic and short-term small studies [137]. The general principles are to avoid hypoglycemia by increasing lower-threshold limits to 90 mg/dl (5 mmol/L). The upper threshold is controversial, with recommendations of 150 to 180 mg/dl (7.2 mmol/L to10 mmol/L).

Patients Taking Oral Medications. Oral antidiabetic medications are usually stopped the day of surgical intervention and resumed once oral food intake is established. Frequently metformin is not resumed until actual hospital dismissal because of its potential for severe adverse events in patients who may be dehydrated, undergo surgical intervention, or use contrast material for radiologic tests. Thiazolidinediones are safe in patients with mild renal impairment but may predispose to edema and congestive heart failure and are frequently stopped during hospitalization. Meglitinides, which have a shorter duration of action, may be safer to use than sulfonylureas. However, both meglitinides and sulfonylureas can be used in the stable hospitalized type 2 DM patient with caution to avoid hypoglycemia. As a replacement, insulin is used for the short term.

Patients Using Insulin. Patients with type 1 DM must have some form of insulin at all time. Patients with type 2 DM can delay insulin injection till after the procedure, if the procedure is short (e.g., endoscopy) and does not interfere with meal timing (e.g., early morning procedure). In most situations of surgical interventions and during severe illness and hospitalization, insulin is provided in a reduced dose to avoid hypoglycemia but in a way to continue adequate control.

In most situations, the patient is fasting, and then meal insulin is discontinued before any intervention, and only basal insulin is provided (1/2–2/3 dose of NPH) until the patient recovers and is able to eat. In patients who have a complicated hospital course, further adjustments of the original regimen are needed. Frequently during an illness, the insulin dose provided is higher than the prehospitalization dosage.

Intravenous Infusion

Continuous intravenous insulin infusion is being used more frequently today especially for critically ill patients [133–135,137]. Several protocols are available, and no evidence suggests the superiority of one regimen to another.

Insulin Sliding Scale

The use of a sliding scale is widespread and is frequently (>25%) the cause of episodic hypoglycemia and excessive hyperglycemia. Sliding scales could be useful if basal insulin or (oral agent) were provided and if sliding scales were adjusted to each individual patient [138]. Sliding scales therefore should be used for a short period only.

REFERENCES

Type 1 Diabetes Mellitus

Etiology, Epidemiology, and Diagnosis

1. (*1C*) **McKinney PA** et al. Perinatal and neonatal determinants of childhood type 1 diabetes. Diabetes Care 1999;22:928–932.

   In this case-controlled study, a higher frequency of neonatal infections was noted to be a risk factor for subsequent development of type 1 DM. Other factors including having a mother with type 1 DM, having an older mother, and preeclampsia during pregnancy were risk factors for the development of diabetes.

2. (*1C*) **Dahlquist G** et al. The epidemiology of diabetes in Swedish children 0–14 years: A six-year prospective study. Diabetologia 1985;28:802–808.

   In this case-controlled study, hospital records of 892 patients with type 1 DM were compared with those of 2,291 controls. Different perinatal events were noted to increase the risk of type 1 DM, including maternal–child blood group, birth stress with cesarean section, and infectious diseases.

3. (*1C*) **Luo DF** et al. Confirmation of three susceptibility genes to insulin-dependent diabetes mellitus: IDDM4, IDDM5 and IDDM8. Hum Mol Genet 1996;5:693–698.

   In this trial, linkage analysis for 265 families with type 1 DM confirmed linkage of IDDM 4, IDDM 5, and IDDM 8 to type 1 DM.

4. (*1C*) **Molbak AG** et al. Incidence of insulin-dependent diabetes mellitus in age groups over 30 years in Denmark. Diabet Med 1994;11:650–655.

   In this historical prospective study cohort of nearly 1 million Danish subjects, 16.2% used insulin for treatment of type 1 DM.

5. (*1B*) **Verge CF** et al. Number of autoantibodies (against insulin, GAD or ICA512/IA2) rather than particular autoantibody specificities determines risk of type I diabetes. J Autoimmun 1996; 9:379–383.

   In this study, insulin antibodies, GAD antibodies, and ICA 512 antibodies were measured in 45 subjects newly diagnosed with type 1 DM, 882 first-degree relatives, and 217 control subjects. ICA 512 antibodies were measured in 45 subjects newly diagnosed with type 1 DM, 882 first-degree relatives, and 217 control subjects. The number of positive antibodies rather than the particular antibody predicted type 1 DM.

6. (*1A*) **Ziegler AG** et al. Autoantibody appearance and risk for development of childhood diabetes in offspring of parents with type 1 diabetes: The 2-year analysis of the German BABYDIAB Study. Diabetes 1999;48:460–468.

   This prospective cohort multicenter follow-up study was undertaken to establish the role of autoantibodies in type 1 DM in children of patients with type 1 DM. A population of 1,353 children was recruited immediately after birth in 1998, and 114 children completed 4-year follow-up testing. Results at birth indicated that none of the children produced autoantibodies except those that had been acquired from their mothers. Antibodies detected at 9 months were present at 2 years. At 2 years, antibodies appeared in 11% of children and 3.5% of children who had more than one antibody. IAAs were most frequently detected and were usually the first antibodies to appear in the circulation. Cumulative risk for type 1 DM at 5 years was 1.8% and was 50% for those children who possessed more than one antibody at the age of 2 years. Diabetes developed in only nine children during the study.

7. (*1C*) **Kulmala P** et al. Prediction of insulin-dependent diabetes mellitus in siblings of children with diabetes: The Childhood Diabetes in Finland Study Group. J Clin Invest 1998;101:327–336.

   In this observational population-based study, combined screening with GAD and IA-2 protein autoantibodies identified 70% of those testing positive in the histochemical ICA test. This study illustrates the difficulties in securing a diagnosis of type 1 DM predisposition through measurement of autoantibodies.

8. (*1B*) **Vardi P** et al. Predictive value of intravenous glucose tolerance test insulin secretion less than or greater than the first percentile in islet cell antibody positive relatives of type 1 (insulin-dependent) diabetic patients. Diabetologia 1991;34:93–102.

   In this study of a high-risk population, in 15 of 17 subjects with intravenous glucose tolerance test scores below the first percentile, type 1 DM developed, whereas in three of 18 with intravenous glucose tolerance test results higher than the first percentile, diabetes developed ($p = 0.001$; OR, 38). The negative predictive value of an intravenous glucose tolerance test result higher than the first percentile was 83%.

9. (*1A*) **Diabetes Prevention Trial: Type 1 Diabetes Study Group**. Effects of insulin in relatives of patients with type 1 diabetes mellitus. N Engl J Med 2002;346:1685–1691.

   This randomized controlled multicenter nonblinded clinical trial studied the effect of injectable insulin in preventing DM in relatives of patients with type 1 DM. Of 84,228 first- and second-degree relatives of patients with type 1 DM, 372 subjects tested positive for multiple antibodies, projecting an increased risk for future diagnosis of type 1 DM. Three hundred thirty-nine of 372 subjects were randomly assigned to receive low-dose subcutaneous Ultralente insulin twice-daily injections and insulin infusion over a period of 4 days once yearly or to undergo observation. DM developed in 69 subjects in the treated group versus 70 subjects in the observation group, indicating no role for injectable insulin for preventing type 1 DM.

10. (*1C*) **Yu L** et al. Diabetes Prevention Trial 1: Prevalence of GAD and ICA512 (IA-2) autoantibodies by relationship to proband. Ann N Y Acad Sci 2002;958:254–258.

    In this study among children of whom both parents had DM, the prevalence of autoantibodies was 8.6%, and in single parents with diabetes, the prevalence was 4%. The children of diabetic fathers had higher antibody prevalence than the children of diabetic mothers.

Treatment

11. (*1A*) **The Diabetes Control and Complications Trial Research Group**. The effect of intensive treatment of diabetes on the development and progression of long-term complications in insulin-dependent diabetes mellitus. N Engl J Med 1993;329:977–986.

    This was a prospective randomized multicenter study with primary end points of microvascular and macrovascular complications. Mean follow-up was 6.5 years. To evaluate the efficacy of intensive insulin therapy in preventing long-term complications in 1,441 patients with type 1 DM, nearly half had no evidence of retinopathy (primary prevention cohort). Patients were assigned to receive intensive insulin with three or more daily injections or insulin pump compared with another group assigned to conventional therapy of daily insulin injections. Intensive insulin therapy reduced the mean risk for developing retinopathy by 76% in the primary prevention group and 54% in the secondary prevention cohort. Intensive insulin therapy reduced microalbuminuria by 39% and proteinuria by 54%. Neuropathy was reduced by 60%. Macrovascular disease end points were not statistically different between the two groups. The most adverse events noted were a twofold to threefold increase in severe hypoglycemia in the arm that received intensive insulin treatment.

12. (*1A*) **Lawson ML** et al. Effect of intensive therapy on early macrovascular disease in young individuals with type 1 diabetes. Diabetes Care 1999;22(suppl 2):B35–B39.

   In this meta-analysis of six studies on the effect of intensive insulin treatment on macrovascular disease in patients with type 1 DM, no significant effect was noted on the number of patients in whom cardiovascular events developed or on mortality rates from cardiovascular disease.

13. (*1A*) **Egger M** et al. Risk of adverse effects of intensified treatment in insulin-dependent diabetes mellitus: A meta-analysis. Diabetes Med 1997;14:919–928.

   In this meta-analysis of 14 studies, 1,028 patients were allocated to intensified insulin treatment and 1,039 patients to conventional treatment. The risk of severe hypoglycemia was mainly due to glycemic goals, as determined by the degree of normalization of glycemia.

14. (*1C*) **DCCT.** Effect of intensive therapy on the microvascular complications of type 1 diabetes mellitus. JAMA 2002;287:2563–2569.

   The writing team of the DCCT summarized the results of the DCCT cohort and succeeding follow up of 7 years in this article, which indicated that intensive insulin should be started early to reach a goal of hemoglobin A_{1c} less than 7%.

15. (*1A*) **Gale EA.** A randomized, controlled trial comparing insulin Lispro with human soluble insulin in patients with type 1 diabetes on intensified insulin therapy: The UK Trial Group. Diabetes Med 2000;17:209–214.

   In this randomized double-blind crossover study of 12 weeks' duration, 93 patients used MDIs of Lispro or regular insulin. NPH insulin was used in both these groups. Lispro insulin was as effective as regular insulin in achieving glycemic control.

16. (*1A*) **Pickup J** et al. Glycaemic control with continuous subcutaneous insulin infusion compared with intensive insulin injections in patients with type 1 diabetes: Meta-analysis of randomised controlled trials. BMJ 2002;324:705.

   This meta-analysis reviews the effects of two different modalities of insulin treatment on glycemic control. Insulin infusion controls blood glucose better than multiple daily injection, but the differences are few.

17. (*1A*) **Tsui E** et al. Intensive insulin therapy with insulin Lispro: A randomized trial of continuous subcutaneous insulin infusion versus multiple daily insulin injection. Diabetes Care 2001;24:1722–1727.

   In this randomized trial, 27 patients were enrolled to receive either MDIs or insulin effusions. The results were similar in relation to glycemic control and quality of life.

18. (*1A*) **Davey P** et al. Clinical outcomes with insulin Lispro compared with human regular insulin. Clin Ther 1997;19:656–674.

   In this meta-analysis, insulin Lispro was compared with regular insulin for outcome events. Results showed that glucose control is better with Lispro and without concurrent increase in hypoglycemia.

19. (*1A*) **Heller SR** et al. Effect of the fast-acting insulin analog Lispro on the risk of nocturnal hypoglycemia during intensified insulin therapy. Diabetes Care 1999;22:1607–1611.

   One hundred sixty-five patients with type 1 DM participated in this randomized crossover open-label study with either Lispro or insulin regular insulin. Glycemic control was equal for both groups. More hypoglycemia episodes occurred with regular insulin.

20. (*2A*) **Zinman B** et al. Effectiveness of human Ultralente versus NPH insulin in providing basal insulin replacement for an insulin Lispro multiple daily injection regimen: A double-blind randomized prospective trial. Diabetes Care 1999;22:603–608.

   In this double-blind randomized clinical trial, Ultralente was compared with NPH as basal insulin in 178 patients. At the end of the study, higher doses of Ultralente were needed to achieve glycemic control. The study suggests that NPH might be superior to Ultralente, but this is a function of the methods in the study, and different management of Ultralente injections might yield different results.

21. (*1C*) **Jones JM** et al. Eating disorders in adolescent females with and without type 1 diabetes: Cross sectional study. BMJ 2000;320:1563–1566.

   This study noted an increase prevalence of eating disorders in 356 girls aged 12 to 19 with type 1 DM compared with 1098 age-matched control (OR, 2.4; $p < 0.001$). Mean hemoglobin A_{1c} was also noted to be higher in diabetic subjects with an eating disorder.

22. (*1A*) **Gilbertson HR** et al. The effect of flexible low glycemic index dietary advice versus measured carbohydrate exchange diets on glycemic control in children with type 1 diabetes. Diabetes Care 2001;24:1137–1143.

Flexible dietary instructions with an emphasis on low-glycemic-index foods improved hemoglobin A_{1c} levels when compared with the standard carbohydrate exchange diet in this randomized, prospective, parallel study of 104 subjects over a 12-month period. The difference in hemoglobin A_{1c} was 8.05 versus 8.61 ($p = 0.05$).

23. (*1C*) **Landt KW** et al. Effects of exercise training on insulin sensitivity in adolescents with type I diabetes. Diabetes Care 1985;8:461–465.

The effects of exercise were studied in nine patients with type 1 DM and six controls. After 12 weeks, significant increases in insulin sensitivity, maximal oxygen uptake, and lean body mass were noted. No significant change was seen in glycated hemoglobin.

24. (*1C*) **Schiffrin A, Parikh S.** Accommodating planned exercise in type I diabetic patients on intensive treatment. Diabetes Care 1985;8:337–342.

In this interventional study, 13 type 1 DM patients receiving intensive insulin were asked to exercise after injecting their insulin. A significant decrease in blood glucose levels of 60 mg/dl was noted reaching a nadir at 45 minutes.

Type 2 Diabetes Mellitus

Etiology

25. (*1C*) **Brancati FL** et al. Body weight patterns from 20 to 49 years of age and subsequent risk for diabetes mellitus: The Johns Hopkins Precursors Study. Arch Intern Med 1999;159:957–963.

In this observational longitudinal study of former medical students, being overweight at the age of 25 predicted the development of diabetes.

26. (*1C*) **Rich-Edwards JW** et al. Birthweight and the risk for type 2 diabetes mellitus in adult women. Ann Intern Med 1999;130:278–284.

In this cohort observational study, among 69,526 women who were observed during follow-up, DM developed in 2,123. Low birth weight was associated with an increased risk of type 2 DM in a reverse J-shaped association.

Treatment

27. (*1A*) **Knowler WC** et al. Reduction in the incidence of type 2 diabetes with lifestyle intervention or metformin. N Engl J Med 2002;346:393–403.

Life-style intervention and metformin reduced the incidence of type 2 DM in patients with elevated fasting glucose measurements (but not determined to have diabetes). Life-style changes were more effective than in findings related to metformin.

28. (*1A*) **UK Prospective Diabetes Study Group (UKPDS 7).** Response of fasting plasma glucose to diet therapy in newly presenting type II diabetic patients. Metabolism 1990;39: 905–912.

This randomized multicenter clinical trial studied the effects of variable interventions on multiple clinical outcomes, including diabetic complications, in newly diagnosed type 2 DM patients in the United Kingdom. The results of 3,044 patients treated with dietary intervention were studied; other UKPDS reports studied varying numbers of patients. A considerable variation was noted in the response to diet in patients with newly diagnosed type 2 DM. Patients with higher glucose concentrations and those who lost more weight responded by greater declines in glucose concentrations. Weight loss of 28% of ideal body weight was required to achieve near-normal glycemia in patients whose fasting plasma glucose levels exceeded 180 mg/dl. Fasting plasma glucose response to diet is determined more by caloric restrictions than by weight loss.

29. (*1A*) **Boule NG** et al. Effects of exercise on glycemic control and body mass in type 2 diabetes mellitus: A meta-analysis of controlled clinical trials. JAMA 2001;286:1218–1227.

A meta-analysis of 14 studies that showed that hemoglobin A_{1c} levels decreased significantly with exercise when compared with results in placebo (7.6% vs. 8.3%), even though no significant change in weight was seen in the exercise group.

30. (*1A*) **UK Prospective Diabetes Study Group (UKPDS 34).** Effect of intensive blood-glucose control with metformin on complications in overweight patients with type 2 diabetes. Lancet 1998;352:854–865.

The use of metformin in overweight patients with type 2 DM reduced mortality, stroke, and diabetes complications, suggesting that metformin is the drug of choice in patients with type 2 DM who are overweight. It is not associated with serious hypoglycemic side effects.

31. **Johansen K.** Efficacy of metformin in the treatment of NIDDM: Meta-analysis. Diabetes Care 1999;22:33–37.

This was a meta-analysis of nine randomized controlled trials comparing metformin with placebo and 10 trials comparing metformin with sulfonylurea. Sulfonylurea and metformin had similar effects on lowering glucose and glycated hemoglobin. Sulfonylurea caused weight gain of 1.7 kg on an average, whereas metformin was associated with a weight loss of 1.2 kg.

32. (*1B*) **Fanghanel G** et al. Metformin's effects on glucose and lipid metabolism in patients with secondary failure to sulfonylureas. Diabetes Care 1996;19:1185–1189.

In a small randomized controlled trial, the effectiveness of metformin and insulin was compared in patients considered to have been failed by sulfonylurea therapy. Metformin effectively reduced hemoglobin

A_{1c} from 12.8% to 8.9%, triglycerides, cholesterol, and body mass index. Insulin treatment was also effective but did not influence body mass index, cholesterol, or hypertension.

33. (*1A*) **UK Prospective Diabetes Study Group (UKPDS 13).** Relative efficacy of randomly allocated diet, sulphonylurea, insulin, or metformin in patients with newly diagnosed non-insulin dependent diabetes followed for three years. BMJ 1995;310:83–88.

Sulfonylurea, insulin, and metformin controlled glucose levels effectively in patients with newly diagnosed type 2 DM in a similar fashion and were superior to diet alone. Sulfonylurea and insulin were associated with weight gain of 3.5 to 4.8 kg over a 3-year period, whereas metformin was not associated with significant weight changes.

34. (*1A*) **UK Prospective Diabetes Study Group (UKPDS 28).** A randomized trial of efficacy of early addition of metformin in sulfonylurea-treated type 2 diabetes. Diabetes Care 1998;21: 87–92.

Adding metformin to the pharmacotherapeutic regimen of 591 subjects taking sulfonylurea reduced glucose effectively and reduced the rates of "marked hyperglycemia" development when compared with findings in patients receiving sulfonylurea as monotherapy.

35. (*1A*) **Blohme G** et al. Glibenclamide and glipizide in maturity-onset diabetes: A double-blind cross-over study. Acta Med Scand 1979;206:263–267.

Sulfonylureas have similar clinical effects on lowering blood glucose.

36. (*1A*) **UK Prospective Diabetes Study Group (UKPDS 33).** Intensive blood-glucose control with sulphonylurea or insulin compared with conventional treatment and risk of complications in patients with type 2 diabetes. Lancet 1998;352:837–853.

This is another publication from the UKPDS group of 3,867 patients with newly diagnosed type 2 DM. Patients were randomly assigned to the intensive arm of the study (i.e., insulin treatment or sulfonylureas, chlorpropamide, glibenclamide, or glipizide) or the conventional arm with diet. Subjects in the intensive group had a higher number of hypoglycemic episodes than did those in the conventional group ($p < 0.0001$). Major hypoglycemic episodes rates were 0.7% with conventional treatment, 1.0% with chlorpropamide, 1.4% with glibenclamide, and 1.8% with insulin per year, respectively. Weight gain was higher in the intensive group (2.9 kg) than in the conventional group ($p < 0.001$). Finally, subjects who took insulin had a greater weight gain (4.0 kg) than those assigned chlorpropamide (2.6 kg) or glibenclamide (1.7 kg). In sum, sulfonylurea and insulin intensive therapy reduced microvascular diabetic complications but not macrovascular disease.

37. (*1A*) **Matthews DR** et al. for the UK Prospective Diabetes Study Group (UKPDS 26). Sulphonylurea failure in non-insulin-dependent diabetic patients over six years. Diabetes Med 1998;15:297–303.

In 1,305 patients newly diagnosed with type 2 DM and started on sulfonylurea, 48% required additional treatment by 6 years, especially patients whose body mass index was less than 30 kg/m^2.

38. (*1A*) **Rosenstock J** et al. Glimepiride, a new once-daily sulfonylurea: A double-blind placebo-controlled study of NIDDM patients: Glimepiride Study Group. Diabetes Care 1996;19: 1194–1199.

Patients with type 2 DM were assigned to glimepiride (8–16 mg) or placebo. Hemoglobin A_{1c} increased from 7.7% to 9.7% in the placebo group but decreased from 7.9% to 8.1% with glimepiride.

39. (*1A*) **Chiasson JL** et al. The efficacy of acarbose in the treatment of patients with non-insulin-dependent diabetes mellitus: A multicenter controlled clinical trial. Ann Intern Med 1994;121:928–935.

Acarbose treatment improved glycemic control in type 2 DM patients who took acarbose monotherapy or in combination with metformin, sulfonylurea, or insulin.

40. (*1A*) **Holman RR** et al. for the UK Prospective Diabetes Study Group (UKPDS 44). A randomized double-blind trial of acarbose in type 2 diabetes shows improved glycemic control over 3 years. Diabetes Care 1999;22:960–964.

When compared with placebo, acarbose monotherapy or combination therapy reduced hemoglobin A_{1c} by 0.2% to 0.5% in patients with type 2 DM over a period of 3 years. Noncompliance with therapy was mainly due to side effects of flatulence and diarrhea.

41. (*1A*) **Wolffenbuttel BH, Landgraf R**. A 1-year multicenter randomized double-blind comparison of repaglinide and glyburide for the treatment of type 2 diabetes: Dutch and German Repaglinide Study Group. Diabetes Care 1999;22:463–467.

Repaglinide's action is similar to that of glyburide in reducing plasma glucose concentrations; adverse effect profile also is similar.

42. (*1A*) **Phillips LS** et al. for the Rosiglitazone Clinical Trials Study Group. Once- and twice-daily dosing with rosiglitazone improves glycemic control in patients with type 2 diabetes. Diabetes Care 2001;24:308–315.

Thiazolidinedione monotherapy reduced hemoglobin A_{1c} and plasma glucose levels effective in patients with type 2 DM.

43. (*1A*) **Yki-Jarvinen H** et al. Comparison of bedtime insulin regimens in patients with type 2 diabetes mellitus: A randomized, controlled trial. Ann Intern Med 1999;130:389–396.

    Combining metformin with bedtime insulin is an effective method of controlling hyperglycemia and is not associated with weight gain compared with findings from other insulin regimens.

44. (*1A*) **Anderson JH Jr** et al. Mealtime treatment with insulin analog improves postprandial hyperglycemia and hypoglycemia in patients with non-insulin-dependent diabetes mellitus: Multicenter Insulin Lispro Study Group. Arch Intern Med 1997;157:1249–1255.

    The use of preprandial insulin Lispro was compared with that of regular insulin in 722 patients with type 2 DM. During Lispro therapy, lower rates of hypoglycemia were noted, although peak glucose values were higher with regular insulin 1 and 2 hours after meals.

45. (*1A*) **Johnson JL** et al. Efficacy of insulin and sulfonylurea combination therapy in type II diabetes: A meta-analysis of the randomized placebo-controlled trials. Arch Intern Med 1996;156:259–264.

    In this meta-analysis of 16 studies, fasting glucose as well as hemoglobin A_{1c} concentrations improved with combination treatment of insulin and sulfonylurea when compared with results derived from insulin monotherapy. Furthermore, smaller doses of insulin were used.

Diabetic Ketoacidosis
Etiology, Epidimiology, and Presentation

46. (*1C*) **Rewers A** et al. Predictors of acute complications in children with type 1 diabetes. JAMA 2002;287:2511–2518.

    In this cohort of 1,243 children with type 1 DM who lived in Denver, Colorado, incidence of ketoacidosis was eight per 100 person-years. In multivariate analysis, the risk for ketoacidosis increased with higher hemoglobin A_{1c} and higher dose of insulin use in older children. Other factors played an important role, such as under insurance coverage and the concurrent presence of psychiatric disorders.

47. (*1C*) **Johnson DD** et al. Diabetic ketoacidosis in a community-based population. Mayo Clin Proc 1980;55:83–88.

    In this community-based case-matched retrospective review of 92 patients with DKA, infection was the main precipitating factor for the episodes.

48. (*1C*) **Faich GA** et al. The epidemiology of diabetic acidosis: A population-based study. Am J Epidemiol 1983;117:551–558.

    The presentation of and precipitating factors for 137 patients with DKA are discussed. Twenty percent of patients were those with newly developed diabetes.

49. (*1C*) **Malone ML** et al. Characteristics of diabetic ketoacidosis in older versus younger adults. J Am Geriatr Soc 1992;40:1100–1104.

    This was a retrospective chart review of 220 cases of DKA. Twenty-seven cases occurred in patients who were older than 65 years. Treatment of DKA in this age group was associated with increased hypoglycemia and higher rates of death.

Treatment

50. (*1B*) **Fisher JN** et al. Diabetic ketoacidosis: Low-dose insulin therapy by various routes. N Engl J Med 1977;297:238–247.

    In this randomized controlled study of 45 patients with DKA, three groups receiving insulin therapy by various routes were compared. When compared with the groups receiving subcutaneous or intramuscular insulin, the group receiving low-dose intravenous insulin had a faster rate of fall of plasma glucose ($p = 0.01$) but no significant change in time to recovery. This route was also more effective initially in reducing ketone levels ($p < 0.05$).

51. (*1B*) **Burghen GA** et al. Comparison of high-dose and low-dose insulin by continuous intravenous infusion in the treatment of diabetic ketoacidosis in children. Diabetes Care 1980;3:15–20.

    In this randomized controlled study, low-dose intravenous insulin was compared with high-dose intravenous insulin (0.1 vs. 1 unit/kg/hr) in 32 patients with DKA. Low-dose insulin resulted in slower rates of glucose decline but was as effective as high-dose insulin in treating DKA and recovery. Furthermore, a lower incidence of significant hypoglycemia was found in patients receiving low-dose insulin.

52. (*1C*) **Carroll P, Matz R**. Uncontrolled diabetes mellitus in adults: Experience in treating diabetic ketoacidosis and hyperosmolar coma with low-dose insulin and uniform treatment regimen. Diabetes Care 1983;6:579–585.

    Retrospective analysis of 275 patients with uncontrolled diabetes who received low-dose insulin regimens and fluid resuscitation with hypotonic solutions, leading to a lower mortality rate than expected. DKA mortality increased in those who were older than 50 years.

53. (*1B*) **Edwards GA** et al. Effectiveness of low-dose continuous intravenous insulin infusion in diabetic ketoacidosis: A prospective comparative study. J Pediatr 1977;91:701–705.

    In this randomized controlled study of 20 pediatric patients, low-dose insulin intravenously was compared with high-dose insulin subcutaneously. No statistical difference was observed in the rate of correction of DKA or reduction of plasma glucose measurements.

54. (*2C*) **Lever E, Jaspan JB**. Sodium bicarbonate therapy in severe diabetic ketoacidosis. Am J Med 1983;75:263–268.

In this retrospective analysis of 95 cases of DKA, the authors found no difference between patients who received bicarbonate therapy (72 cases) and those who did not (22 cases).

55. (*1B*) **Morris LR** et al. Bicarbonate therapy in severe diabetic ketoacidosis. Ann Intern Med 1986;105:836–840.

In this randomized controlled trial, 10 patients with DKA were treated with bicarbonate and 11 were not. No significant difference was seen in outcome or benefits.

56. (*1C*) **Glaser N** et al. Risk factors for cerebral edema in children with diabetic ketoacidosis: The Pediatric Emergency Medicine Collaborative Research Committee of the American Academy of Pediatrics. N Engl J Med 2001;344:264–269.

In this case-matched report of 61 children with DKA, cerebral edema was associated with lower partial pressures of arterial carbon dioxide and higher levels of serum urea nitrogen. Treatment with bicarbonate was associated with increased rates of cerebral edema.

57. (*1B*) **Fisher JN, Kitabchi AE**. A randomized study of phosphate therapy in the treatment of diabetic ketoacidosis. J Clin Endocrinol Metab 1983;57:177–180.

In this randomized controlled study, 15 patients with DKA received phosphate treatment and were compared with another 15 patients who did not receive phosphate treatment. No statistical difference was found in serum electrolytes, 2,3-DPG levels, or recovery from DKA. Phosphate treatment resulted in hypocalcemia.

58. (*1C*) **Rosenbloom AL**. Intracerebral crises during treatment of diabetic ketoacidosis. Diabetes Care 1990;13:22–33.

In this report of 69 cases of intracerebral complications after DKA, most of the patients were children younger than 5 years. Pathologic findings varied and included localized brain edema, hemorrhage, thrombosis, and infection.

59. (*1C*) **Krane EJ** et al. Subclinical brain swelling in children during treatment of diabetic ketoacidosis. N Engl J Med 1985;312:1147–1151.

Computed tomography scans from six children who received treatment for DKA showed evidence of subclinical brain swelling during therapy.

Hyperosmolar Coma

60. (*1C*) **Wachtel TJ** et al. Predisposing factors for the diabetic hyperosmolar state. Arch Intern Med 1987;147:499–501.

In this case-controlled study of 135 patients with hyperosmolar coma who were matched to randomly selected patients with diabetes, predictors of the development of hyperosmolar coma were female gender, newly diagnosed diabetes, and acute infection.

61. (*1C*) **Gale EA** et al. Severely uncontrolled diabetes in the over-fifties. Diabetologia 1981;21:25–28.

In this observational study of 317 patients admitted to hospital with severely uncontrolled diabetes and hyperglycemia, 43% of patients older than 50 years died as a result. About 30% of patients had not previously been diagnosed with diabetes.

62. (*1C*) **Khardori R, Soler NG**. Hyperosmolar hyperglycemic nonketotic syndrome: Report of 22 cases and brief review. Am J Med 1984;77:899–904.

In this observational study of 22 patients with hyperosmolar coma, the mortality rate was 36%.

63. (*1C*) **Wachtel TJ** et al. Hyperosmolarity and acidosis in diabetes mellitus: A three-year experience in Rhode Island. J Gen Intern Med 1991;6:495–502.

This retrospective chart review study described features of 278 subjects in Rhode Island who were diagnosed with hyperosmolar coma over a 3-year period. Infection was the most frequent precipitating factor (27%). Mortality rates were 12%, and mortality was associated with older age, higher osmolality, and residing in a nursing home.

64. (*1C*) **Fulop M** et al. Hyperosmolar nature of diabetic coma. Diabetes 1975;24:594–599.

In this observational study of 47 patients with hyperosmolar coma, obtundation and impaired consciousness were related to the severity of hyperglycemia regardless of the degree of ketoacidosis.

Treatment

65. (*1C*) **Keller U** et al. Course and prognosis of 86 episodes of diabetic coma: A five year experience with a uniform schedule of treatment. Diabetologia 1975;11:93–100.

In this small descriptive study, 58 episodes of severe diabetic ketoacidotic coma and of 28 episodes of non-ketotic coma (total 86) are compared. The non-ketotic patients were older. A comparison of the age groups of survivors and those patients who died within 72 hrs showed an increase in mortality with age. On admission, blood glucose, osmolarity and blood urea were higher in the fatal cases. Blood urea was the most important indicator of a fatal outcome. The response of blood glucose to insulin was impaired in the subsequently fatal cases. Early mortality was 14% in the ketotic and 29% in the non-ketotic cases. The most frequent causes of death were circulatory failure.

66. *(1C)* **To LB, Phillips PJ.** Hyperosmolar non-ketotic diabetic coma: Less sodium in therapy? Anaesth Intensive Care 1980;8:349–352.

   Retrospective observational study of 18 patients with hyperosmolar coma showing elevated serum sodium concentration with standard therapy. The use of dextrose infusion is recommended to avoid electrolyte abnormalities.

67. *(1B)* **Rosenthal NR, Barrett EJ.** An assessment of insulin action in hyperosmolar hyperglycemic nonketotic diabetic patients. J Clin Endocrinol Metab 1985;60:607–610.

   In this experimental study, rates of glucose decline after administration of insulin and fluids were less than those in nondiabetic subjects, suggesting a state of insulin resistance in hyperosmolar coma.

68. *(1C)* **Bendezu R** et al. Experience with low-dose insulin infusion in diabetic ketoacidosis and diabetic hyperosmolarity. Arch Intern Med 1978;138:60–62.

   In this comparative observational study, low-dose insulin injections resulted in a satisfactory decrease of serum glucose in patients with hyperosmolar coma as well as DKA. Patients with hyperosmolar coma were more sensitive to insulin than were DKA patients.

Hypoglycemia

Etiology and Diagnosis

69. *(1A)* **Brunelle BL** et al. Meta-analysis of the effect of insulin Lispro on severe hypoglycemia in patients with type 1 diabetes. Diabetes Care 1998;21:1726–1731.

   In this meta-analysis of eight trials, 2,576 patients with type 1 DM were included. Insulin Lispro treatment was associated with less severe hypoglycemia than was that with regular insulin (3.1% vs. 4.4% of patients) and (102 vs. 131 episodes; $p = 0.024$).

70. *(1A)* **Home PD** et al. Insulin Aspart vs human insulin in the management of long-term blood glucose control in type 1 diabetes: A randomized controlled trial. Diabetes Med 2000;17:762–770.

   In this multicenter randomized open-label study, 1,070 patients were randomly assigned to receive the insulin Aspart or human insulin. Insulin Aspart improved levels of glycated hemoglobin and postprandial glucose but not preprandial glucose levels. Insulin Aspart treatment was associated with less severe nocturnal hypoglycemia (1.3% vs. 3.4%; $p < 0.05$) as well as less hypoglycemia after a meal (1.8% vs. 5%; $p < 0.005$).

71. *(1A)* **MacLeod KM** et al. A comparative study of responses to acute hypoglycemia induced by human and porcine insulins in patients with type 1 diabetes. Diabetes Med 1996;13:346–357.

   In a double-blind crossover trial, the effects of insulin ("human engineered" vs. animal derived)-induced hypoglycemia on physiologic as well as counter-regulatory hormonal responses were compared in 40 patients with type 1 DM. The magnitude and pattern of response of counter-regulatory hormones to hypoglycemia induced by either of these insulins were indistinguishable, as were the scores of autonomic and neural glycopenic symptoms.

72. *(1C)* **Fischer KF** et al. Hypoglycemia in hospitalized patients: Causes and outcomes. N Engl J Med 1986;315:1245–1250.

   Unblinded retrospective cohort study of 94 hospital patients. The predictors of hypoglycemia were missing meals, renal and hepatic disease, infections, shock, burns, cancer, and pregnancy.

73. *(1C)* **Feher MD** et al. Hypoglycaemia in an inner-city accident and emergency department: A 12-month survey. Arch Emerg Med 1989;6:183–188.

   A missed meal accounted for 52% of all precipitating causes of hypoglycemia in a 12-month survey in this inner-city emergency department practice report.

74. *(1C)* **Muhlauser I** et al. Risk factors of severe hypoglycemia in adult patients with type I diabetes: A prospective population-based study. Diabetologia 1998;41:1274–1282.

   This was a prospective observational study of 669 patients with type 1 DM and hypoglycemia. Predictors of hypoglycemia were prior severe hypoglycemia (HR, 1.9), goal of glycemic control (HR, 0.07), and impaired awareness, among other factors.

75. *(1C)* **Davis EA** et al. Hypoglycemia: Incidence and clinical predictors in a large population-based sample of children and adolescents with IDDM. Diabetes Care 1997;20:22–25.

   In this observational trial, rates of hypoglycemia were higher in children younger than 6 years and were higher in those who had tight glucose control (hemoglobin A_{1c} <7%; $p < 0.001$).

76. *(1B)* **Gold AE** et al. Frequency of severe hypoglycemia in patients with type 1 diabetes with impaired awareness of hypoglycemia. Diabetes Care 1994;17:697–703.

   In this small prospective comparative trial, 29 patients with type 1 DM who had impaired awareness were compared with 31 type 1 DM patients with intact awareness. Sixty-six percent of patients with such awareness had severe hypoglycemia compared with 26% of patients from the other group ($p < 0.01$).

77. *(1C)* **Stephenson JM** et al. Is autonomic neuropathy a risk factor for severe hypoglycemia? The EURO-DIAB IDDM Complications Study. Diabetologia 1996;39:1372–1376.

   In this European study of more than 3,000 diabetic patients, combined autonomic deficit in heart rate and blood pressure responses to standing were associated with a modest increase in the risk of severe hypoglycemia.

78. (*1A*) **Diabetes Control and Complications Trial Research Group.** Hypoglycemia in the Diabetes Control and Complications Trial. Diabetes 1997;46:271–286.

In this DCCT study, there were 3,788 episodes of severe hypoglycemia, and 1,027 of these episodes resulted in seizures or coma. The relative risk for coma or seizure was 3.0 for intensive therapy. This increased risk persisted for each year during the follow-up period of 9 years. Intensive treatment was also associated with an increased risk of multiple episodes within the same patient. Within each treatment group (intensive vs. conventional), the number of previous episodes of hypoglycemia was a good predictor of risk of future episode and so was the current glycated hemoglobin level.

79. (*1A*) **Diabetes Control and Complications Trial Research Group.** Effect of intensive diabetes treatment on the development and progression of long-term complications in adolescents with insulin-dependent diabetes mellitus. J Pediatr 1994;125:177–188.

This analysis from the DCCT group focused on 195 patients with type 1 DM between the ages of 13 to 17 years. In this report, a threefold increase of severe hypoglycemia was found in the intensively treated group.

80. (*1C*) **Berger W** et al. The relatively frequent incidence of severe sulfonylurea-induced hypoglycemia in the last 25 years in Switzerland: Results of 2 surveys in Switzerland in 1969 and 1984. Schweiz Med Wochenschr 1986;116:145–151.

In this observational study, the incidence of oral agent–induced hypoglycemia was 0.22 to 0.24 per 1,000 patients. Use of chlorpropamide or glibenclamide was associated with higher frequency of hypoglycemia than was use of tolbutamide.

81. (*1A*) **Landgraf R** et al. A comparison of repaglinide and glibenclamide in the treatment of type 2 diabetic patients previously treated with sulphonylureas. Eur J Clin Pharmacol 1999;55:165–171.

In this randomized controlled study of 195 patients with type 2 DM, no significant difference in adverse events including hypoglycemia was seen between the groups using repaglinide and glibenclamide.

Treatment

82. (*1B*) **Slama G** et al. The search for an optimized treatment of hypoglycemia: Carbohydrates in tablets, solution, or gel for the correction of insulin reactions. Arch Intern Med 1990;150:589–593.

In this French study, hypoglycemia was induced in 41 patients with type 1 DM. Blood glucose concentrations at 10 minutes were similar for glucose, sucrose, or polysaccharide treatment. Treatment with glucose tablets did not produce results that differed from those found with glucose solution. Fruit juice and glucose gel did not raise glucose levels effectively at 10 minutes.

83. (*1B*) **Wiethop BV, Cryer PE.** Alanine and terbutaline in treatment of hypoglycemia in IDDM. Diabetes Care 1993;16:1131–1136.

In this study, oral glucose and subcutaneous glucagon increased plasma glucose concentrations in hypoglycemic type 1 DM patients quickly over 30- to 60-minute periods, but this glucose increase was transient. Glucose levels increased to nearly 11 mmol/L.

84. (*1C*) **Palatnick W** et al. Clinical spectrum of sulfonylurea overdose and experience with diazoxide therapy. Arch Intern Med 1991;151:1859–1862.

This was a retrospective study of 40 episodes of oral agent–induced hypoglycemia. Six patients had severe, resistant hypoglycemia that responded to intravenous diazoxide.

85. (*1C*) **Fanelli CS** et al. Long-term recovery from unawareness, deficient counterregulation, and lack of cognitive dysfunction during hypoglycemia, following institution of rational, intensive insulin therapy in IDDM. Diabetologia 1994;37:1265–1276.

In this study, glycemic goals were relaxed in 21 patients with type 1 DM with hypoglycemia unawareness. This action resulted in an increase of hemoglobin A_{1c} by 1% over 1 year and reduced the frequency of hypoglycemia significantly.

86. (*1C*) **Northam EA** et al. Neuropsychological profiles of children with type 1 diabetes 6 years after disease onset. Diabetes Care 2001;24:1541–1546.

In this Australian study, patients with type 1 DM were followed up prospectively after the onset of disease. Neuropsychological tests were performed at 2 and 6 years after diagnosis. The results of a 6-year follow-up of 90 diabetic patients indicated that the neuropsychological profiles are affected by severe hypoglycemia, particularly in very young children.

87. (*1B*) **Detlofson I** et al. Oral bedtime cornstarch supplementation reduces the risk for nocturnal hypoglycaemia in young children with type 1 diabetes. Acta Paediatr 1999;88:595–597.

In this randomized controlled study, bedtime snacks reduced episodes of hypoglycemia by 64% in 14 preschool children.

Complications of Diabetes

Cardiovascular Disease

88. (*1C*) **Stamler J** et al. Diabetes, other risk factors, and 12-year cardiovascular mortality for men screened in the Multiple Risk Factor Intervention Trial. Diabetes Care 1993;16:434–444.

In this observational study, 12% of 5,163 men who took diabetes medications died of cardiovascular disease over a period of 12 years compared with 6% of men who did not take diabetic medications.

89. (*1A*) **Stratton IM** et al. (UKPDS 35). Association of glycaemia with macrovascular and microvascular complications of type 2 diabetes: Prospective observational study. BMJ 2000;321:405–412.

    In this report from UKPDS, hemoglobin A_{1c} reduction by 1% led to a reduction of 14% for MI.

90. (*1C*) **Agewall S** et al. Usefulness of microalbuminuria in predicting cardiovascular mortality in treated hypertensive men with and without diabetes mellitus: Risk Factor Intervention Study Group. Am J Cardiol 1997;80:164–169.

    In this small study, microalbuminuria predicted cardiovascular disease in diabetic patients.

91. (*1B*) **Hansson L** et al. Effects of intensive blood-pressure lowering and low-dose aspirin in patients with hypertension: Principal results of the Hypertension Optimal Treatment (HOT) randomised trial. HOT Study Group. Lancet 1998;351:1755–1762.

    This randomized controlled study used felodipine to lower blood pressure. In a subgroup of patients with diabetes, cardiovascular events were reduced by 51% when the diastolic blood pressure was 80 mm Hg or lower compared with the diabetic group with diastolic blood pressure above 80 and below 90 mm Hg.

92. (*1A*) **Lindholm LH** et al. Cardiovascular morbidity and mortality in patients with diabetes in the Losartan Intervention for Endpoint Reduction in Hypertension Study (LIFE): A randomised trial against atenolol: The LIFE Study Group. Lancet 2002;359:1004–1010.

    In this study, 1,195 patients with diabetes and hypertension were randomly assigned to receive atenolol or losartan. Mortality from all causes and mortality from cardiovascular disease were significantly lower in the losartan group, by 61% and 63%, respectively.

93. (*1A*) **Heart Outcomes Prevention Evaluation (HOPE) Study Investigators**. Effects of ramipril on cardiovascular and microvascular outcomes in people with diabetes mellitus: Results of the HOPE study and MICRO-HOPE substudy. Lancet 2000;355:253–259.

    In this randomized study, 3,577 diabetic patients with or without preexisting cardiovascular disease were assigned to ramipril, 10 mg/day. After 4.5 years of follow-up, ramipril lowered the risk of MI by 22%, stroke by 33%, overt nephropathy by 24%, and cardiovascular death by 37%.

94. (*1B*) **Pyorala K** et al. Cholesterol lowering with simvastatin improves prognosis of diabetic patients with coronary heart disease: A subgroup analysis of the Scandinavian Simvastatin Survival Study (4S). Diabetes Care 1997;20:614–620.

    In this subgroup analysis of the 4S study, 202 diabetic patients with hypercholesterolemia were randomly assigned to simvastatin treatment, which reduced cardiovascular events.

95. (*1B*) **Rubins HB** et al. Gemfibrozil for the secondary prevention of coronary heart disease in men with low levels of high-density lipoprotein cholesterol: Veterans Affairs High-Density Lipoprotein Cholesterol Intervention Trial Study Group. N Engl J Med 1999;341:410–418.

    In this study, 627 diabetic men and 1,904 nondiabetic men were randomly assigned to gemfibrozil or placebo. After 5.1 years of follow-up, a relative reduction of 24% was noted in the combined incidence of stroke, cardiovascular death, and nonfatal MI.

96. (*1B*) **Goldberg RB** et al. Cardiovascular events and their reduction with pravastatin in diabetic and glucose-intolerant myocardial infarction survivors with average cholesterol levels: Subgroup analyses in the Cholesterol and Recurrent Events (CARE) Trial: The CARE Investigators. Circulation 1998;98:2513–2519.

    In this subgroup analysis of the CARE trial, 586 patients with diabetes were randomly assigned to pravastatin or placebo. The group using pravastatin reduced the absolute risk of cardiovascular event by 8%.

97. (*1A*) **Malmberg K** et al. Randomized trial of insulin-glucose infusion followed by subcutaneous insulin treatment in diabetic patients with acute myocardial infarction (DIGAMI study): Effects on mortality at 1 year. J Am Coll Cardiol 1995;26:57–65.

    In this randomized controlled study, 620 patients were randomly assigned to receive insulin infusion followed by subcutaneous insulin for a period of 3 months or conventional diabetes treatment soon after diagnosis of acute MI. The relative mortality rate was reduced by 29% in the group using insulin infusion at 1 year.

98. (*1A*) **Bypass Angioplasty Revascularization Investigation (BARI) Investigators**. Comparison of coronary bypass surgery with angioplasty in patients with multivessel disease. N Engl J Med 1996;335:217–225.

    Among diabetic patients with multivessel cardiac disease, revascularization with coronary artery bypass graft had a better 5-year survival rate than did angioplasty (80.6% vs. 65.5%; $p = 0.003$).

Eye Disease

99. (*1A*) **Chaturvedi N** et al. Effect of lisinopril on progression of retinopathy in normotensive people with type 1 diabetes. Lancet 1998;351:28–31.

    In this randomized controlled study, 220 patients with type 1 DM and retinopathy were randomly assigned to receive lisinopril versus placebo and observed during 2 years of follow-up. Lisinopril use was associated with a 50% reduction of progression of retinopathy.

100. (*1A*) **Chew EY** et al. Effects of aspirin on vitreous/preretinal hemorrhage in patients with diabetes mellitus: ETDRS Report no. 20. Arch Ophthalmol 1995;113:52–55.

The ETDRS was a randomized controlled study designed to assess the benefit of laser panretinal photocoagulation in reducing severe visual loss in 3,711 patients with nonproliferative or mild proliferative diabetic retinopathy. During intervention, patients were randomly assigned to receive aspirin, 650 mg/day, or placebo. In addition, one eye was assigned to early treatment with photocoagulation, and the other eye served as control in each patient. Results showed that vitreous or preretinal hemorrhage occurred in 39% of eyes assigned to aspirin and 37% assigned to placebo ($p = 0.3$). The conclusion was that aspirin therapy caused no harm.

101. (*1A*) **Early Treatment Diabetic Retinopathy Study Research Group**. Early photocoagulation for diabetic retinopathy: ETDRS Report no. 9. Ophthalmology 1991;98(suppl):766–785.

This is another report from the ETDRS demonstrating that focal photocoagulation is effective in macular edema.

102. (*1A*) **Diabetic Retinopathy Study.** Photocoagulation treatment of proliferative diabetic retinopathy: The second report of Diabetic Retinopathy Study findings. Ophthalmology 1978;85: 82–106.

The DRS was a randomized controlled study of laser (xenon and argon) panretinal photocoagulation in the prevention of severe visual loss. This study provided evidence of benefit for laser treatment in patients with diabetic proliferative retinopathy.

103. (*1A*) **Ferris F.** Early photocoagulation in patients with either type I or type II diabetes. Trans Am Ophthalmol Soc 1996;94:505–537.

In this analysis of the ETDRS, patients with type 2 DM and older diabetic patients benefited from scatter photocoagulation if they were diagnosed with severe nonproliferative retinopathy or early proliferative retinopathy.

104. (*1C*) **Kohner EM** et al. (UKPDS 52). Relationship between the severity of retinopathy and progression to photocoagulation in patients with type 2 DM in the UKPDS. Diabetes Med 2001;18: 178–184.

Another report from the UKPDS demonstrating that few patients with type 2 DM without retinopathy would progress to significant retinopathy requiring photocoagulation after 3 to 6 years of follow-up.

Diabetic Neuropathy

105. (*1C*) **Dyck PJ** et al. The prevalence by staged severity of various types of diabetic neuropathy, retinopathy, and nephropathy in a population-based cohort: The Rochester Diabetic Neuropathy Study. Neurology 1993;43:817–824.

The prevalence of neuropathy in 380 patients with type 1 and type 2 DM residing in Rochester, Minnesota, was examined in this study.

106. (*1A*) **Dyck PJ** et al. The Rochester Diabetic Neuropathy Study: Reassessment of tests and criteria for diagnosis and staged severity. Neurology 1992;42:1164–1170.

In this report of the Rochester Diabetic Neuropathy Study, nerve conduction and quantitative autonomic testing were found to be most sensitive and objective in detection of neuropathy.

107. (*2A*) **Nicolucci A** et al. A meta-analysis of trials on aldose reductase inhibitors in diabetic peripheral neuropathy: The Italian Study Group: The St. Vincent Declaration. Diabetes Med 1996;13:1017–1026.

In this meta-analysis of 13 randomized clinical trials comparing the effects of aldose reductase inhibitors with placebo, as measured by nerve conduction studies, a significant reduction in decline was noted for the median nerve motor velocities but not peroneal motor, median sensory, or sural sensory velocities. Other results, benefits, and adverse effects were unclear.

108. (*1B*) **Argoff CE** et al. Consensus Guidelines: Treatment planning and options. Mayo Clin Proc 2006;81(4, suppl):S12–S25.

In this review of clinical trials, the authors divide medical treatment of painful diabetic neuropathy to first-tier and second-tier treatments.

109. (*1A*) **Backonja M** et al. Gabapentin for the symptomatic treatment of painful neuropathy in patients with diabetes mellitus: A randomized controlled trial. JAMA 1998;280:1831–1836.

In this randomized controlled study, 165 patients were assigned to gabapentin or placebo. The use of gabapentin reduced daily pain scores more than did placebo.

110. (*1A*) **Zhang WY** et al. The effectiveness of topically applied capsaicin: A meta-analysis. Eur J Clin Pharmacol 1994;46:517–522.

In this meta-analysis, capsaicin was better than placebo in treating diabetic neuropathy (OR, 2.74; CI, 1.73–4.3).

Renal Disease

111. (*1C*) **Warram J** et al. Progression of microalbuminuria to proteinuria in type 1 diabetes: Nonlinear relationship with hyperglycemia. Diabetes 2000;49:94–100.

In this study, 279 type 1 DM patients with microalbuminuria were observed for a period of 4 years. The rate of progression increased steeply at levels of hemoglobin A_{1c} between 7.5% and 8.5% but continues to increase at a slower rate after that.

112. (*1A*) **United Kingdom Prospective Diabetes Study Group** (UKPDS 39). Efficacy of atenolol and captopril in reducing the risk of macrovascular complications in type 2 diabetes. BMJ 1998;317:713–720.

   In this report, 758 patients were allocated to tight blood pressure control and 390 patients to conventional blood pressure treatment. The tight blood pressure control group used captopril or atenolol. Captopril treatment did not differ from that using atenolol in relation to controlling blood pressure, macrovascular disease, retinopathy, and hypoglycemia. The group using β-blockers gained 2 kg over an 8-year period in comparison with results in the group using captopril.

113. (*1A*) **United Kingdom Prospective Diabetes Study Group (UKPDS 38).** Tight blood pressure control and risk of macrovascular and microvascular complications in type 2 diabetes. BMJ 1998;317:703–713.

   In this report, tight blood pressure control of 144/82 mm Hg was associated with 44% less stroke, 37% less microvascular disease, and 32% reduction in death related to diabetes compared with conventional blood pressure control of 154/87 mm Hg.

114. (*1A*) **Brenner BM** et al. Effects of losartan on renal and cardiovascular outcomes in patients with type 2 diabetes and nephropathy. N Engl J Med 2001;345:861–869.

   More than 1,500 patients with type 2 DM were assigned to receive losartan or placebo. After 3.4 years, a 28% risk reduction in end-stage renal disease was seen with the use of losartan.

115. (*1A*) **Lewis EJ** et al. Renoprotective effect of the angiotensin-receptor antagonist irbesartan in patients with nephropathy due to type 2 diabetes. N Engl J Med 2001;345:851–860.

   More than 1,700 patients with type 2 DM and hypertension were assigned to receive irbesartan or amlodipine or placebo. After a period of 2.6 years, the irbesartan group had better renal outcomes as measured by doubling creatinine levels and diagnoses of end-stage renal disease. The effect of irbesartan was independent of that of lowering blood pressure.

116. (*1A*) **Lewis EJ** et al. The effect of angiotensin-converting-enzyme inhibition on diabetic nephropathy: The Collaborative Study Group. N Engl J Med 1993;329:1456–1462.

   Four hundred nine patients with type 1 DM were assigned to receive either placebo or captopril. After a 3-year follow-up, serum creatinine levels doubled in 25 patients taking captopril and 43 patients taking placebo. Captopril treatment was associated with 50% reduction in the risk of renal end points.

117. (*1A*) **Pedrini MT** et al. The effect of dietary protein restriction on the progression of diabetic and nondiabetic renal diseases: A meta-analysis. Ann Intern Med 1996;124:627–632.

   In this meta-analysis of five studies and 108 type 1 DM patients, low-protein diets significantly reduced the risk of progression to renal failure and death. Low-protein diets also slowed the progression of urinary microalbuminuria.

Intensive Glycemic Management

118. (*1B*) **Wagner VM** et al. Severe hypoglycaemia, metabolic control and diabetes management in children with type 1 diabetes in the decade after the Diabetes Control and Complications Trial: A large-scale multicenter study. Eur J Pediatr 2005;164:73–79.

   In this large-scale multicenter study, the incidence of hypoglycemia and glycemic control were investigated in 6,309 children with type 1 diabetes. Young children had more severe hypoglycemic events (31.2/100 patient years) as compared with older children (19.7; 21.7/100 patient years; $p < 0.05$), independent of the treatment regimen. Significant predictors of hypoglycemia were younger age ($p < 0.0001$), longer diabetes duration ($p < 0.0001$), higher insulin dose/kg per day ($p < 0.0001$), injection regimen ($p < 0.0005$), and center experience ($p < 0.05$).

119. (*1B*) **Plank J** et al. Systematic review and meta-analysis of short-acting insulin analogues in patients with diabetes mellitus. Arch Intern Med. 2005;165:1337–1344.

   This evidence based meta-analysis compares the effect of treatment with short-acting insulin analogues versus regular insulin on glycemic control, hypoglycemic episodes, quality of life, and diabetes-specific complications. Forty-two randomized controlled trials assessed the effect of analogues versus regular insulin in 7,933 patients with type 1 diabetes mellitus, type 2 diabetes mellitus, and gestational diabetes mellitus. The difference between A(1c) values obtained using analogues and regular insulin was minimal: -0.12% for adult patients with type 1 diabetes mellitus and -0.02% for patients with type 2 diabetes mellitus. No differences between treatments were observed in children with type 1 diabetes, pregnant women with type 1 diabetes mellitus, and women with gestational diabetes.

120. (*1B*) **Bode B** et al. Comparison of insulin aspart with buffered regular insulin and insulin lispro in continuous subcutaneous insulin infusion: A randomized study in type 1 diabetes. Diabetes Care 2002;25:439–444.

   In this study, 146 adult patients with type 1 were randomly assigned to insulin pump treatment with insulin aspart, regular insulin, or lispro for 16 weeks in an open-label, randomized, parallel-group study. Treatment groups had similar baseline A(1c) and after 16 weeks of treatment, A_{1c} values were relatively unchanged from baseline. The rates of hypoglycemic episodes (blood glucose <50 mg/dl) per patient per month were also similar.

121. (*1A*) **Ratner RE** et al. Less hypoglycemia with insulin glargine in intensive insulin therapy for type 1 diabetes: U.S. Study Group of Insulin Glargine in Type 1 Diabetes. Diabetes Care. 2000;23:639–643.

This multicenter randomized parallel-group study compared insulin glargine with NPH human insulin in subjects with type 1 diabetes who had been previously treated with multiple daily injections of NPH insulin and regular insulin. In a total of 534 well-controlled type 1 diabetic subjects, a small and insignificant change A_{1c} levels was noted with insulin glargine (−0.16%) compared with NPH insulin (−0.21%). After the 1-month titration phase, significantly fewer subjects receiving insulin glargine experienced symptomatic hypoglycemia (39.9% vs. 49.2%).

122. (*1B*) **De Leeuw I** et al. Insulin detemir used in basal-bolus therapy in people with type 1 diabetes is associated with a lower risk of nocturnal hypoglycaemia and less weight gain over 12 months in comparison to NPH insulin. Diabetes Obes Metab 2005;7:73–82.

In this multicentre, open-label, parallel-group study, 308 people were randomized to twice-daily insulin detemir or NPH insulin as the basal component of basal-bolus therapy over a period of 12 months. Glycemic control improved in both groups with HbA(1c) decreasing by 0.64 and 0.56% point in the insulin detemir and NPH insulin groups. No significant difference was apparent between treatments in terms of A(1c). Episodes of nocturnal hypoglycemia during (months 2–12) was 32% lower in the detemir group ($p = 0.02$). After 12 months, baseline-adjusted mean body weight was slightly but significantly lower in the insulin detemir group than in the NPH insulin group ($p < 0.001$).

123. (*1B*) **Pickup J** et al. Glycaemic control with continuous subcutaneous insulin infusion compared with intensive insulin injections in patients with type 1 diabetes: Meta-analysis of randomized controlled trials. BMJ 2002;324:705.

In this meta-analysis of 12 randomized controlled trials. 301 people with type 1 diabetes were allocated to insulin infusion, and 299 were allocated to insulin injections. Mean blood glucose concentration was lower in people receiving continuous subcutaneous insulin infusion compared with those receiving insulin injections, equivalent to a difference of 1.0 mmol/l. The percentage of glycated hemoglobin was also lower in people receiving insulin infusion, equivalent to a difference of 0.51%. Blood glucose concentrations were less variable during insulin infusion. This improved control during insulin infusion was achieved with an average reduction of 14% in insulin dose, equivalent to 7.58 units/day, indicating a small difference in glycemic control.

124. (*1B*) **Ratner RE** et al. Amylin replacement with pramlintide as an adjunct to insulin therapy improves long-term glycaemic and weight control in type 1 diabetes mellitus: A 1-year, randomized controlled trial. Diabetes Med 2004;21:1204–1212.

In a double-blind, placebo-controlled, parallel-group, multicenter study, 651 patients with type 1 diabetes were randomized to mealtime injections of pramlintide or placebo, in addition to their insulin therapy, for a year. Addition of pramlintide (60 μg 3 times daily or 4 times daily) to insulin led to significant reductions in A(1c) from baseline to week 52 of 0.29% ($p < 0.011$) and 0.34% ($p < 0.001$), compared with a 0.04% reduction in placebo group, and was accompanied by a small but significant reduction in body weight from baseline to week 52 of 0.4 kg in pramlintide treatment groups, compared with a 0.8-kg gain in body weight in the placebo group.

125. (*1B*) **Hollander P** et al. Addition of pramlintide to insulin therapy lowers HbA_{1c} in conjunction with weight loss in patients with type 2 diabetes approaching glycaemic targets. Diabetes Obes Metab 2003;5:408–414.

In this pooled post hoc analysis of two randomized trials, investigators showed that adjunctive therapy with pramlintide resulted in significant reductions in both HbA_{1c} and body weight from baseline to week 26 (−0.43% and −2.0 kg differences from placebo, respectively; both $p < 0.001$). These changes were achieved without a concomitant increase in the overall rate of severe hypoglycemic events.

126. (*1A*) **Buse JB** et al. Effects of exenatide (exendin-4) on glycemic control over 30 weeks in sulfonylurea-treated patients with type 2 diabetes. Diabetes Care 2004;27:2628–2635.

This study evaluated the ability of exenatide to improve glycemic control in patients with type 2 diabetes after maximally effective doses of a sulfonylurea failed as monotherapy. In a multicenter placebo-controlled, blinded study, the investigators showed that exenatide significantly reduced A(1c) (by −0.86%) in patients with type 2 diabetes for whom maximally effective doses of a sulfonylurea failed, and that exenatide was associated with (−1.6 kg) weight loss.

127. (*1A*) **Chiasson JL** et al. Acarbose treatment and the risk of cardiovascular disease and hypertension in patients with impaired glucose tolerance: the STOP-NIDDM trial. JAMA. 2003; 290:486–494.

In this multicenter double-blind, placebo-controlled, randomized trial, a total of leaving 1,368 patients were studied for 3.3 years (Patients were randomized to receive either placebo ($n = 715$) or 100 mg of acarbose 3 times a day ($n = 714$). Three hundred forty-one patients (24%) discontinued their participation prematurely, 211 in the acarbose-treated group and 130 in the placebo group. Decreasing postprandial hyperglycemia with acarbose was associated with a 49% relative risk reduction in the development of cardiovascular events and a 2.5% absolute risk reduction. Acarbose was also associated with a 34% relative risk reduction in the incidence of new cases of hypertension. Even after adjusting for major risk factors, the reduction in the risk of cardiovascular events associated with acarbose treatment was still statistically significant.

128. (*1C*) **Umpierrez GE** et al. Hyperglycemia: An independent marker of in-hospital mortality in patients with undiagnosed diabetes. J Clin Endocrinol Metab 2002: March;87(3):978–982.

In this study, the medical records of 2,030 consecutive adult patients admitted to a community teaching hospital were reviewed for glucose levels, length of stay, and outcome. Hyperglycemia was present in 38% of patients admitted to the hospital, of whom 26% had a known history of diabetes, and 12% had no history of diabetes before the admission. Newly discovered hyperglycemia was associated with higher in-hospital mortality rate (16%) compared with those patients with a history of diabetes (3%) and subjects with normoglycemia (1.7%; both $p < 0.01$). In addition, new hyperglycemic patients had a longer length of hospital stay, a higher admission rate to an intensive care unit, and were less likely to be discharged to home, frequently requiring transfer to a transitional care unit or nursing home facility.

129. (*1B*) **Rassias AJ** et al. Insulin infusion improves neutrophil function in diabetic cardiac surgery patients. Anesth Analg 1998:88:1011–1016.

In this small study of 26 patients, the investigators tested the effect of an insulin infusion on perioperative neutrophil function in diabetic patients scheduled for coronary artery bypass surgery and found that a continuous insulin infusion and glucose control during surgery improves white cell function in diabetic patients and may increase resistance to infection after surgery.

130. (*1C*) **Levitan EB** et al. Is nondiabetic hyperglycemia a risk factor for cardiovascular disease? A meta-analysis of prospective studies. Arch Intern Med 2004;164:2147–2155.

In this meta-analysis of 38 prospective reports, cardiovascular disease incidence or mortality was an end point, and blood glucose levels were measured prospectively. Blood glucose level was determined to be a risk marker for CVD among apparently healthy individuals without diabetes.

131. (*1C*) **Bolk J** et al. Impaired glucose metabolism predicts mortality after a myocardial infarction. Int J Cardiol 2001;79:207–214.

In this prospective follow-up trial of 336 consecutive patients with acute myocardial infraction followed up for 14 months, blood glucose was a determinant of mortality. One-year mortality rate was 19.3% and increased to 44% in patients with glucose levels >11.1 mmol/l. The mortality was higher in diabetic patients than in nondiabetic patients (40 vs. 16%; $p < 0.05$). Multivariate analysis revealed an independent effect of glucose level on mortality.

132. (*1C*) **Capes SE** et al. Stress hyperglycaemia and increased risk of death after myocardial infarction in patients with and without diabetes: A systematic overview. Lancet 2000;355:773–778.

In this meta-analysis, the relative risks of in-hospital mortality and congestive heart failure in hyperglycemic and normoglycemic patients with and without diabetes were evaluated by performing a meta-analysis of 15 studies. The authors found that patients without diabetes who had glucose concentrations more than or equal to range of 6.1 to 8.0 mmol/L had a 3.9-fold higher risk of death than did patients without diabetes who had lower glucose concentrations. Glucose concentrations higher than values in the range of 8.0 to 10.0 mmol/L on admission were associated with increased risk of congestive heart failure or cardiogenic shock in patients without diabetes. In patients with diabetes who had glucose concentrations more than or equal to a range from 10.0 to 11.0 mmol/L, the risk of death was moderately increased (1.7), indicating that stress hyperglycemia with myocardial infarction is associated with an increased risk of in-hospital mortality in patients with and without diabetes.

133. (*1B*) **Furnary AP** et al. Continuous intravenous insulin infusion reduces the incidence of deep sternal wound infection in diabetic patients after cardiac surgical procedures. Ann Thorac Surg 1999;67:352–360.

In this prospective comparative study of diabetic patients who underwent open heart surgical procedures, 968 patients were treated with sliding-scale-guided intermittent subcutaneous insulin, and 1,499 were patients treated with a continuous intravenous insulin infusion in an attempt to maintain a blood glucose level of less than 200 mg/dl. Compared with subcutaneous insulin injections, continuous intravenous insulin infusion induced a significant reduction in perioperative blood glucose levels, which led to a significant reduction in the incidence of deep sternal wound infection in the continuous intravenous insulin infusion group [0.8% (12 of 1,499)] versus the intermittent subcutaneous insulin injection group [2.0% (19 of 968); $p = 0.01$]. Multivariate logistic regression revealed that continuous intravenous insulin infusion induced a significant decrease in the risk of deep sternal wound infection ($p = 0.005$; relative risk, 0.34).

134. (*1B*) **Fath-Ordoubadi F, Beatt KJ**. Glucose-insulin-potassium therapy for treatment of acute myocardial infarction: an overview of randomized placebo-controlled trials. Circulation 1997;96: 1152–1156

This meta-analysis of nine studies with total of 1,932 patients revealed that using insulin infusion reduces hospital mortality from 21% (205 of 972 patients) in the placebo group to 16.1% (154 of 956) in the treatment group. The proportional mortality reduction was 28% (CI, 10% to 43%). The number of lives saved per 1,000 patients treated was 49.

135. (*1B*) **van den Berghe G** et al. Intensive insulin therapy in the critically ill patients. N Engl J Med 2001;345:1359–1367.

In this landmark prospective, randomized, controlled study, ICU patients were randomly assigned to receive intensive insulin therapy [maintenance of blood glucose at a level between 80 and 110 mg/dl (4.4 and 6.1 mmol/L)] or conventional treatment [infusion of insulin only if the blood glucose level exceeded

215 mg/dl (11.9 mmol/L)] and maintenance of glucose at a level between 180 and 200 mg/dl (10.0 and 11.1 mmol/L). At 12 months, with a total of 1,548 patients enrolled, intensive insulin therapy reduced mortality during intensive care from 8.0% with conventional treatment to 4.6% ($p < 0.04$). The benefit of intensive insulin therapy was attributable to its effect on mortality among patients who remained in the intensive care unit for more than 5 days (20.2% with conventional treatment, as compared with 10.6% with intensive insulin therapy; $p = 0.005$). The greatest reduction in mortality involved deaths due to multiple-organ failure with a proven septic focus. Intensive insulin therapy also reduced overall in-hospital mortality by 34%, bloodstream infections by 46%, acute renal failure requiring dialysis or hemofiltration by 41%, the median number of red cell transfusions by 50%, and critical-illness polyneuropathy by 44%, and patients receiving intensive therapy were less likely to require prolonged mechanical ventilation and intensive care.

136. (*1B*) **Pittas AG** et al. Insulin therapy for critically ill hospitalized patients: A meta-analysis of randomized controlled trials. Arch Intern Med 2004;164:2005–2011.

In this meta-analysis of 35 randomized controlled trials, insulin therapy decreased short-term mortality by 15% [relative risk (RR), 0.85]. In subgroup analyses, insulin therapy also decreased mortality in the surgical intensive care unit (RR, 0.58), when the aim of therapy was glucose control (RR, 0.71), and in patients with diabetes mellitus (RR, 0.73).

137. (*1B*) **Furnary AP** et al. Continuous insulin infusion reduces mortality in patients with diabetes undergoing coronary artery bypass grafting. J Thorac Cardiovasc Surg 2003;125:1007–1021.

In this comparative trial, patients with diabetes undergoing coronary artery bypass grafting ($n = 3,554$) were treated aggressively with either subcutaneous insulin (between 1987 and 1991) or with continuous insulin infusion (between 1992 and 2001) for hyperglycemia. Observed mortality with continuous insulin infusion (2.5%; $n = 65/2,612$) was significantly lower than with subcutaneous insulin (5.3%; $n = 50/942$; $p < 0.0001$). Likewise, glucose control was significantly better with continuous insulin infusion (177 ± 30 mg/dl vs. 213 ± 41 mg/dl; $p < 0.0001$).

138. (*1C*) **Dickerson LM** et al. Glycemic control in medical inpatients with type 2 diabetes mellitus receiving sliding scale insulin regimens versus routine diabetes medications: A multicenter randomized controlled trial. Ann Fam Med 2003;1:29–35.

In this study of 153 hospitalized patients with type 2 DM, the investigators used an insulin sliding-scale regimen that was adjusted to individual patients and was accompanied by antidiabetic agent for background/basal coverage. In this form, insulin sliding scale did not perform better than standard treatment, and no significant differences were found between the group treated with conventional treatment and the group treated with sliding scale combined with some form of antidiabetic basal coverage. Although this is a small study, it shows that insulin sliding scale can be used safely in certain situations.

Lipid Disorders

Francis Q. Almeda

Coronary heart disease (CHD) is the leading cause of death in the United States, and despite major advances in cardiovascular care, the cardiac event rates remain significant. Dyslipidemia is a major risk factor for the development and progression of atherosclerotic cardiovascular disease (ASCVD) and remains a major health issue in contemporary clinical practice [1]. The diagnosis and treatment of patients with lipid disorders has been shown to reduce significantly the risk of future cardiac events. The intensity of risk-reduction therapy should be adjusted the individual's absolute risk [2], and thus the identification of the patient's overall cardiovascular risk status is the central component for the optimal treatment of individuals with dyslipidemia.

Lipid disorders can be classified into primary (genetic or inherited) (Table 7.1) or secondary (due to disease or environmental factors). Important secondary factors that result in altered lipid metabolism include hypothyroidism, diabetes mellitus, renal disease, obstructive liver disease, alcohol intake, and various medications, and the identification and modification of these secondary causes should be aggressively pursued.

LIPOPROTEIN METABOLISM

Lipoproteins are large complexes that transport lipids [mainly cholesterol esters, triglycerides (triacylglycerol; TAG), and fat-soluble vitamins] to and from the vasculature to various body tissues. The plasma lipoproteins are divided into five main classes based on their relative densities: chylomicrons, very low density lipoproteins (VLDLs), intermediate-density lipoproteins (IDLs), low-density lipoproteins (LDLs), and high-density lipoproteins (HDLs).

Lipoprotein metabolism occurs through two basic mechanisms, which include the transport of dietary lipids to the liver and peripheral tissues (exogenous pathway), and the production and delivery of hepatic lipids into the circulation and peripheral tissues (endogenous pathway) [3]. In the exogenous pathway, dietary cholesterol is acted on by the intestinal cells to form cholesterol esters through the addition of fatty acids. TAGs from the diet are hydrolyzed by pancreatic lipases within the intestine and emulsified with bile acids to form micelles. Longer-chain fatty acids are incorporated into TAGs and complexed with other particles such as cholesterol esters and phospholipids to form chylomicrons (which have a high concentration of TAGs). These particles are acted on by lipoprotein lipase along the capillary endothelium, and the TAGs are hydrolyzed, releasing free fatty acids, most of which are taken up by adjacent adipocytes or myocytes,

Table 7.1. Inherited Lipid Disorders

Condition	Mechanisms/Characteristics
Familial combined hypercholesterolemia (FCHL)	The most common primary lipid disorder may affect ≤2% of U.S. population. Autosomal dominant. Increased secretion of apo B-100 with resulting in varying patterns of high LDL with moderate elevations of TAG and low HDL. Significantly increased risk of atherosclerotic cardiovascular disease (ASCVD). Common comorbidities include diabetes, hypertension, and obesity
Familial hypertriglyceridemia (FHTG)	Relatively common (one in 500). Autosomal dominant. Usually with moderately to severely elevated TAG (250 mg/dl–1,000 mg/dl) with mildly increased cholesterol (<250 mg/dl) with low HDL due mainly to increased production and impaired clearance of VLDL, although more severe form has elevated chylomicrons
Familial hypercholesterolemia (FH)	Occurs in one in 500. Deficient or defective LDL receptor resulting in reduced clearance and accumulation of LDL with normal TAG. Autosomal dominant. Heterozygous FH (LDL range, 325–450 mg/dl). Homozygous FH with very high LDL (500–1,000 mg/dl). Clinical clues include tendon xanthomas, childhood CHD, arcus cornea in young patients, premature ASCVD
Primary (familial) hypoalphalipoproteinemia	Most common genetic cause of low HDL. HDL <10th percentile with normal cholesterol and TAG levels after secondary causes of low HDL are excluded. Increased risk of premature ASCVD
Familial defective Apo B-100	Occurs in one in 1,000. Autosomal dominant. Moderate elevation in LDL with normal TAG. Mutant apo B-100 poorly recognized by LDL receptor. Palmar and tuberoeruptive xanthomas, premature ASCVD. Clinically resembles heterozygous FH
Familial dysbetalipoproteinemia (FDBL)	Occurs in one in 10,000. Mixed hyperlipidemia due to increased chylomicrons and VLDL remnants due to defective apolipoprotein E. Autosomal dominant. Tendon xanthomas, premature ASCVD
Familial chylomicronemia syndrome (FCS)	Occurs in ~1 in 1,000,000. Autosomal recessive. Genetic deficiency of lipoprotein lipase or cofactor ApoC-II resulting in extremely high TAG (>1,000 mg/dl) due to chylomicronemia. Recurrent pancreatitis, lipemia retinalis, eruptive xanthomas, hepatomegaly. Usually *without* premature ASCVD
Tangier disease	Rare disease manifested by very low HDL due to mutations in the gene *ABCA1* results in rapid clearance of HDL from the circulation. Patients have cholesterol accumulation in the reticuloendothelial system with hepatomegaly and pathognomonic enlarged yellowish orange tonsils
LCAT deficiency	Rare disorder of low HDL due to lecithin/cholesterol acyltransferase deficiency. Increased catabolism of HDL. Corneal opacities due to accumulation of cholesterol in lens ("fish-eye disease")

Table 7.2. Updated ATP III LDL-C Goals and Cut Points for Therapeutic Life-style Changes and Drug Therapy in Different Risk Categories

Risk Category	LDL-C Goal (mg/dl)	Initiate TLC (mg/dl)	Consider Drug Therapy (mg/dl)
High risk: CHD or CHD risk equivalents (10-year risk, >20%)[a]	<100 mg/dl (optimal goal <70 mg/dl)[b]	≥100 mg/dl[c]	≥100 mg/dl (<100 in selected high-risk populations)[b]
Moderately high risk: 2+ risk factors (10-year risk, 10–20%)[d]	<130 mg/dl	≥130 mg/dl	≥130 mg/dl (100–129, consider drug options)[e]
Moderate risk: 2+ risk factors (10-year risk, <10%)	<130 mg/dl	≥130 mg/dl	≥160 mg/dl
Low risk: 0–1 risk factors	<130 mg/dl	≥160 mg/dl	≥190 mg/dl (160–189, LDL-lowering drug optional)

[a] CHD includes established coronary artery disease (history of myocardial infarction, unstable or stable angina, coronary revascularization, or evidence of clinically significant myocardial ischemia). CHD equivalents include diabetes and evidence of noncoronary atherosclerosis (peripheral arterial disease, abdominal aortic aneurysm, carotid artery disease, transient ischemic attacks or stroke).

[b] Very high risk favors the optional LDL-C goal of 70 mg/dl, and in patients with high triglycerides and low HDL.

[c] In individual at high risk or moderately high risk with lifestyle-related risk factors (i.e., obesity, physical inactivity, elevated triglyceride, low HDL, metabolic syndrome), aggressive therapeutic life-style changes to modify these risk factors is advisable regardless of the LDL level.

[d] Risk factors include: age (men >45 years, and women >55 years), hypertension (BP >140/90 mm Hg or taking antihypertensive medication), smoking, low HDL (<40 mg/dl), and family history of premature CAD (CHD in male first-degree relative <55 years; CHD in female first-degree relative <65 years).

[e] For moderately high-risk individuals, if the LDL is 100–129 mg/dl at baseline or on TLC, initiation of an LDL-lowering drug to achieve an LDL of <100 mg/dl is a therapeutic option.

and the remaining particles (chylomicron remnants) are transported to the liver. In the endogenous pathway, VLDL is transformed into IDL and then into LDL through hepatic metabolism. VLDL particles are similar to chylomicrons, but have a higher ratio of cholesterol to TAGs and contain apolipoprotein B-100. The TAG of VLDL is hydrolyzed by lipoprotein lipase, and the particles continue to become smaller and more dense and transform into IDL, which is composed of similar amounts of cholesterol and TAG. The hepatic cells remove approximately half of VLDL remnants and IDL. The remainder of IDL is modified by hepatic lipase to form LDL. LDL is composed of a core of primarily cholesterol esters, surrounded by a surface of phospholipids, free cholesterol, and apolipoprotein B. The majority of circulating LDL is cleared through LDL-mediated endocytosis in the liver. Modified (oxidized) plasma LDL accumulates in the intima and is acted on by activated macrophages (foam cells) and through complex mechanisms involving cytokines, growth factors, smooth cell proliferation, and inflammation, and results in atheroma formation [4]. The process of transferring cholesterol from peripheral cells to the liver for removal from the body by biliary secretion is called reverse cholesterol transport. The role of HDL in enhancing reverse cholesterol transport is one of the mechanisms by which HDL protects against the process of atherosclerosis. The major protein of HDL is apo A1.

The major lipid abnormalities of clinical significance result in an alteration in the levels of LDL, HDL, and TAG, and these disorders are the primary focus of this chapter. Other associated abnormalities that have been investigated include abnormal levels of serum homocysteine and lipoprotein (a), although the data surrounding these and other emerging risk factors remain controversial [5].

LOW-DENSITY LIPOPROTEIN (LDL) CHOLESTEROL

Trials

The largest body of evidence exists for improved outcomes with LDL lowering, and thus LDL remains the major therapeutic target for intervention [2]. Large epidemiologic studies such as the Seven Countries Study [6] confirmed the association of total serum cholesterol and coronary heart disease. In addition, the Multiple Risk Factor Intervention Trial [7] demonstrated that this relation was continuous and graded, without a threshold level. Large, placebo-controlled, randomized trials confirmed the benefit of LDL lowering on reducing long-term cardiac event rates [8–10].

Primary Prevention Trials

The central principle of management of the patient without established atherosclerotic vascular disease is that the intensity of risk reduction should be commensurate with the individual's absolute cardiovascular risk (Table 7.2). The major risk factors (exclusive of LDL cholesterol) include age older than 45 years in men and older than 55 years in women, cigarette smoking, hypertension (defined as ≥140/90 mm Hg or on antihypertensive medication), low HDL cholesterol (<40 mg/dL), and a family history of premature coronary heart disease in first-degree relative (younger than 55 years in male relative, and younger than 65 years in female relative [2]. The LDL cholesterol is not included among the risk factors because the reason for assessing these risk factors is to treat the LDL. A high HDL (≥60 mg/dL) is regarded as a "negative" risk factor and removes one other risk factor from the total count.

The patient's risk is estimated first by determining the number of risk factors. The first group comprises patients with no to one risk factors. Traditionally, this group has been assigned to a low-risk category (10-year risk of CHD, <10%), and the recommended LDL goal has been <160 mg/dL. However, a very high LDL (>190 mg/dL) may warrant consideration of drug therapy to reduce long-term risk. In addition, a single powerful risk factor (strong family history of premature CHD, heavy cigarette smoking, very low HDL, poorly controlled hypertension) favors the use of drugs to reduce the LDL.

The second group of patients comprises those with two or more risk factors. The 10-year risk of a cardiac event is assessed by using the Framingham scoring, which takes into account the patient's age, gender, HDL, blood pressure, smoking status, and family history of premature ASCVD, and may be calculated by using tables or hand-held and Internet-based online calculators (www.nhlbi.nih.gov/guidelines/cholesterol). Framingham scoring will stratify persons with multiple risk factors into those with a 10-year risk of CHD of more than 20%, 10% to 20%, or less than 10%. The LDL goal of patients with multiple (2+) risk factors and a 10-year risk of 10% to 20% has traditionally been less than 130 mg/dL [2], but an LDL goal of less than 100 mg/dL is a therapeutic option based on updated clinical guidelines [11], and drug therapy (in addition to therapeutic life-style changes) should be considered to achieve this goal. Patients with multiple risk factors that confer a risk for a major cardiac event of more than 20% over a 10-year period are at highest risk and are treated as if they had established cardiovascular disease.

Importantly, a patient's risk may be affected by other factors not included in major factors outlined earlier. Other risk factors that should be taken into consideration include obesity, sedentary life-style, and an atherogenic diet, which are excellent targets for clinical intervention. Other emerging risk factors such as lipoprotein (a), homocysteine, pro-inflammatory markers such as high-sensitivity C-reactive protein, and impaired fasting glucose further guide the intensity of risk reduction in selected individuals. In addition, LDL subclasses may be measured through nuclear magnetic resonance (NMR) spectroscopy, and the detection of smaller denser LDL particles may provide incremental information on cardiovascular risk [12]. Furthermore, the metabolic syndrome is a constellation of interrelated metabolic risk factors with underlying insulin resistance that imparts an especially high risk for the development of ASCVD and diabetes [11].

The WOSCOPS Trial [13] enrolled middle-aged men with hypercholesterolemia (mean total cholesterol, 272 mg/dL) and no history of myocardial infarction (MI) to treatment with pravastatin and found a significant reduction in death and nonfatal MI by 31% compared with placebo over a mean follow-up of 4.9 years. The ASCOT-LLA Trial [14] evaluated treatment with atorvastatin in hypertensive patients with modest hypercholesteremia (total cholesterol, <240 mg/dL) compared with placebo. After median follow-up of 3.3 years, the trial was stopped prematurely because of a highly significant 36% reduction in fatal CHD and nonfatal MI, which became apparent in the first year of follow-up. The ALLHAT Trial (15) was a similar study that evaluated the administration of pravastatin in the treatment of older, hypertensive, moderately hypercholesterolemic (mean total cholesterol, 244 mg/dL, and mean LDL, 148 mg/dL) patients with one additional risk factor compared with placebo with a mean follow-up 4.8 years. The results of this trial showed that no statistically significant differences in mortality or CHD event rates existed, although this may have been due to the high rate of nonstudy statin in the usual-care group or the modest differential in total cholesterol and LDL between the pravastatin and usual-care group compared with prior statin trials. The AFCAPS/TeXCAPS Trial (16) enrolled patients without CHD and with average serum cholesterol levels (mean total cholesterol, 221 mg/dL, and mean LDL, 150 mg/dL) and below-average HDL (mean HDL, 36 mg/dL) levels to lovastatin and demonstrated a reduction in the first acute major coronary event (MI, unstable angina, or sudden cardiac death) by 37% (16). Taken in aggregate, these landmark clinical trials (10,13–16) suggest that lipid-lowering therapy in intermediate- to high-risk patients without established ASCVD with moderate hypercholesterolemia is beneficial and is associated with lower adverse major cardiac event rates on follow-up.

Secondary Prevention Trials

The highest-risk group includes those patients with established cardiovascular disease or a "CHD risk equivalent." This group comprises patients with known coronary artery disease, other clinical forms of atherosclerotic vascular disease, including peripheral vascular disease, carotid artery disease, abdominal aortic aneurysm, and diabetes mellitus, and patients with multiple risk factors that confer a risk for a major cardiac event of more than 20% over a 10-year period. The identification of subclinical atherosclerotic disease such as high coronary calcification, significant carotid intimal medial thickness, or significant atherosclerotic burden on CT angiography likewise warrants aggressive and intensive lipid lowering.

The 4S Trial (8) was the first trial to demonstrate a reduction in total mortality (30% relative-risk reduction) in middle-aged patients with high cholesterol (mean total cholesterol, 272 mg/dL, and mean LDL, 190 mg/dL) with established CHD treated with simvastatin compared with placebo, in addition to reducing major coronary events and coronary revascularization, over an average of 5.4 years. The CARE (10) trial extended these findings and to patients with established CHD and "average" cholesterol levels (mean total cholesterol, 209 mg/dL, and mean LDL, 139 mg/dL) and demonstrated a 24% relative-risk reduction in the primary end points (mortality and major cardiac event rates and stroke). The LIPID Trial (9) was the largest trial of secondary prevention and similarly demonstrated a 24% reduction in CHD mortality, as well as total mortality and fatal and nonfatal MI. The Heart Protection Study (17) demonstrated a reduction in all-cause mortality with treatment with simvastatin in a wide range of high-risk patients (coronary artery disease, occlusive arterial disease, or diabetes), irrespective of their baseline LDL level. Importantly, a significant reduction was noted in nonfatal MI, stroke, and coronary and noncoronary revascularization, and the risk reductions were similar and significant, even in patients with a "low" baseline LDL level (<116 mg/dL), suggesting that lower is better. In summary, these large randomized clinical trials clearly demonstrated that lipid-lowering therapy with statins in patients with established ASCVD resulted in a highly significant reduction in mortality and cardiac events over a wide range of LDL values.

How Low Should You Go?

The Heart Protection Study (17) and the PROVE IT Trial (18) showed incremental 22% and 16% reductions in risk for adverse cardiac events with LDL levels reduced to less than 100 mg/dL. The Treat To New Targets Trial (TNT) (19) demonstrated a 22% relative and a 2.2% absolute risk reduction of more major cardiac events (including death from CHD, nonfatal MI, resuscitation after a cardiac arrest, and fatal or nonfatal stroke) in the group receiving high-dose atorvastatin compared with the low-dose group. The mean LDL in the high-dose group was 77 mg/dL compared with 101 mg/dL in the low-dose group. Overall, these data suggest that no clear-cut identifiable threshold exists for LDL level for risk reduction and that "lower is better." Based on these recent trials demonstrating reduced cardiovascular event rates with lower LDL levels, the current recommendation for optimal LDL is less than 70 mg/dL in patients at very high risk (11). The factors that place a patient at very high risk include established ASCVD and CHD equivalents, multiple major risk factors, and severe and poorly controlled risk factors (i.e., smoking). No major safety issues have been identified thus far with reducing LDL to the range of 50 to 70 mg/dL [20].

Treatment Options

Dietary Modification

Life-style and dietary modification remain crucial, and reduced intake of saturated fat and cholesterol, increased physical activity, and weight control for all patients is recommended. All patients should be advised to adopt therapeutic life-style changes including reduced intake of saturated fats (<7% of total calories) and cholesterol (<200 mg/d), increased intake of soluble fiber (10–25 g/day), weight reduction, and increased physical activity. Dietary modification and should be a mainstay of any LDL lowering strategy; however, the average LDL reduction from diet alone is in the range of 5% to 10% [21], and compliance with a strict diet remains problematic in the clinical setting.

Statins (3-Hydroxy-3-Methylglutaryl Coenzyme A Reductase Inhibitors)

Statins reduce serum LDL levels through intracellular inhibition of the rate-limiting step in cholesterol production, which reduces cholesterol biosynthesis in the liver and upregulates LDL-C receptors to increase clearance of LDL-C from the blood. The statins reduce the LDL by 18% to 55%, increase HDL by 5% to 15%, and reduce TAG by 7% to 30% (Table 7.3). At the current available doses, rosuvastatin and atorvastatin are the most potent statins, followed in order of LDL-reducing potency by simvastatin, lovastatin, pravastatin, and fluvastatin. Each doubling of a statin dose achieves an approximately 6% additional reduction in serum LDL (the "rule of 6s"). A large meta-analysis involving 14 randomized placebo-controlled trials involving 90,056 patients showed that lowering LDL-cholesterol levels by 39 mg/dL (1 mmol/L) with statin therapy significantly reduces the 5-year risk of major coronary events, coronary revascularization, and stroke by 21% [22]. This benefit emerged early, was sustained, and was related mainly to the individual's absolute risk and to the absolute reduction in LDL-cholesterol levels achieved.

Statin Therapy in High-Risk Populations

Statins have been shown to be beneficial in a wide range of high-risk populations including acute coronary syndromes [18,23,24], diabetics [25], the elderly [26], and in patients with moderate chronic renal disease [27]. Surprisingly, statin therapy had a

Table 7.3. FDA-Approved Drugs for Treating Lipoprotein Abnormalities

Drugs	Lipid Effects	Adverse Effects/Drug Interactions
Statins Pravastatin (40–80 mg qhs) Lovastatin (20–80 mg qhs) Fluvastatin (20–80 mg qhs) Simvastatin (20–80 mg qhs) Atorvastatin (10–80 mg qhs) Rosuvastatin (10–40 mg qhs)	LDL: ↓18–55% HDL: ↑5–15% TAG: ↓7–30%	Increased risk of myopathy with itraconazole, ketoconazole, erythromycin, clarithromycin, erythromycin, HIV protease inhibitors, nefazodone, amiodarone, verapamil, or large large quantities of grapefruit juice (>1 quart daily); may raise hepatic transaminase levels
Cholesterol-absorption inhibitor Ezetimibe (10 mg qd)	LDL: ↓15–20% HDL: ↑2–5% TAG: ↓3–8%	Side effects include headache and diarrhea; myopathy and hepatitis rare
Fibric acids Gemfibrozil (600 mg b.i.d.) Fenofibrate (48–145 mg or 43–130 mg qd)	LDL: ↓5–20% HDL: ↑10–20% TAG: ↓20–55%	Side effects include rash and dyspepsia; potentiates the action of warfarin; contraindicated in patients with gallstones or severe renal insufficiency/hemodialysis; variable effects of the serum LDL, and may increase LDL
Nicotinic acids Immediate-release (100 mg t.i.d. to 2 g t.i.d.) Sustained-release (250 mg b.i.d. to 1.5 g b.i.d.) Extended-release (500 mg qhs to 2 g qhs)	LDL: ↓5–20% HDL: ↑15–35% TAG: ↓20–50%	Most common side effect is flushing; potentiates the action of warfarin; may precipitate acute gout and esophageal reflux, hyperglycemia
Bile acid sequestrants Cholestyramine (4–24 g/day) Colestipol (5–40 g/day) Colesevelam (3,750–4,375 mg qd)	LDL: ↓15–30% HDL: ↑3–5% TAG: ↑3–10%	Common side effects include nausea, constipation, and bloating; associated with increased TAG levels
Fish oils Omega-3 fatty acid (3–12 g)	LDL: ↑45% HDL: ↑9% TAG: ↓45%	Associated with increased LDL level; side effects include dyspepsia and fishy aftertaste

neutral effect of cardiovascular outcomes in a large trial involving diabetic patients receiving hemodialysis [28], and future randomized trails will address the issue of statin therapy in severe chronic kidney disease.

Pleiotropic Effects of Statins
Although treatment with statins has resulted in major reductions in cardiac event rates, the amount of plaque regression demonstrated has been modest at most [29,30] raising the possibility that the beneficial effects extend over and beyond LDL lower-

ing. The pleiotropic effects of statins include anti-inflammatory, anti-thrombotic, immunomodulatory, and vascular effects, although the precise mechanisms and magnitude of these non–LDL-lowering properties in reducing cardiac risk remain elusive [31].

Safety Issues
Statins are generally well tolerated; however, common minor side effects include muscle and joint aches ($\leq$5%), fatigue, dyspepsia, and headaches. More serious side effects such as severe myositis with generalized muscle pain and weakness and elevated creatine kinase (rarely leading to rhabdomyolysis and acute renal failure) or severe hepatitis may occur infrequently. Adverse drug interactions should be carefully monitored (Table 7.3), particularly at higher doses and in elderly patients with low body weight, and patients with impaired renal function or receiving combination therapy with fibrates and/or nicotinic acid [32]. Liver transaminases should be checked before starting therapy and with increases in dosage. High elevations of liver transaminases (>3 times the upper limit of normal) are exceedingly rare, and usually resolve completely after discontinuing the statin. Milder increases in liver-function tests (1 to 3 times the upper limit of normal) require close monitoring, but do not necessarily require stopping the drug in the absence of symptoms [33].

Ezetimibe (Zetia)
Ezetimibe acts through inhibition of intestinal cholesterol absorption in the small intestine, leading to a reduction in hepatic cholesterol stores and increasing clearance of cholesterol from the blood. As monotherapy, ezetimibe effectively decreases LDL by 15% to 20% [34]. The combination of absorption pathway in the small intestine with ezetimibe and a statin results in dual inhibition through inhibition of the production pathway and the production pathway in the liver, respectively, reducing the LDL by as much as an additional 25%, with potentially fewer side effects [35].

Bile Acid Sequestrants (Resins)
Bile acid sequestrants act through binding bile acids in the intestine, resulting in increased excretion in the stool, stimulating greater intrahepatic cholesterol utilization for bile acid synthesis. This results in upregulation of the LDL receptor, which enhances clearance of LDL in the bloodstream. In general, resins reduce LDL by 15% to 30%. The available bile-acid sequestrants include cholestyramine, colesevelam, and colestipol. Treatment with cholestyramine has been associated with a reduction in progression of atherosclerosis compared with control [36]. Because resins are not systemically absorbed, they are extremely safe, but are associated with side effects such as nausea, constipation, and bloating. Other medications should be taken either 1 hour before or 4 hours after the resins because of binding and decreased absorption (i.e., warfarin, digoxin). Resins may significantly increase the TAG level and should be avoided in patients with hypertriglyceridemia.

Nicotinic Acid and Fibric Acids
Nicotinic acid and fibric acid modestly reduce LDL (approximately 5% to 20%) and are used mainly as therapies to reduce TAG and increase LDL and are discussed in detail later in the chapter under Treatment Options for HDL/TAG.

Combination Therapy
Even with the most potent statins, achieving the target LDL is often challenging with monotherapy. Higher doses of statins are associated with higher-risk myopathy and hepatotoxicity. Combination therapy with a statin with ezetimibe has a synergistic mechanism of action by inhibiting dual pathways. Because of the increasing prevalence of diabetes and insulin resistance with several metabolic abnormalities, combination therapy is often the optimal approach for achieving the desired results by targeting multiple lipoprotein particles and metabolic pathways [37]. Thus combination therapy

with a statin and niacin [38,39] or a statin and a fibrate [40], or all three together, may the preferred strategy, particularly with markedly abnormal HDL and TAG levels, although safety issues remain a concern.

Nonpharmacologic Strategies

LDL apheresis involves the direct removal of LDL from the plasma and may be the preferred option in severe drug-resistant or refractory hyperlipidemia. Partial ileal bypass surgically depletes the enterohepatic supply of bile acids resulting in upregulation of the of the LDL receptor in the liver, increasing LDL clearance, and may be an option in patients with severely elevated LDL and normal TAG refractory to maximal medical management who are not candidates for LDL apheresis.

HIGH-DENSITY LIPOPROTEIN (HDL) CHOLESTEROL AND TRIGLYCERIDES (TAG)

Although LDL remains the primary lipid-lowering priority, low HDL and high TAG have been associated with increased cardiac risk and are potential targets for therapeutic intervention. A meta-analysis [41] that suggested that a TAG elevation of 89 mg/dL is associated with a 14% risk in coronary risk in men and 37% risk in women after adjustment for HDL, although other studies have not found independent risk [42]. TAG has great variability and may be affected by recent weight change, exercise status, or consumption of carbohydrates or alcohol, and medications such as estrogen and isotretinoin. The recommended TAG goal is less than 150 mg/dL [2]. "Non-HDL" is equal to total cholesterol minus the HDL and represents the spectrum of atherogenic apolipoprotein B (apo-B)-carrying lipoproteins including VLDL, chylomicron remnants, VLDL remnants, IDL, lipoprotein (a), and LDL. If TAG levels are 200 mg/dL or more, non-HDL is a secondary target of treatment after the LDL goal has been achieved. The non-HDL goal is 30 mg/dL higher than the specified goal for LDL (Table 7.2). If the TAG levels are 500 mg/dL or more, then treatment of TAG takes priority over LDL reduction because of the desire to reduce the risk of acute pancreatitis.

Epidemiologic data clearly suggest that a low HDL may be a significant risk factor comparable to and independent of an elevated LDL [43]. A low HDL has been defined as less than 40 mg/dL in men and less than 50 mg/dL in women. A "high" HDL is more than 60 mg/dL, although the classification of the "optimal" HDL will continue to evolve.

Pooled data from several studies estimate a 2% to 3% reduction in cardiovascular risk for every 1-mg/dL increase in HDL [44]. The potential mechanisms of action whereby HDL delays the development and progression of atherosclerosis include reverse cholesterol transport, anti-inflammatory activity, and antioxidant effects [45]. Limited data exist on the benefits of elevating HDL through pharmacologic intervention, although this may be because currently available agents achieve only moderate increases in HDL. The metabolic syndrome and diabetes mellitus, because of their similar pathophysiology, are associated with low HDL and high TAG, and are relatively common causes of these disorders. The genetic disorders resulting in elevated TAG and low HDL are outlined in Table 7.1.

Treatment Options

Therapeutic Lifestyle Changes

HDL levels have been shown to increase with weight reduction, regular aerobic exercise, modest alcohol consumption, and smoking cessation. Typically, one may expect a 1-mg/dL increase in HDL for every 3-kg weight loss. Regular aerobic exercise may increase HDL by 10% to 20% in sedentary adults.

Nicotinic Acid (Niacin)

Nicotinic acid, or niacin, is a B-complex vitamin that increases HDL 15% to 35% and decreases TAG by 20% to 50%. Niacin increases HDL through metabolic pathways that increase the pre-B, apo A-I–rich HDL particles, which is the cardioprotective subfraction of HDL. The Coronary Drug Project showed that treatment with niacin reduced the risk of nonfatal MI, even after 15 years of follow-up [46]. The most common side effect is cutaneous flushing, and this may be diminished by increasing the dose gradually, prescribing the drug with meals or at bedtime, and by taking aspirin or ibuprofen 30 minutes beforehand. The major adverse side effect of niacin is hepatotoxicity.

Fibric Acids (Fibrates)

Fibrates are agonists of PPARα, which is a nuclear receptor involved in the modulation of lipid and carbohydrate metabolism. Fibrates increase hydrolysis of TAG by enhancing lipoprotein lipase activity, increase clearance of TAG-rich lipoproteins from the plasma, and decrease the rate of release of free fatty acids from adipocytes. Fibrates are the most effective agents for reducing TAG (20% to 55%), and also effectively increase HDL (10% to 20%). These agents have variable effects of the serum LDL, and treated patients with hypertriglyceridemia may have an increase in their LDL. Fibrates are the drug of choice in patients with severe hypertriglyceridemia (more than 1,000 mg/dL). The common side effects and adverse interactions of fibrates are outlined in Table 7.3.

Fibrates have been shown to be beneficial in both primary prevention [47] and in patients with established CHD [42]. The VA-HIT Trial compared treatment with gemfibrozil with that with placebo in men with established CAD and average LDL levels (less than 140 mg/dL) and low HDL (less than 40 mg/dL), After a mean follow up of 5 years, gemfibrozil decreased TAG levels by 31% and increased HDL by 6%, whereas levels of LDL remained quantitatively unchanged. A relative risk reduction of 22% was seen in CHD death and nonfatal MI. Surprisingly, fenofibrate failed to reduce the primary end point (CHD death or nonfatal MI) significantly compared with placebo in 9,795 diabetic patients in the Fenofibrate Intervention and Event Lowering in Diabetes (FIELD) trial, although the authors suggested that the higher rate of starting statin therapy in patients allocated to placebo might have attenuated a moderately larger treatment benefit [48].

Statins

Statins typically result in only a modest increase in HDL, and this effect appears to be independent of LDL-reducing capacity. Simvastatin (8% to 16% increase), rosuvastatin (8% to 14%), and pravastatin (2% to 12%) are the most potent HDL-raising agents, whereas atorvastatin, fluvastatin, and lovastatin increase HDL up to 9%. Treatment with statins results in a modest decrease in serum TAG of approximately 7% to 30%. The greater the efficacy of statins in reducing LDL, the greater the effect on lowering the TAG.

Fish Oils

Fish oils contain a high concentration of polyunsaturated fatty acids and have been shown to reduce plasma triglycerides up to 45%, although they may be associated with increased LDL levels. Omega-3-acid ethyl esters (Omacor) are available as an adjunct to diet for the reduction of very high TAG levels (≥500 mg/dL) in adults. The mechanism of action is poorly defined but may involve the inhibition of acyl CoA:1,2-diacylglycerol acyltransferase and increased peroxisomal β-oxidation in the liver.

New Treatment Options for Increasing HDL

Several new and exciting therapies for reducing HDL are currently undergoing intense investigation. Cholesterol Ester Transfer Protein (CETP) inhibition is the most promising new therapy and consists of inhibiting CETP, a plasma glycoprotein produced in the liver that circulates in the bloodstream bound to HDL that facilitates transfer of cholesterol esters between lipoproteins. CETP activity is potentially atherogenic and results in the net transfer of cholesterol esters from HDL to VLDL and LDL, thereby decreasing the concentration of HDL and increasing the concentration of LDL. Pharmacologically inhibiting CETP has been shown to increase the reverse cholesterol transport to the liver by increasing HDL and enhancing the hepatic uptake of cholesterol via scavenger receptor B-1 (SRB-1) [49]. CETP inhibition with a molecule known as JTT-705 (which results in irreversible binding to the protein) resulted in a significant 28% increase in HDL levels in combination with pravastatin in 152 patients [50]. Similarly, in human subjects with low HDL levels, CETP inhibition with the potent and selective torcetrapib resulted in significantly increased HDL levels (from 46% to 106%) and reduced LDL levels when administered as monotherapy or when given in combination with a statin [51]. Other novel therapies under investigation include direct infusions of plasma-derived or synthetic apolipoprotein A-1, and agents that augment the expression of scavenger receptors.

LIPOPROTEIN (A)

Lipoprotein (a) or Lp (a) is a lipoprotein similar to LDL in lipid and protein concentration, but is composed of two protein particles, apolipoprotein (Apo) B-100 and apolipoprotein (a) [52]. The precise role of Lp (a) in the pathogenesis and progression of atherosclerosis remains controversial [5], but potential mechanisms of Lp (a) include binding to proinflammatory oxidized phospholipids [53], decreased nitric oxide synthesis, increased leukocyte adhesion and smooth muscle proliferation, and inhibition of the fibrinolytic system. However, substantial uncertainty remains regarding the role of Lp (a) in clinical practice, although an elevated level might warrant more-aggressive treatment in patients who have high-risk family histories but few other risk factors. Statins do not decrease Lp (a) levels, and statin therapy may increase in Lp(a) approximately 30%. Niacin currently is the only available lipid-lowering drug that significantly reduces the plasma levels of Lp (a).

HOMOCYSTEINE

An elevated level of homocysteine has been implicated as a risk factor for coronary atherosclerosis, although the precise pathophysiology behind this association remains undefined [5]. Treatment of hyperhomocysteinemia with folic acid and vitamin has shown mixed results in terms of reducing subsequent cardiac events. However, a recent large randomized trial enrolling 3,749 patients (NORVIT Trial [54]) showed that the combination of high-dose vitamin B_6 and folic acid reduced homocysteine levels by 28% but was associated with an increased the risk of stroke and MI.

FUTURE DIRECTIONS

Although the mean total cholesterol levels in adults in the United States have progressively declined, significant population segments still have cholesterol concentrations near or at the level of increased risk [55]. The increasing prevalence of obesity, metabolic syndrome, and diabetes mellitus will fuel the need for comprehensive therapeutic strategies for dealing with multiple lipid and metabolic disorders. LDL cholesterol will remain the main target for intervention; however, new treatment options for increasing HDL cholesterol will continue to evolve rapidly. The proper identification of the patients at increased risk for the development and progression of ASCVD and the optimal goals for therapy will continue to be the major focus of the basic and clinical trials in the future.

REFERENCES

1. *(1C+)* **Carroll MD** et al. Trends in serum lipids and lipoproteins of adults, 1960–2002. JAMA 2005;294:1773–1781.

   This study analyzed data from the National Health and Nutrition Examination Surveys (NHANES) and found that between 1988 and 1994 and 1999 and 2002, total serum cholesterol levels of adults decreased from 206 mg/dl to 203 mg/dl (5.26 mmol/L; $p = 0.009$), and LDL levels decreased from 129 mg/dl to 123 mg/dl ($p < 0.001$), with greater decreases demonstrated in men 60 years or older and in women 50 years or older.

2. **National Cholesterol Education Program (NCEP) Expert Panel on Detection, Evaluation, and Treatment of High Blood Cholesterol in Adults (Adult Treatment Panel III).** Executive summary of the third report. JAMA 2001;285:2486–2497.

   This third ATP summarized the current recommendations for the diagnosis and treatment of hypercholesterolemia, with emphasis on the intensive management of LDL cholesterol in high-risk populations (goal LDL ≤100 mg/dl) and primary prevention in patients with multiple risk factors.

3. **Levine GN** et al. Cholesterol reduction in cardiovascular disease: Clinical benefits and possible mechanisms. N Engl J Med 1995;332:512–521.

   This article comprehensively reviews the pathophysiology, diagnosis, and treatment of hypercholesterolemia.

4. **Ross R.** Atherosclerosis: An inflammatory disease. N Engl J Med 1999;340:115–126.

   This article reviews the role of inflammation in the development and progression atherosclerosis.

5. **Hackam DG, Anand SS.** Emerging risk factors for atherosclerotic vascular disease: A critical review of the evidence. JAMA 2003;290:932–940.

   This article reviewed the epidemiologic, basic science, and clinical trial evidence surrounding C-reactive protein, lipoprotein(a), fibrinogen, and homocysteine, and found limited data regarding the additive yield of screening for these factors over that of current validated global risk-assessment strategies.

6. *(1B)* **Verschuren WM** et al. Serum total cholesterol and long-term coronary heart disease mortality in different cultures: Twenty-five-year follow-up of the seven countries study. JAMA 1995;274:131–136.

   This study evaluated the relation of total cholesterol and mortality baseline in 12,467 middle-aged men in seven countries. By using a linear approximation, a 20-mg/dl increase in total cholesterol corresponded to an increase in CHD mortality risk of 12%.

7. *(1A)* **Stamler J** et al. Is relationship between serum cholesterol and risk of premature death from coronary heart disease continuous and graded? Findings in 356,222 primary screenees of the Multiple Risk Factor Intervention Trial (MRFIT). JAMA 1986;256:2823–2828.

   This trial examined the relation of serum cholesterol and long-term mortality in a cohort of 356,222 middle-aged men and demonstrated a continuous, graded, strong relation between serum cholesterol and 6-year age-adjusted CHD death rate in all subgroups.

8. *(1A)* **The Scandinavian Simvastatin Survival Study (4S).** Randomised trial of cholesterol lowering in 4444 patients with coronary heart disease. Lancet 1994;344:1383–1389.

   This large, randomized placebo-controlled trial evaluated the effect of cholesterol lowering with simvastatin on mortality and morbidity in 4,444 patients with CHD. After 5.4 years of follow-up, simvastatin produced favorably altered total cholesterol (-25%), LDL cholesterol (-35%), and HDL ($+8\%$). The relative risk of death in the simvastatin group was 0.70 (12% vs. 8%; 95% CI, 0.58–0.85; $p = 0.0003$), with a 37% reduction ($p < 0.00001$) in the risk of undergoing myocardial revascularization.

9. *(1A)* **The Long-Term Intervention with Pravastatin in Ischaemic Disease (LIPID) Study Group.** Prevention of cardiovascular events and death with pravastatin in patients with coronary heart disease and a broad range of initial cholesterol levels. N Engl J Med 1998;339: 1349–1357.

   This large, randomized, placebo-controlled trial compared the effects of pravastatin (40 mg/day) in 9,014 patients (aged 31–75 years) with established CHD. After 6.1 years of follow-up, a 22% relative risk reduction in overall mortality was found in the pravastatin group compared with placebo (11% vs. 14.1%; 95% CI, 13–31%; $p < 0.001$), lower MI (29% relative risk reduction, $p < 0.001$), lower stroke (19% relative risk reduction, $p = 0.048$), and lower coronary revascularization (20% relative risk reduction, $p < 0.001$).

10. *(1A)* **Sacks FM** et al. The effect of pravastatin on coronary events after myocardial infarction in patients with average cholesterol levels: Cholesterol and Recurrent Events Trial investigators. N Engl J Med 1996;335:1001–1009.

    This large, randomized, placebo-controlled trial compared pravastatin (40 mg/day) with placebo in 4,159 patients (3,583 men and 576 women) with myocardial infarction who had "average" cholesterol levels (mean total cholesterol, 209 mg/dl; mean LDL, 139 mg/dl). A 24% relative risk reduction occurred in the pravastatin group compared with placebo in fatal coronary event or nonfatal MI (10.2% vs.13.2%; 95% CI, 9%–36%; $p = 0.003$), less coronary bypass surgery (7.5% vs. 10%, $p = 0.005$), and less coronary angioplasty (8.3% vs. 10.5%; $p = 0.01$), and 31% relative risk reduction in stroke ($p = 0.03$).

11. **Grundy SM** et al. Implications of recent clinical trials for the National Cholesterol Education Program Adult Treatment Panel III guidelines. Circulation 2004;110:227–239.

    This consensus article summarizes the latest recommendations based on recent trials since the publication of the 2001 ATP Guidelines. The goal of LDL of a patient at very high risk is less than 70 mg/dl. In addition, an LDL goal of <100 mg/dl in moderately high risk individuals (2+ risk factors and a 10-year risk of 10%–20%) is a therapeutic option.

12. *(2C)* **Rosenson RS** et al. Relations of lipoprotein subclass levels and low-density lipoprotein size to progression of coronary artery disease in the Pravastatin Limitation of Atherosclerosis in the Coronary Arteries (PLAC-I) trial. Am J Cardiol 2002;90:89–94.

    In this study, lipoprotein subclass analyses were performed on frozen plasma samples from 241 participants in the PLAC-1 Trial by using an automated nuclear magnetic resonance technique. Within treatment groups, CAD progression was most strongly related to the LDL particle number (placebo) and levels of small HDL (pravastatin). In logistic regression models that adjusted for chemically determined lipid levels and other covariates, a small LDL level of 30 mg/dl (median) or more was associated with a ninefold increased risk of CAD progression ($p < 0.01$) in the placebo group.

13. *(1A)* **Shepherd J** et al. Prevention of coronary heart disease with pravastatin in men with hypercholesterolemia: West of Scotland Coronary Prevention Study Group. N Engl J Med 1995;333: 1301–1307.

This large, randomized, placebo-controlled trial evaluated the treatment with pravastatin (40 mg/day) in 6,595 men (aged 45 to 64 years) with moderate hypercholesterolemia and no history of myocardial infarction. After 4.9 years, pravastatin reduced plasma cholesterol levels by 20% and LDL levels by 26%. There was a 31% relative-risk reduction of coronary events (nonfatal MI or death from coronary heart disease) compared with placebo (95% CI, 17%–43%; $p < 0.001$), less nonfatal myocardial infarctions (31% reduction; $p < 0.001$), and lower death from all cardiovascular causes (32% reduction; $p = 0.033$).

14. *(1A)* **Sever PS** et al. Prevention of coronary and stroke events with atorvastatin in hypertensive patients who have average or lower-than-average cholesterol concentrations, in the Anglo-Scandinavian Cardiac Outcomes Trial–Lipid Lowering Arm (ASCOT-LLA): A multicentre randomised controlled trial. Lancet 2003;361:1149–1158.

This large, randomized, placebo-controlled study assessed the benefits of cholesterol reduction in the primary prevention of CHD in hypertensive patients who were not conventionally deemed to be dyslipidemic. In this trial, a subset of 10,305 with nonfasting total cholesterol concentrations of 252 mg/dl or less were randomly assigned to atorvastatin (10 mg/day) or placebo. Treatment was stopped early after a median follow-up of 3.3 years because of a significantly lower event rate (nonfatal myocardial infarction and fatal CHD) in the atorvastatin group compared with placebo (hazard ratio, 0.64; 95% CI, 0.50–0.83; $p = 0.0005$), which emerged in the first year of follow-up. In addition, fatal and nonfatal strokes were lower in the atorvastatin group ($p = 0.024$).

15. *(1A)* The Antihypertensive and Lipid-Lowering Treatment to Prevent Heart Attack Trial (ALL-HAT-LLT). Major outcomes in moderately hypercholesterolemic, hypertensive patients randomized to pravastatin vs usual care. JAMA 2002;288:2998–3007.

This randomized, nonblinded study assessed the effect of pravastatin compared with usual care on all-cause mortality in 10,355 older moderately hypercholesterolemic, hypertensive participants with at least one additional CHD risk factor. The mean age was 66 years; mean total cholesterol was 224 mg/dl; mean LDL-C was 146 mg/dl; HDL was 48 mg/dl; and TAG was 152 mg/dl. After 4.8 years of follow-up, all-cause mortality was similar for the two groups [relative risk (RR), 0.99; 95%CI, 0.89–1.11; $p = 0.88$]. These results may be due to the modest differential in total cholesterol (9.6%) and LDL-C (16.7%) between pravastatin and usual care compared with prior statin trials supporting cardiovascular disease prevention.

16. *(1A)* **Downs JR** et al. Primary prevention of acute coronary events with lovastatin in men and women with average cholesterol levels: Results of AFCAPS/TexCAPS. Air Force/Texas Coronary Atherosclerosis Prevention Study. JAMA 1998;279:1615–1622.

This was a large, randomized, placebo-controlled study evaluating the effect of lovastatin (20–40 mg/day) in 5,608 men and 997 women without evident CHD with average total cholesterol and LDL and below-average HDL. The mean total cholesterol level was 221 mg/dl, mean LDL-C level was 150 mg/dl, mean HDL-C was 36 mg/dl for men and 40 mg/dl for women, and median TAG level was 158 mg/dl. After an average follow-up of 5.2 years, lovastatin significantly reduced the incidence of a first major coronary event (fatal or nonfatal MI, unstable angina, or sudden cardiac death) [relative risk (RR), 0.63; 95% CI, 0.50–0.79; $p < 0.001$], myocardial infarction (RR, 0.60; 95% CI, 0.43–0.83; $p = 0.002$), unstable angina (RR, 0.68; 95% CI, 0.49–0.95; $p = 0.02$), coronary revascularization procedures (RR, 0.67; 95% CI, 0.52–0.85; $p = 0.001$).

17. *(1A)* MRC/BHF Heart Protection Study of cholesterol lowering in 20,536 high-risk individuals: A randomised placebo-controlled trial. Lancet 2002;360:7–22.

This large, randomized, placebo-controlled trial evaluated the effects of simvastatin (40 mg/daily) in 20,536 subjects (aged 40–80 years) with coronary disease, other occlusive arterial disease, or diabetes, irrespective of their baseline LDL level. All-cause mortality was significantly reduced (12.9% vs.14.7%; $p = 0.0003$), because of a highly significant 18% reduction in the coronary death rate (5.7% vs. 6.9%; $p = 0.0005$). A significant reduction in adverse events was found, even in those who presented with an initial LDL cholesterol below 116 mg/dl.

18. *(1A)* **Cannon CP** et al. Intensive versus moderate lipid lowering with statins after acute coronary syndromes. N Engl J Med 2004;350:1495–1504.

This large, randomized trial enrolled 4,162 patients with an acute coronary syndrome within the preceding 10 days and compared treatment with pravastatin (40-mg/day standard therapy) with atorvastatin (80-mg/day intensive therapy). After a mean follow-up of 24 months, the median LDL achieved during treatment with pravastatin was 95 mg/dl compared with 62 mg/dl with the high-dose atorvastatin group ($p < 0.001$). A 16% relative risk reduction was noted in the rates of the primary end point (composite of death from any cause, myocardial infarction, documented unstable angina requiring rehospitalization, coronary revascularization, and stroke) in the atrovastatin group compared with the pravastatin group (22.4% vs. 26.3%; 95% CI, 5%–26%; $p = 0.005$). The study did not meet the prespecified criterion for equivalence but did identify the superiority of the more intensive regimen.

19. *(1A)* **LaRosa JC** et al. Intensive lipid lowering with atorvastatin in patients with stable coronary disease. N Engl J Med 2005;352:1425–1435.

This was a large, randomized trial which prospectively evaluated the efficacy and safety of lowering LDL cholesterol levels below 100 mg/dl in patients with stable CHD. The 10,001 subjects were randomly assigned to double-blind therapy and received 10 mg or 80 mg of atorvastatin per day. After a median of 4.9 years, the mean LDL levels were 77 mg/dl in the 80-mg atorvastatin treatment group, and 101 mg/dl in the 10-mg atorvastatin treatment group. The incidence of persistent elevations in liver aminotransferase levels was 0.2% in the low-dose group and 1.2% high-dose group ($p < 0.001$). The primary event (occurrence of a first major cardiovascular event, defined as death from CHD, nonfatal non–procedure-related myocardial infarction, resuscitation after cardiac arrest, or fatal or nonfatal stroke) occurred in 8.7% receiving 80 mg of atorvastatin, as compared with 10.9% receiving 10 mg of atorvastatin (22% relative reduction in risk (hazard ratio, 0.78; 95 CI, 0.69–0.89; $p < 0.001$). No difference was seen between the two treatment groups in overall mortality.

20. **O'Keefe JH Jr** et al. Optimal low-density lipoprotein is 50 to 70 mg/dl: lower is better and physiologically normal. J Am Coll Cardiol 2004;43:2142–2146.

This article concisely reviews the recent randomized trial data supporting reduced atherosclerosis progression and coronary heart disease events with lowering LDL to less than 70 mg/dl. The authors emphasize that no major safety concerns have surfaced in studies that lowered LDL to this range of 50 to 70 mg/dl.

21. *(2B)* **Hunninghake DB** et al. The efficacy of intensive dietary therapy alone or combined with lovastatin in outpatients with hypercholesterolemia. N Engl J Med 1993;328:1213–1219.

In this trial, 111 outpatients with moderate hypercholesterolemia were treated with the NCEP Step 2 diet (low in fat and cholesterol) and lovastatin (20 mg/day), both alone and together. The LDL level was reduced by a mean of 5% (95% confidence interval, 3%–7%) during the low-fat diet compared with the high-fat diet ($p < 0.001$). With lovastatin therapy as compared with placebo, the reduction was 27%, whereas the combination of diet and drug therapy resulted in a mean LDL reduction of 32%.

22. *(1A)* **Baigent C** et al. Efficacy and safety of cholesterol-lowering treatment: Prospective meta-analysis of data from 90,056 participants in 14 randomised trials of statins. Lancet 2005;366: 1267–1278.

This is a prospective meta-analysis of data from 90,056 individuals in 14 randomized trials involving statin therapy. A 12% proportional reduction in all-cause mortality occurred per mmol/L reduction in LDL cholesterol [rate ratio (RR) 0.88; 95% CI, 0.84–0.91; $p < 0.0001$], a 19% reduction in coronary mortality (0.81; 0.76–0.85; $p < 0.0001$), lower rates of myocardial infarction or coronary death (0.77; 0.74–0.80; $p < 0.0001$), and lower rates of coronary revascularization (0.76; 0.73–0.80; $p < 0.0001$), fatal or nonfatal stroke (0.83; 0.78–0.88; $p < 0.0001$). The proportional reduction in major vascular events differed significantly ($p < 0.0001$) according to the absolute reduction in LDL cholesterol achieved. These benefits were significant within the first year, but were greater in subsequent years.

23. *(1A)* **Schwartz GG** et al. Effects of atorvastatin on early recurrent ischemic events in acute coronary syndromes: the MIRACL study: a randomized controlled trial. JAMA 2001;285:1711–1718.

This large, randomized, placebo-controlled trial enrolled 3,086 patients with an acute coronary syndrome to treatment with atorvastatin (80 mg/day) initiated within 24 to 96 hours. At 16 weeks follow-up, a reduction in adverse cardiac events was noted (death, nonfatal acute MI, cardiac arrest with resuscitation, or recurrent symptomatic myocardial ischemia with objective evidence and requiring emergency rehospitalization) in the atorvastatin group compared with placebo [14.8% vs. 17.4%, relative risk (RR), 0.84; 95% CI, 0.70–1.00; $p = 0.048$], which was driven mainly by recurrent symptomatic ischemia. In the atorvastatin group, the mean LDL declined from 124 mg/dl to 72 mg/dl; however, elevated liver transaminases (>3 times) were more common than in the placebo group (2.5% vs. 0.6%; $p < 0.001$).

24. *(1A)* **de Lemos JA** et al. Early intensive vs a delayed conservative simvastatin strategy in patients with acute coronary syndromes: phase Z of the A to Z trial. JAMA 2004;292:1307–1316.

This large, randomized trial compared the early initiation of an intensive simvastatin regimen (40 mg/day for 1 month and then 80 mg/day) with delayed initiation of a less-intensive regimen (placebo for 4 months and then 20 mg/day) in 4,497 patients with an acute coronary syndrome. Although the primary end point was not achieved, the early initiation of an aggressive simvastatin regimen resulted in a favorable trend toward reduction of major cardiovascular events.

25. *(1A)* **Colhoun HM** et al. Primary prevention of cardiovascular disease with atorvastatin in type 2 diabetes in the Collaborative Atorvastatin Diabetes Study (CARDS): Multicentre randomised placebo-controlled trial. Lancet 2004;364:685–696.

This large, randomized, placebo-controlled trial evaluated the effectiveness of atorvastatin (10 mg/day) for primary prevention of major cardiovascular events in 2,838 patients with type 2 diabetes without high concentrations of LDL-cholesterol. After a median follow-up of 3.9 years, a 37% relative risk reduction in cardiovascular events was seen in the atorvastatin group compared with placebo (95% CI, 0.52–0.17; $p = 0.001$).

26. *(1A)* **Shepherd J** et al. Pravastatin in elderly individuals at risk of vascular disease (PROS-PER): A randomised controlled trial. Lancet 2002;360:1623–1630.

This randomized trial enrolled 5,804 elderly patients (70–82 years) with a history of, or risk factors for, vascular disease to pravastatin (40 mg/day; $n = 2,891$) or placebo. After a mean follow-up of 3.2 years, a reduction in the primary end point (composite of coronary death, nonfatal myocardial infarction, and fatal or nonfatal stroke) in the pravastatin group compared with placebo (hazard ratio, 0.85; 95% CI, 0.74–0.97; $p = 0.014$).

27. *(1B)* **Tonelli M** et al. Effect of pravastatin in people with diabetes and chronic kidney disease. J Am Soc Nephrol 2005;16:3748–3754.

This study evaluated the effect of pravastatin (40 mg/day) on reducing the incidence of first or recurrent cardiovascular events (myocardial infarction, coronary death, or percutaneous/surgical coronary revascularization) in patients with non–dialysis-dependent stage 2 or 3 chronic kidney disease (CKD) and concomitant diabetes, by using data from three randomized trials of pravastatin, 40 mg daily, versus placebo. After a median follow-up of 64 months, the adjusted incidence of the primary outcome was lowest in individuals with neither CKD nor diabetes (15.2%), intermediate in individuals with only CKD (18.6%) or only diabetes (21.3%), and highest in individuals with both characteristics (27.0%).

28. *(2A)* **Wanner C** et al. Atorvastatin in patients with type 2 diabetes mellitus undergoing hemodialysis. N Engl J Med 2005;353:238–248.

This was a large, randomized, double-blind, placebo-controlled trial evaluating the effect of treatment with atorvastatin (20 mg/day) in 1,255 subjects with type 2 diabetes mellitus receiving hemodialysis. After a median follow-up of 4 years, no significant difference was found in the primary end point (composite of death from cardiac causes, nonfatal MI, and stroke) in the atorvastatin group compared with placebo (relative risk, 0.92; 95 CI, 0.77–1.10; $p = 0.37$). This failure of statins in reducing the risk of cardiac event rates may have related to the need for starting treatment earlier, the need for longer follow up, the high risk of death from other causes in hemodialysis patients (such as electrolyte imbalances or infection), or the differences in the nature of atherosclerosis in hemodialysis patients. The ongoing Study of Heart and Renal Protection (SHARP) trial will study the benefit of combination therapy with simvastatin and ezetimibe compared with placebo in approximately 9,000 subjects with advanced kidney disease, and the Study to Evaluate the Use of Rosuvastatin in Subjects on Regular Hemodialysis: An Assessment of Survival and Cardiovascular Events (AURORA) will compare treatment with rosuvastatin with placebo in 2,700 hemodialysis patients and will help to clarify this issue in the future.

29. *(2B)* **Brown G** et al. Regression of coronary artery disease as a result of intensive lipid-lowering therapy in men with high levels of apolipoprotein B. N Engl J Med 1990;323:1289–1298.

This angiographic trial enrolled 120 men with hypercholesterolemia treated with lovastatin (20 mg, b.i.d) and colestipol (10 g, t.i.d); niacin (1 g, 4 times a day), and colestipol (10 g, t.i.d.); or conventional therapy with placebo. Intensive lipid-lowering therapy reduced the frequency of progression of coronary lesions, increased the frequency of regression, and reduced the incidence of cardiovascular events.

30. *(1A)* **Nissen SE** et al. Effect of intensive compared with moderate lipid-lowering therapy on progression of coronary atherosclerosis: A randomized controlled trial (REVERSAL). JAMA 2004; 291:1071–1080.

This study compared the effect of regimens designed to produce intensive lipid lowering or moderate lipid lowering on coronary artery atheroma burden and progression, intensive lipid-lowering treatment with atorvastatin (mean LDL, 79 mg/dl), and reduced progression of coronary atherosclerosis compared with pravastatin (mean LDL, 110 mg/dl). Compared with baseline values, patients treated with atorvastatin had no change in atheroma burden, whereas patients treated with pravastatin showed progression of coronary atherosclerosis.

31. *(1B)* **Robinson JG** et al. Pleiotropic effects of statins: Benefit beyond cholesterol reduction? A meta-regression analysis. J Am Coll Cardiol 2005;46:1855–1862.

This article reviewed the data from five diet, three bile acid sequestrant, one surgery, and 10 statin trials, with 81,859 participants, and found that the regression lines for nonstatin and statin trials were similar and consistent with a one-to-one relation between LDL-C lowering and CHD and stroke reduction over 5 years of treatment.

32. **Rosenson RS.** Current overview of statin-induced myopathy. Am J Med 2004;116:408–416.

This article reviews the risk factors associated with statin-induced myopathy and emphasizes the pharmacokinetic properties of the various agents and the proper selection and identification of patients at risk for myotoxic effects.

33. **Pasternak RC** et al. ACC/AHA/NHLBI Clinical advisory on the use and safety of statins. Circulation 2002;106:1024–1028.

This consensus statement summarizes the recommendations concerning the various safety issues surrounding the proper utilization of statins in clinical medicine.

34. **Brown WV.** Cholesterol absorption inhibitors: Defining new options in lipid management. Clin Cardiol 2003;26:259–264.

This article reviews the pharmacokinetics and pharmacodynamics of ezetimibe and summarizes the results from available clinical trials.

35. *(1B)* **Ballantyne CM** et al. Dose-comparison study of the combination of ezetimibe and simvastatin (Vytorin) versus atorvastatin in patients with hypercholesterolemia: The Vytorin Versus Atorvastatin (VYVA) study. Am Heart J 2005;149:464–473.

This randomized study compared the combination of ezetimibe/simvastatin with atorvastatin across dose ranges in 1,902 patients and found that at each milligram-equivalent statin dose comparison, and averaged across doses, ezetimibe/simvastatin provided greater LDL reductions (47%–59%) than atorvastatin (36%–53%).

36. *(1B)* **Watts GF** et al. Effects on coronary artery disease of lipid-lowering diet, or diet plus cholestyramine, in the St Thomas' Atherosclerosis Regression Study (STARS). Lancet 1992;339: 563–569.

   This trial assessed the efficacy of dietary reduction and diet and cholestyramine on angiographic end-points in men with CHD90, and found that dietary change alone slowed overall progression and increased overall regression of coronary artery disease, and diet plus cholestyramine was additionally associated with a net increase in coronary lumen diameter.

37. **Rosenson RS.** The rationale for combination therapy. Am J Cardiol 2002;90:2K–7K.

   This article reviews the rationale for the use of combination therapy in the treatment of dyslipidemia, highlighting management strategies emphasizing the use of combination therapy involving statins in conjunction with niacin, fibric-acid derivatives, or bile acid resins or intestinal inhibitors of active cholesterol transport.

38. **Levy DR, Pearson TA.** Combination niacin and statin therapy in primary and secondary prevention of cardiovascular disease. Clin Cardiol 2005;28:317–320.

   This article reviews the impact of lipid-modifying combination therapy with niacin plus a statin on achieving lipid goals and improving clinical outcomes.

39. *(1B)* **Brown BG** et al. Simvastatin and niacin, antioxidant vitamins, or the combination for the prevention of coronary disease. N Engl J Med 2001;345:1583–1592.

   This trial evaluated simvastatin–niacin and antioxidant–vitamin therapy, alone and together, for cardiovascular protection in 160 patients with coronary disease and low plasma levels of HDL. This study showed that simvastatin plus niacin provides marked clinical and angiographically measurable benefits.

40. *(1B)* **Pauciullo P** et al. Efficacy and safety of a combination of fluvastatin and bezafibrate in patients with mixed hyperlipidaemia (FACT study). Atherosclerosis 2000;150:429–436.

   This randomized trial assessed the effect of fluvastatin (40 mg), bezafibrate (400 mg), fluvastatin (20 mg) + bezafibrate (400 mg), or fluvastatin (40 mg) + bezafibrate (400 mg) for 24 weeks in 333 patients with CAD and mixed hyperlipidemia. Bezafibrate alone and fluvastatin+bezafibrate combinations resulted in greater increases in HDL and decreases in TAG compared with fluvastatin alone ($p < 0.001$).

41. *(1B)* **Hokanson JE, Austin MA.** Plasma triglyceride level is a risk factor for cardiovascular disease independent of high-density lipoprotein cholesterol level: A meta-analysis of population-based prospective studies. J Cardiovasc Risk 1996;3:213–219.

   This meta-analysis evaluated the magnitude of the association between triglyceride and cardiovascular disease in the general population, and found that triglyceride is a statistically significant risk factor in men (RR, 1.14; 95% CI, 1.05–1.28) and in women (RR, 1.37; 95% CI, 1.13–1.66) for cardiovascular disease, independent of HDL cholesterol.

42. *(1A)* **Rubins HB** et al. Gemfibrozil for the secondary prevention of coronary heart disease in men with low levels of high-density lipoprotein cholesterol: Veterans Affairs High-Density Lipoprotein Cholesterol Intervention Trial Study Group. N Engl J Med 1999;341:410–418.

   This large, randomized trial in 2,531 men with coronary heart disease and hypercholesterolemia with low HDL (HDL ≤40 mg/dl and an LDL ≤140 mg/dl) compared gemfibrozil (1,200 mg/day) and placebo. After a median follow-up of 5.1 years, a 22% relative risk reduction in the gemfibrozil group was found in the primary end point (nonfatal myocardial infarction or coronary death (17.3% vs. 21.7%; 95% CI, 7%–35%; $p = 0.006$).

43. *(1B)* **Gordon T** et al. High density lipoprotein as a protective factor against coronary heart disease: The Framingham Study. Am J Med 1977;62:707–714.

   This trial evaluated the association of lipoprotein values, including fasting TAG, HDL, and LDL in 2,815 men and women (ages 49 to 82) on cardiac event rates, and found the major potent lipid risk factor was HDL, which had an inverse association with the incidence of coronary heart disease ($p < 0.001$).

44. *(1A)* **Gordon DJ** et al. High-density lipoprotein cholesterol and cardiovascular disease: Four prospective American studies. Circulation 1989;79:8–15.

   This study analyzed the data from four prospective large trials and found that a 1-mg/dl increase in HDL was associated with a significant coronary heart disease risk reduction of 2% in men and 3% in women.

45. **Shah PK** et al. Exploiting the vascular protective effects of high-density lipoprotein and its apolipoproteins: An idea whose time for testing is coming, part II. Circulation 2001;104: 2498–2502.

   This article reviews the pathophysiology and mechanisms behind the potential vascular protective effects of HDL.

46. *(1A)* **Canner PL** et al. Fifteen year mortality in Coronary Drug Project patients: Long-term benefit with niacin. J Am Coll Cardiol 1986;8:1245–1255.

   This trial evaluated the efficacy and safety of five lipid-lowering drugs in 8,341 men with established CHD. With a mean follow-up of 15 years, nearly 9 years after termination of the trial, mortality from all causes in each of the drug groups, except for niacin, was similar to that in the placebo group. Mortality in the niacin group was 11% lower than that in the placebo group (52% vs. 58.2%; $p = 0.0004$).

47. *(1A)* **Huttunen JK** et al. The Helsinki Heart Study: Central findings and clinical implications. Ann Med 1991;23:155–159.

This article elaborates on the main findings and clinical implications of the Helsinki Heart Study, which was a controlled primary prevention evaluating the efficacy of gemfibrozil in lowering LDL, raising HDL, and reducing subsequent adverse cardiac events.

48. *(2A)* **Keech A** et al. Effects of long-term fenofibrate therapy on cardiovascular events in 9795 people with type 2 diabetes mellitus (the FIELD study): Randomised controlled trial. Lancet 2005;366:1849–1861.

This large, randomized, placebo-controlled trial evaluated the effect of fenofibrate on cardiovascular disease events in 9,795 patients (aged 50–75 years) with type 2 diabetes mellitus. After 5 years, no difference was found in overall mortality [6.6% in the placebo group and 7.3% in the fenofibrate group (p = 0.18)]. Although fenofibrate did not significantly reduce the risk of the primary outcome of coronary events, it did reduce total cardiovascular events, mainly because of fewer nonfatal MIs and revascularizations (RR, 0.79; CI, 0.68–0.93; p = 0.003).The higher rate of starting statin therapy in patients assigned to placebo may have attenuated a larger treatment benefit.

49. **Barter PJ, Kastelein JJ.** Targeting cholesteryl ester transfer protein for the prevention and management of cardiovascular disease. J Am Coll Cardiol 2006;47:492–499.

This review article summarizes the current basic science and clinical data on cholesteryl ester transfer protein (CETP) inhibitors (JTT-705 and torcetrapib) and their role in the treatment of low HDL.

50. *(1B)* **Kuivenhoven JA** et al. Effectiveness of inhibition of cholesteryl ester transfer protein by JTT-705 in combination with pravastatin in type II dyslipidemia. Am J Cardiol 2005;95: 1085–1088.

This randomized, double-blind, placebo-controlled trial evaluated the use of the CETP inhibitor JTT-705 (300 or 600 mg) combined with pravastatin (40 mg) in 155 patients with dyslipidemia. Four weeks of treatment with JTT-705 600 mg led to a 30% decrease in CETP activity (p < 0.001), a 28% increase in HDL cholesterol (p < 0.001), and a 5% decrease in LDL cholesterol (p < 0.03).

51. *(1A)* **Brousseau ME** et al. Effects of an inhibitor of cholesteryl ester transfer protein on HDL cholesterol. N Engl J Med 2004;350:1505–1515.

This was a single-blind, placebo-controlled trial evaluating the effects of torcetrapib (120 mg daily or twice a day), a potent inhibitor of CETP, on plasma lipoprotein levels in 19 subjects with low levels of HDL cholesterol (<40 mg/dl), nine of whom were also treated with 20 mg of atorvastatin daily. Treatment with 120 mg of torcetrapib daily increased plasma concentrations of HDL cholesterol by 61% (p < 0.001) and 46% (p = 0.001) in the atorvastatin and nonatorvastatin cohorts, respectively, and treatment with 120 mg twice daily increased HDL cholesterol by 106% (p < 0.001).

52. **Deb A, Caplice NM.** Lipoprotein(a): New insights into mechanisms of atherogenesis and thrombosis. Clin Cardiol 2004;27:258–264.

This review discusses the structure of Lp(a) in relation to its biochemical actions, summarizes the current data on various pathophysiologic mechanisms of Lp(a)-induced vascular disease, and the role of cell and tissue-specific effects in promoting atherosclerosis.

53. **Tsimikas S** et al. Oxidized phospholipids, Lp(a) lipoprotein, and coronary artery disease. N Engl J Med 2005;353:46–57.

This study measured levels of oxidized LDL and Lp(a) lipoprotein in 504 patients immediately before coronary angiography and found that circulating levels of oxidized LDL are strongly associated with angiographically documented coronary artery disease, particularly in patients 60 years of age or younger. These data suggest that the atherogenicity of Lp(a) lipoprotein may be mediated in part by associated proinflammatory oxidized phospholipids.

54. *(2A)* Preliminary Results of the Norwegian Vitamin Trial (NORVIT) presented at the European Society of Cardiology Congress in Stockholm, Sweden; September 2005.

This large, randomized, placebo-controlled trial evaluated various combinations of high-dose vitamin B_6 and folic acid in 3,749 MI survivors. The results revealed that the combination of vitamin B_6 and folic acid, as well as folic acid alone, effectively lowered homocysteine levels by 28%, without any improvement in clinical outcomes. The risk of stroke and MI was 18% in the placebo group, which was similar to both the folic-acid–only group and the vitamin-B_6–only group. By contrast, in the combination group, 23% of patients had a fatal or nonfatal stroke or MI, a statistically significant absolute increase of 5%, compared with the other treatment arms (p = 0.029).

55. *(1C+)* **Arnett DK** et al. Twenty-year trends in serum cholesterol, hypercholesterolemia, and cholesterol medication use: The Minnesota Heart Survey, 1980–1982 to 2000–2002. Circulation 2005;112:3884–3891.

This study examined the 20-year trends in cholesterol, hypercholesterolemia, lipid-lowering drug use, and cholesterol awareness, treatment, and control from Minnesota Heart Survey (MHS). The results showed that although hypercholesterolemia prevalence continued to fall, significant population segments still have cholesterol concentrations near or at the level of increased risk.

Obesity and Nutrition

Jeffrey I. Mechanick and Elise M. Brett

DEFINITION

Obesity is a chronic disease diagnosed when an adult person has a body mass index (BMI) of 30 to 34.9 (class I), 35 to 39.9 (class II), more than 40 (class III, "extreme obesity"), more than 50 (class IV, "superobesity"), or more than 60 kg/M² ("super-super obesity"). BMI is not a direct measure of adiposity but rather a derived value correlated with total body fat and risk for certain complications. BMI is calculated as the weight in kilograms, divided by the height in meters, squared. Alternatively, one can calculate the weight in pounds, divide by the height in inches, squared, and multiply by 703. Risks for cardiovascular disease (CVD), type 2 diabetes (T2DM), and hypertension are further defined by subgrouping overweight (25–29.9 kg/m²) or obese BMI categories into those with increased abdominal obesity by waist circumference: more than 102 cm (40 inches) for men and 88 cm (35 inches) for women; or waist-to-hip ratio: more than 0.9 for men and more than 0.85 for women. In pediatric and adolescent persons, BMI percentiles for ages 5 to 17 years are used. "At risk" persons are those between the 85th and 95th percentiles, and "overweight" persons are above the 95th percentile [1]. However, the U.S. Preventive Services Task Force concludes that insufficient evidence exists "to recommend for or against routine screening for overweight in children and adolescents as a means to prevent adverse health outcomes" [2].

EPIDEMIOLOGY

More than 1.7 billion persons worldwide are overweight or obese [3]. The prevalence of overweight or obesity among U.S. adults during 2001 through 2002 is 65.7%; obesity, 30.6%; and class III obesity, 5.1%, with women generally having a higher prevalence of obesity compared with men [4]. The prevalence of children or adolescents at risk for overweight or obesity during the same time period is 31.5%, and overweight, 16.5% [4]. No racial or ethnic differences in prevalence rates exist among men, but among women, the prevalence rates are greatest among non-Hispanic black women (49.0%) > Mexican-American women (38.4%) > non-Hispanic white women (30.7%) [4]. No evidence suggests that these rates are decreasing [4]. The 30-year risks of being overweight are more than 91% for men and 73% for women, for being obese are more than 47% for men and 38% for women, and for having class III obesity or more are more than 4% for men and 6% for women [5]. Increasing BMI is associated with the prevalence of T2DM, heart disease, hypertension, dyslipidemia, asthma, arthritis, certain cancers (colon, cervix, breast, prostate, and lung), venous thromboembolic disease, sleep apnea, and poor general health [6,7]. Obesity, but not overweight, is associated with excess mortality (111,909 deaths associated with obesity) in 2000 in the United States [8]. Weight reduction, in addition to increased physical activity, decreases the risk of T2DM in prediabetic patients [9], and trials are under way to determine the effects of weight reduction on the prevention of cardiovascular disease [10].

Irrespective of BMI, the accumulation of fat in the abdomen, pancreas, liver, and muscle is strongly associated with the metabolic complications of obesity [11], hypertension [12], and CVD [13]. Depending on the definition used, visceral obesity is part of the "metabolic" or "insulin-resistance" syndrome, along with hypertension, impaired glucose regulation, dyslipidemia, and other biomarkers for prothrombotic and proinflammatory states [14]. Metabolic syndrome is a univariate predictor of coronary heart disease (odds ratio, 2.07) [15]. Metabolic syndrome also predicts development of T2DM, and weight reduction of 3 to 6 kg by life-style change or medication (orlistat or metformin) reduces the risk for T2DM [9,16,17]. The overall prevalence of metabolic syndrome among Americans older than 50 years is 44% [15]. The definition, implications, and even semantics of this syndrome have been recently challenged [18,19].

ETIOLOGY

Obesity is the result of certain genetic and environmental factors that result in positive energy balance (calorie consumption > energy expenditure). Heritability accounts for 30% to 70% of the variation in body mass within a population, but consistently replicated common genetic variants have not been associated with common obesity [20–22]. Genetic factors determine set-points for appetite, intermediary metabolism, and physical activity behavior. Environmental factors that produce a state of energy surfeit consist of (1) prenatal factors; (2) availability of inexpensive, palatable, energy-dense foods; (3) large portion sizes; (4) social, economic, ethnic, and cultural pressures to overconsume food; (5) media advertising; and (6) sedentary life style [23]. It has been proposed that increased consumption of energy-dense foods (relatively low in water content [dry], high in fat content and particularly found in "fast foods") is a major contributor to the obesity epidemic. One theory suggests that humans have a weak ability to recognize high-energy-density foods and to downregulate the bulk of food ingested to avoid consumption of excess calories [24]. However, a critical review of the data concluded that a causal relation has not been clearly demonstrated [25]. Similarly, high-fat diets have not been shown to cause excess body fat in the general population [26], although genetically susceptible individuals may exist [27]. Interestingly, breakfast consumption, especially those including a ready-to-eat cereal, has been shown to correlate with lower BMI and lower risk of obesity in women, as compared with skipping breakfast [28]. Ruxton et al. [29] asserted that a breakfast meal high in fiber and low in fat represents a beneficial nutritional profile and decreased risk for obesity, but longitudinal studies are required to confirm this association.

PATHOPHYSIOLOGY

Appetite centers in the paraventricular nucleus, arcuate nucleus, and lateral hypothalamus play a central role in allowing overconsumption of calories. Ghrelin is orexigenic (stimulates appetite), is produced by the stomach, and has a dominant role over leptin, which is anorexigenic (inhibits appetite) and is produced by adipose cells. In the arcuate nucleus, adenosine monophosphate–activated protein kinase, Agouti-related protein, neuropeptide Y, γ-aminobutyric acid, and galanin inhibit the satiety centers of the arcuate and paraventricular nuclei and stimulate the feeding center of the lateral hypothalamus, which also decreases energy expenditure. Peptides in the arcuate nucleus satiety center include proopiomelanocortin, α-melanocyte–stimulating hormone, cocaine- and amphetamine-related transcript, and neurotensin. Gut hormones, such as insulin, glucagon-like peptide 1 (GLP-1), peptide YY, and cholecystokinin inhibit the feeding centers, activate the satiety centers, and increase energy expenditure. Polymorphisms that affect secretion or signal transduction of any of these pathways can influence the body composition set-point.

Once environmental factors exploit a genetically determined predisposition in body composition, creating obesity, an inflammatory state ensues. Adipokines (interleukin-6, tumor necrosis factor-α, leptin, and adiponectin) are products from adipose tissue that contribute to an inflammatory state with obesity. Hyperinsulinemia, which leads to decreased cardioprotection, is also associated with obesity and a proinflammatory state [30].

TREATMENT

The initial goal of therapy is to identify and treat associated cardiovascular risk factors (high blood pressure, elevated glucose, dyslipidemia) and to prevent further weight gain. Then a realistic goal for weight loss should be determined. In general, an initial goal of 10% weight loss over a 6-month period with maintenance of lean body mass is feasible and reduces risk. Typically, faster weight loss occurs with diuresis during the first 2 weeks, followed by slower weight loss. By 6 months, weight loss plateaus, and patients may become discouraged. Patients should be reminded of the metabolic changes occurring with weight loss and the need for a maintenance program.

Therapeutic Life-style Changes

The nonpharmacologic and nonsurgical management of obesity involves behavioral modification, healthy eating, and increased physical activity. This should be first-line therapy for obesity and continued throughout a person's life not only to enhance other therapies, but also promote general health. In obese adolescents, modest life-style–only changes are associated with a redistribution of body composition, improved insulin sensitivity, and decreased markers of inflammation [31].

Behavioral

Behavioral therapy is an essential requirement for all weight-management interventions. Patients learn how to overcome obstacles and improve long-term adherence to life-style changes through behavioral therapy. Strategies include healthy eating, increased physical activity, recognizing unhealthy life-style patterns, self-monitoring (keeping logs), stress reduction, stimulus identification and control, setting goals and offering rewards, problem solving, and social support. In adolescents with a mean BMI of 37.6 ± 3.3 kg/m^2, behavioral therapy favorably redistributed body composition in the absence of weight loss while also improving insulin sensitivity and reversing the inflammatory state [31]. In a meta-analysis of randomized studies of children, behavioral family-based treatment led to sustained weight loss [32]. Other benefits of behavioral therapy include improved biomarkers of vascular inflammation [33,34]. Behavioral therapy can induce a 5% to 10% weight loss and is more effective at 1, but not 5 years, compared with a very low calorie diet [35–37]. Behavior therapies also improve the weight-loss response to pharmacotherapy [35,38,39]. Weight gain can be expected with discontinuation of behavioral therapy. Sequential behavioral therapy for weight control after a program for smoking cessation may have superior results compared with concurrent weight-control and smoking-cessation interventions [40].

Healthy Eating and Nutrition

Patients with obesity should be encouraged to restrict calories while following basic principles of healthy eating. For most patients, reducing intake by 500 kcal/day leads to a 0.5- to 1-pound weight loss per week and is associated with no increased risk. Diets should be low in saturated fat (<10% total calories) and dietary cholesterol (<300 mg/day) with minimal *trans*-fatty acids and the majority of dietary fat consumed as monounsaturated fatty acids (MUFA), to decrease the risk of atherosclerosis [41]. The incorporation of larger portions of low–energy-dense foods, such as fruits and vegetables, provides essential fiber and phytonutrients, while maintaining satiety and restricting energy intake [42]. The consumption of caloric beverages with a standard meal is best avoided, as they do not increase satiety and only increase calories consumed [43].

The optimal macronutrient distribution for weight loss has been frequently debated and remains controversial. It is most likely that one approach will not suit all patients. Four randomized controlled studies demonstrated greater weight loss at 6 months, but not by 1 year, with low-carbohydrate diets [44–48]. A plant-based (vegan), low-fat diet, without any prescribed limits on portion size or energy intake, was associated with greater weight loss (-5.8 kg vs. -3.8 kg) compared with a control diet [49]. In a meta-analysis, low-fat diets were not found to be superior to calorie-restricted diets [50]. Although no metabolic advantage for weight loss has been demonstrated, some studies suggest that diets higher in protein (25%–30%) may increase satiety and result in lower caloric intake in a free-living environment [51,52]. The mechanism for the satiating effect of dietary protein is unclear and is not related to postprandial ghrelin secretion, as previously thought [53]. One study showed a greater decrease in triglycerides and reduced fat mass with a high-protein, low-fat diet relative to a conventional high-carbohydrate, low-fat diet, but total weight loss was equivalent after 12 weeks [54]. Weight loss (2.1–3.3 kg over a 1-year period) was comparable among various commercially available diets: Atkins (carbohydrate restriction), Zone (macronutrient balance), Weight Watchers (calorie restriction) and Ornish (fat restriction); successful weight loss was associated with adherence and cardiac risk factor reduction [55].

Very-low-calorie diets (VLCD; <800 kcal/day) or "protein-supplemented modified fasts" and low-calorie diets (LCD; 800–1,500 kcal/day) are associated with comparable rates of weight loss, although more weight is lost initially with VLCDs. In a large, multicenter study [56] involving 1,389 patients followed-up for at least 1 year on a VLCD providing 600–800 calories per day, mean weight loss was -6.9 ± 2.6 kg at day 30, -12.3 ± 5.3 kg at day 90, and -13.1 ± 8.0 kg at 12 months. The weight loss was primarily fat mass, as determined by bioimpedance analysis [56]. VLCDs require protein sources of high nutritional value and supplementation of vitamins and micronutrients, including sodium, potassium, calcium, iron, and magnesium. VLCDs are safest when monitored by a physician as part of a comprehensive weight-reduction program. VLCDs are contraindicated in pregnancy and lactation, major psychiatric disease, severe systemic disease, and type 1 diabetes.

Another popular strategy in obesity treatment is the use of commercial meal replacements (liquids or bars). Meal replacements serve as both a nutritional and a behavioral strategy, as they provide calorie- and portion-controlled meals, generally fortified with vitamins and minerals, and they eliminate the need to make food choices. They are typically used to replace one or two meals daily. A meta-analysis of six controlled trials found that subjects on a diet plan that included liquid meal replacements lost 2.54 kg more at 3 months and 2.44 kg more at 1 year than did those on a reduced-energy food-based plan [57].

High-protein diets deliver a marked acid load to the kidney and thereby increase the risk for bone loss and kidney stones [58,59], although high-dose calcium supplementation during short-term calorie restriction can attenuate bone resorption [60]. High protein consumption can also accelerate chronic kidney disease (CKD) and should be avoided in patients with baseline elevated creatinine and used with caution in patients at high risk for CKD, such as those with diabetes or hypertension [61].

The risk for metabolic bone disease can be further increased by a concomitant vitamin D deficiency. 25-Hydroxyvitamin D levels have been shown to correlate inversely with the percentage of body fat [62], and prevalence rates for vitamin D deficiency (25-OH vitamin D, <16 ng/mL) up to 62% have been demonstrated with a BMI $\geq$ 40 kg/m^2 [63]. This is thought to be due to sequestration of 25-OH vitamin D in fat, possibly in conjunction with reduced sun exposure. Consideration should be given to the need for calcium and vitamin D supplementation while dieting, and depending on the degree of calorie restriction, other micronutrient supplementation may be necessary to prevent deficiencies.

Last, no strong evidence supports the routine use of dietary supplements in the management of obesity. Dietary supplements purported to induce weight loss, including bitter orange (*Citrus aurantium*), chromium picolinate, linoleic acid, chitosan, calcium, *Garcinia cambogia*, glucomannan, guar gum, β-hydroxymethylbutyrate, pyruvate, yerba mate, and yohimbe show little evidence of benefit [64]. Ephedra (Ma huang) demonstrated short-term efficacy, but its sale has been prohibited in the United States since 2004 because of an unacceptable risk of myocardial infarction, stroke, seizures, and death. Functional foods that may facilitate weight loss and decrease oxidative stress are generally plant based and high in fiber and polyphenols.

Physical Activity

All patients must be encouraged to participate in daily physical activity, including a minimum of 30 minutes of exercise every day, or on most days, of the week [65]. Additional physical activity may be necessary to increase energy expenditure in overweight or obese individuals to lose weight. Weight loss induced by physical activity each day, without calorie restriction, is more effective than calorie restriction–induced weight loss with respect to truncal obesity and insulin resistance in men [66]. Over a period of 8 months, high-quantity and vigorous-intensity exercise (20 miles jogging per week) can decrease mean body mass by 3.5 kg and mean fat mass by 4.9 kg (with an increase in lean body mass of 1.4 kg), compared with low-amount and moderate-intensity exercise (12 miles walking per week; equivalent to 30 min a day), which can decrease mean body mass by 1.3 kg and mean fat mass by 2.0 kg (with an increase in lean body mass of 0.7 kg) [67]. When coupled with dietary advice, life-style changes including physical activity can result in weight reductions of 4.5 kg by 1 year and 3.5 kg by 3 years [68]. Greater amounts of exercise with an energy-expenditure goal of 2,500 kcal/week, produce weight losses at 6, 12, and 18 months of 9.0, 8.5, and 6.7 kg, compared with less exercise with an energy-expenditure goal of 1,000 kcal/week, producing weight losses of 8.1, 6.1, and 4.1 kg, respectively [69]. In sedentary women who increased physical activity and adhered to a 1,200- to 1,500-calorie, 20% to 30% fat diet, less than 150 minutes/week exercise resulted in 4.7% weight loss; 150 to 200 minutes/week, in 9.5%; and more than 200 minutes/week, 13.6% [70].

PHARMACOTHERAPY

Antiobesity medications are indicated in those patients for whom therapeutic life-style changes have failed and who have a BMI of 27 kg/m^2 or more (with comorbidities) or 30 kg/m^2 or more (without comorbidities). The amount of weight loss anticipated from antiobesity medication is only up to about 5 kg at 1 year, but this has still been associated with CVD and T2DM risk reduction. The choice of agents depends on individual patient factors (side effects), and these must be discussed with the patient. A Cochrane review determined that sufficient evidence existed only for sibutramine and orlistat for statistically significant weight loss for at least 1 year [71]. These are the only medications currently approved for long-term management of obesity, including weight loss and weight maintenance.

Sibutramine

Sibutramine is an appetite suppressant with combined norepinephrine and serotonin reuptake inhibition. Sibutramine (10–15 mg daily) with life-style changes has been found to induce an increased 4.45-kg weight loss, compared with placebo, at 1 year in overweight and obese patients [72,73]. Adverse effects include headache, dry mouth, palpitations, hypertension, nervousness, and insomnia.

Orlistat

Orlistat is a lipase inhibitor, which decreases the absorption of fat. Based on a meta-analysis of 50 studies, the pooled mean increased weight loss for orlistat (120 mg po, TID) and lifestyle changes, compared with placebo, was 2.59 kg at 6 months and 2.89 kg at 12 months [73]. Orlistat plus life-style changes can decrease the risk for T2DM in patients with impaired glucose tolerance [17]. Adverse effects include diarrhea, flatulence, bloating, abdominal pain, and dyspepsia. Vitamin supplementation at night is recommended because of malabsorption of fat-soluble vitamins (A, D, E, and K). Although the usual dose is 120 mg PO before each meal TID, to minimize these adverse effects, only 120 mg PO daily may be taken preceding the meal containing the most fat. In addition, concomitant use of fiber or psyllium can reduce adverse effects due to malabsorption [74].

FUTURE DIRECTIONS

The anticonvulsant medication, topiramate (25–600 mg daily) results in decreased food intake and is associated with a 6% to 17% weight loss after 14 to 60 weeks of use [75–78]. Topiramate may be most effective for those patients with obesity and binge-eating disorder [78,79]. Adverse effects include paresthesia, cognitive changes, depression, and nervousness. The cannabinoid-1 receptor blocker, rimonabant, also decreases food intake and awaits FDA approval for use as an antiobesity drug. When combined with a hypocaloric diet for a 1-year period, rimonabant was associated with a decrease of 3.4 kg (5 mg daily) and 6.6 kg (20 mg daily), and improvements of cardiovascular risk factors: waist circumference, HDL-c, triglycerides, insulin resistance, and prevalence of the metabolic syndrome [80].

BARIATRIC SURGERY

Surgical management of class III obesity is more effective than conventional management [81]. Bariatric surgery is indicated in those adults with a BMI greater than 40 kg/m^2, where expected benefit outweighs risk, or a BMI more than 35 kg/m^2 with one or more comorbidities, where expected benefit outweighs risk. Laparoscopic bariatric procedures are safe, effective, and preferred, mainly because of shortened hospital stays and an earlier return to normal activity [82,83]. Restrictive bariatric surgical procedures, associated with reduction in obesity-related comorbidities, include the laparoscopic adjustable gastric banding (LAP-BAND) and laparoscopic Roux-en-Y gastric bypass (RGB). This LAP-BAND procedure is associated with 44% to 68% loss of excess weight at 4 years [84,85], although 30% may fail to lose more than 30% of their excess weight [86]. The RGB is associated with a 63% loss of excess weight at 1 year and 71% at 2 years [87]. One study comparing 456 RGBs with 805 LAP-BANDs performed at two different institutions demonstrated greater excess weight loss at 18 months with RGB (74.6% vs. 40.4%) but with higher early postoperative complication rates (4.2% vs. 1.7%) [88]. The biliopancreatic diversion with duodenal switch (BPD-DS) is a combined restrictive and malabsorptive procedure associated with greater long-term loss of excess weight (61%–77% within 3 years) but at the expense of greater complication and nutritional-deficiency rates [83,89,90].

REFERENCES

1. *(1C+)* **Rosner B** et al. Percentiles for body mass index in U.S. children 5 to 17 years of age. J Pediatr 1998;132:211–222.

   In this meta-review of observational data, standardized height and weight measurements from 66,772 children from nine large epidemiologic studies were used to construct BMI distribution tables.

2. (1A) **U.S. Preventive Services Task Force.** Screening and interventions for overweight in children and adolescents: Recommendation statement. http://www.guideline.gov/summary/summary.aspx?doc_id=7155&nbr=4287&string=obesity (accessed on 11/6/2005).

   This evidence-based clinical practice guideline posted on the National Guideline Clearinghouse website details the lack of conclusive evidence regarding screening for overweight in pediatrics.

3. **Deitel M.** Overweight and obesity worldwide now estimated to involve 1.7 billion people. Obes Surg 2003;13:329–330.

   This is a commentary on the 2003 World Health Organization and International Association for the Study of Obesity report in which the prevalence of obesity is increasing. In epidemiologic studies, overweight/obesity was ranked number 10 among global risks affecting disease, disability, and death rates.

4. *(1C+)* **Hedley AA** et al. Prevalence of overweight and obesity among US children, adolescents, and adults, 1999–2002. JAMA 2004;291:2847–2850.

   This is a probability sample from the NHANES involving 4,115 adults and 4,018 children in 1999–2000 and 3,290 adults and 4,258 children in 2001–2002.

5. *(1C+)* **Vasan RS** et al. Estimated risks for developing obesity in the Framingham Heart Study. Ann Intern Med 2005;143:473–480.

   This is a prospective cohort study of 4,117 (59% women) white participants followed up from 1971 through 2001.

6. *(1C)* **Mokdad AH** et al. Prevalence of obesity, diabetes, and obesity-related health risk factors, 2001. JAMA 2003;289:76–79.

   Random-digit telephone survey of 195,005 adults participating in the BRFSS.

7. *(1C)* **Stein PD** et al. Obesity as a risk factor in venous thromboembolism. Am J Med 2005;118: 978–980.

   Observational study from the database of the National Hospital Discharge Survey. In obese patients, an increased relative risk of deep venous thrombosis (2.50) and pulmonary embolus (2.21) was found in men and women, with greatest impact at younger than 40 years.

8. *(1C+)* **Flegal KM** et al. Excess deaths associated with underweight, overweight, and obesity. JAMA 2005;293:1861–1867.

   Data from the NHANES I (1971–1975; 210,563 person-years), II (1976–1980; 122,772 person-years), and III (1988–1994; 124,245 person-years) were analyzed to estimate relative risks of mortality associated with BMI.

9. *(1A)* **Knowler WC** et al. Reduction in the incidence of type 2 diabetes with lifestyle intervention or metformin. N Engl J Med 2002;346:393–403.

   This is a PRCT involving 3,234 nondiabetic persons with impaired glucose regulation receiving either life-style changes (with >7% reduction in body weight and >150 minutes/week physical activity) or metformin, 850 mg PO BID and a mean follow-up of 2.8 years. Life-style changes reduced the incidence of T2DM by 58%, and metformin, by 31%, compared with the placebo group.

10. **Ryan DH** et al. Look AHEAD (action for health in diabetes): Design and methods for a clinical trial of weight loss for the prevention of cardiovascular disease in type 2 diabetes. Control Clin Trials 2003;24:610–628.

    This is a description of a randomized intensive life-style intervention study of approximately 5,000 male and female subjects with T2DM and BMI 25 kg/m^2 or greater. The main end point is time to incidence of a major CVD event.

11. *(2C)* **Kissebah AH** et al. Relation of body fat distribution to metabolic complications of obesity. J Clin Endocrinol Metab 1982;54:254–260.

    Women with upper- versus lower-body-segment obesity underwent glucose tolerance testing, lipid profiling, and fat cell analysis. Abdominal fat cell size correlated with glucose and insulin levels.

12. *(1C)* **Blair D** et al. Evidence for an increased risk for hypertension with centrally located body fat and the effect of race and sex on this risk. Am J Epidemiol 1984;119:526–540.

    Observational data from the First Health and Nutrition Examination Survey (1971–1974) were used to correlate peripheral and central fat with blood pressure in 5,506 participants.

13. (1C) **Larsson B** et al. Abdominal adipose tissue distribution, obesity, and risk of cardiovascular disease and death: 13 year follow up of participants in the study of men born in 1913. Br Med J 1984;288:1401–1404.

    Observational study of 792 54-year-old men for 13 years in which an increased occurrence of stroke and ischemic heart disease was noted in association with increased waist-to-hip circumference ratio.

14. **Mensah GA** et al. Obesity, metabolic syndrome, and type 2 diabetes: Emerging epidemics and their cardiovascular implications. Cardiol Clin 2004;22:485–504.

    This is a review of metabolic syndrome with an abundance of charts and tables.

15. *(1C)* **Alexander CM** et al. NCEP-defined metabolic syndrome, diabetes, and prevalence of coronary heart disease among NHANES III participants age 50 years and older. Diabetes 2003;52:1210–1204.

    Observational study designed to quantify the increased prevalence of CVD in patients with metabolic syndrome with or without T2DM.

16. *(1A)* **Tuomilehto J** et al. Prevention of type 2 diabetes mellitus by changes in lifestyle among subjects with impaired glucose tolerance. N Engl J Med 2001;344:1343–1350.

    This is a PRCT involving 522 middle-aged overweight subjects with impaired glucose tolerance receiving life-style changes (weight reduction, decreased dietary total and saturated fat, increased fiber, and increased physical activity) or no intervention. The main end point was development of T2DM, and glucose-tolerance tests were performed annually. The cumulative incidence of T2DM was 11% in the intervention group and 23% in the control group (58% risk reduction).

17. *(1A)* **Torgerson JS** et al. XENical in the prevention of diabetes in obese subjects (XENDOS) study: A randomized study of orlistat as an adjunct to lifestyle changes for the prevention of type 2 diabetes in obese patients. Diabetes Care 2004;27:155–161.

    This is a 4-year PRCT of 3,305 patients undergoing life-style changes and receiving either orlistat, 120 mg PO t.i.d., or placebo, with main end points being time to onset of T2DM and change in body weight. Benefits were greater in the orlistat-treated group.

18. **Kahn R** et al. The metabolic syndrome: Time for a critical appraisal. Diabetes Care 2005;28: 2289–2304.

   This is a review of the data regarding metabolic syndrome with a conclusion that the syndrome does not exist as currently defined. Specific practical recommendations are provided.

19. **Grundy SM** et al. Diagnosis and management of the metabolic syndrome. Circulation 2005;112: epub ahead of print.

   This is an executive summary of the American Heart Association/National Heart, Lung, and Blood Institute position on the metabolic syndrome as a predictor of CVD.

20. **Lyon HN** et al. Genetics of common forms of obesity: A brief overview. Am J Clin Nutr 2005;82(suppl):215S–217S.

   This is a review of the current status of genetic research and methods used to determine associations with obesity. At present, the genetics are too complex to tease out specific associations.

21. *(1C)* **Allison DB** et al. The heritability of body mass index among an international sample of monozygotic twins reared apart. Int J Obes Relat Metab Disord 1996;20:501–506.

   This is a meta-analysis of observational data from 53 pairs of monozygotic twins reared apart, demonstrating that 70% of the variance in BMI can be attributed to genetic variation.

22. *(1C+)* **Stunkard AJ** et al. The body mass index of twins who have been reared apart. N Engl J Med 1990;322:1483–1487.

   This is a meta-analysis of observational data from identical and fraternal twins reared apart or together, demonstrating substantial genetic and minimal childhood environmental influences on BMI.

23. *(1C)* **Laitinen J** et al. Family social class, maternal body mass index, childhood body mass index, and age at menarche as predictors of adult obesity. Am J Clin Nutr 2001;74:287–294.

   This is a Finnish observational study of 2,876 male and 3,404 female subjects demonstrating predictive power of low social class, high maternal BMI before pregnancy, high BMI during adolescence, and early menarche on adult obesity.

24. *(1C)* **Prentice AM** et al. Fast foods, energy density and obesity: A possible mechanistic link. Obes Rev 2003;4:187–194.

   This is a literature review of clinical studies demonstrating "passive overconsumption" of calories derived from fast foods, approximately 65% higher than in typical British diets, which challenges normal human appetite-control systems, especially in children and adolescents.

25. *(2C)* **Drewnowski A** et al. Dietary energy density and body weight: Is there a relationship? Nutr Rev 2004;62:403–413.

   In this review of the literature, insufficient longitudinal cohort or prospective epidemiologic studies demonstrated a causal association between dietary energy density and obesity risk, even though a link is supported by the findings of several cross-sectional epidemiologic studies.

26. *(1B)* **Willett WC.** Dietary fat plays a major role in obesity: No. Obes Rev 2002;3:59–68.

   In between-population and within-population cross-sectional epidemiologic studies, an association of dietary fat occurs with the prevalence of obesity. Some short-term small, randomized prospective studies even support this association, but a meta-analysis of long-term trials (>1 year) fails to demonstrate this association. Moreover, during a time period in the United States when the percentage of energy consumed derived from fat has decreased, the prevalence of obesity has substantially increased. Thus focusing on dietary fat intake as a priority in the dietary management of obesity may be a "serious distraction."

27. *(2C)* **Blundell JE** et al. Resistance and susceptibility to weight gain: Individual variability in response to a high-fat diet. Physiol Behav 2005;86:614–622.

   In this small observational study, biologic vulnerability for obesity due to a high-fat diet is associated with symptoms that may be part of a "thrifty phenotype": Weak satiety response to fatty meals, preference for high-fat foods, and a strong hedonic attraction to palatable foods and eating.

28. *(1C)* **Song WO** et al. Is consumption of breakfast associated with body mass index in US adults? J Am Diet Assoc 2005;105:1373–1382.

   In this analysis of data from the NHANES 1999–2000 involving 4,218 participants (2,097 men and 2,121 women), inclusion of a ready-to-eat cereal in the breakfast meal was associated with a decreased odds ratio (0.70) for BMI of 25 kg/m^2 or more and inverse association with BMI ($r = -0.37$; $p < 0.01$) in women, but not in men.

29. **Ruxton CH** et al. Breakfast: A review of associations with measures of dietary intake, physiology and biochemistry. Br J Nutr 1997;78:199–213.

   In this review of the literature, the association of breakfast and nutritional status is discussed.

30. **Dandona P** et al. Metabolic syndrome. Circulation 2005;111:1448–1454.

   This is a review of the competing roles of obesity and insulin resistance in the pathogenesis of metabolic syndrome.

31. *(1B)* **Balagopal P** et al. Lifestyle-only intervention attenuates the inflammatory state associated with obesity: A randomized controlled study in adolescents. J Pediatr 2005;146:342–348.

In this small PRCT of only 15 obese adolescents, increased physical activity and calorie restriction for 3 months was associated with decreased C-reactive protein, fibrinogen, and interleukin-6 levels.

32. *(1A)* **Epstein LH** et al. Ten-year outcomes of behavioral family-based treatment for childhood obesity. Health Psychol 1994;13:373–383.

Based on a metareview of four randomized studies of obese children, at 10 years, 34% had decreased their percentage overweight by more than 20%. Thirty percent of patients were not obese. The role of family and friend support for eating and activity habits is emphasized.

33. *(1B)* **Lindahl B** et al. Improved fibrinolysis by intense lifestyle intervention: A randomized trial in subjects with impaired glucose tolerance. J Intern Med 1999;246:105–112.

In this randomized trial of 186 obese patients with impaired glucose tolerance, sustained benefits in fibrinolysis biomarkers was observed with behavioral therapy compared with usual care.

34. *(1B)* **Esposito K** et al. Effect of weight loss and lifestyle changes on vascular inflammatory markers in obese women: A randomized trial. JAMA 2003;289:1799–1804.

In this randomized, single-blind trial of 120 premenopausal nondiabetic obese women adhering to a low-energy Mediterranean diet and increased physical activity and losing more than 10% of their weight, biomarkers for vascular inflammation and insulin resistance were reduced.

35. *(1B)* **Wadden TA** et al. Treatment of obesity by very low calorie diet, behavior therapy, and their combination: A five-year perspective. Int J Obes 1989;13(suppl 2):39–46.

In this randomized controlled study of 76 obese women, behavioral therapy, with (32%) or without (36%) a very-low calorie diet, maintained weight loss at 1 (10.6 and 6.6 kg, respectively) but not at 5 years. At 1 year, more weight loss was found with the combination of behavioral and diet therapy compared with behavioral or diet therapy alone.

36. *(1B)* **Munsch S** et al. Evaluation of a lifestyle change programme for the treatment of obesity in general practice. Swiss Med Wkly 2003;133:148–154.

This is a prospective, randomized study of 122 patients from 14 general practices in Switzerland, consisting of 16 group sessions of 90 minutes each with integrated cognitive behavioral therapy.

37. **Foster GD** et al. Behavioral treatment of obesity. Am J Clin Nutr 2005;82:230S–235S.

This is a review of clinical data on behavioral treatments for obesity.

38. *(1B)* **Wadden TA** et al. Benefits of lifestyle modification in the pharmacologic treatment of obesity: A randomized trial. Arch Intern Med 2001;161:218–227.

In this randomized trial of 53 obese women, sibutramine alone, sibutramine plus life-style modification, and sibutramine, life-style, and portion-controlled diet induced a 4.1%, 10.8%, and 16.5% weight loss, respectively.

39. *(1B)* **Hoeger KM** et al. A randomized, 48-week, placebo-controlled trial of intensive lifestyle modification and/or metformin therapy in overweight women with polycystic ovary syndrome: A pilot study. Fertil Steril 2004;82:421–429.

This is a PRCT limited by recruitment, dropout, and compliance. Patients treated with both life-style changes and metformin lost more weight than those with either intervention alone.

40. *(1B)* **Spring B** et al. Randomized controlled trial for behavioral smoking and weight control treatment: Effect of concurrent versus sequential intervention. J Consult Clin Psychol 2004;72:785–796.

This randomized trial of 315 female smokers found that weight control added to the last, versus the first, 8 weeks of a 16-week smoking cessation was associated with a more lasting and stable weight-suppression effect.

41. **Institute of Medicine.** Dietary, functional, and total fiber: Dietary reference intakes for energy, carbohydrate, fiber, fat, fatty acids, cholesterol, protein, and amino acids. Washington, DC, National Academy Press, 2002:265–334.

This is an official evidence-based resource with tables for easy referencing. The website can be navigated to access information about all aspects of dietary guidelines: http://www.iom.edu/report.asp?id=4340 (Accessed on October 30, 2005).

42. *(1C)* **Ello-Martin JA** et al. The influence of food portion size and energy density on energy intake: Implications for weight management. Am J Clin Nutr 2005;82(1 suppl):236S–241S.

Review of controlled prospective clinical studies concluding that low–energy-dense foods intake suppresses appetite and limits calorie consumption for up to 2 days.

43. *(1C)* **DellaValle DM** et al. Does the consumption of caloric and non-caloric beverages with a meal affect energy intake? Appetite 2005;44:187–193.

In this study, 44 women were observed eating lunch over a 6-week course in which different beverages were provided. When caloric beverages were consumed with lunch, the total energy intake was on average 104 ± 16 kcal greater, without any effect on satiety, than when noncaloric beverages were consumed.

44. *(1B)* **Foster GD** et al. A randomized trial of a low-carbohydrate diet for obesity. N Engl J Med 2003;348:2082–2090.

This 1-year randomized multicenter controlled trial of 63 obese men and women demonstrated greater weight loss at 3 and 6 months (about 4% difference in weight), but not by 1 year, of a low-carbohydrate, high-protein, high-fat diet compared with a conventional low-calorie, high-carbohydrate, low-fat diet.

45. *(1B)* **Yancy WS** et al. A low-carbohydrate, ketogenic diet versus a low-fat diet to treat obesity and hyperlipidemia. Ann Intern Med 2004;140:769–777.

This is a randomized controlled trial of 120 overweight hyperlipidemic subjects over 24 weeks demonstrating greater weight loss (−12.9% vs. −6.7%) and adherence (76% vs. 57%) of a low-carbohydrate diet (<20 g carbohydrate initially) compared with a low-fat diet (<30% fat calories, <300 mg daily cholesterol, 500–1,000 kcal/day energy deficit). Greater improvements in hypertriglyceridemia and low HDL levels were also observed in the low-carbohydrate group.

46. *(1B)* **Brehm BJ** et al. A randomized trial comparing a very low carbohydrate diet and a calorie-restricted low fat diet on body weight and cardiovascular risk factors in healthy women. J Clin Endocrinol Metab 2003;88:1617–1623.

In this randomized controlled trial of 53 healthy obese subjects over a 6-month period, greater weight loss (8.5 vs. 3.9 kg) and fat-mass loss (4.8 vs. 2.0 kg) was observed with an ad libitum low-carbohydrate diet versus a calorie-restricted diet with 30% of calories as fat. No differences were found between the groups of calories consumed, lipids, fasting glucose, insulin, or blood pressure, although the low-carbohydrate group had higher β-hydroxybutyrate levels.

47. *(1B)* **Samaha FF** et al. A low-carbohydrate as compared with a low-fat diet in severe obesity. N Engl J Med 2003;348:2074–2081.

In this randomized controlled trial of 79 obese subjects (39% with diabetes and 43% with metabolic syndrome) over a 6-month period, greater weight loss (−5.8 vs. −1.9 kg) was observed with a low-carbohydrate diet compared with a calorie-restricted low-fat diet. Improvements in hypertriglyceridemia and insulin resistance were greater in the low-carbohydrate group.

48. *(1B)* **Stern L** et al. The effects of low-carbohydrate versus conventional weight loss diets in severely obese adults: One-year follow-up of a randomized trial. Ann Intern Med 2004;140: 778–785.

This study reports the 1-year follow-up data from the study by Samaha FF, et al. (2003). Weight-loss differences at 6 months were not present at 1 year, although lipid and glycemic status (A_{1c} levels) remained better in the low-carbohydrate group.

49. (1B) **Barnard ND** et al. The effects of a low-fat, plant-based dietary intervention on body weight, metabolism, and insulin sensitivity. Am J Med 2005;118:991–997.

In this randomized controlled study of 64 overweight postmenopausal women over a 14-week period, an ad libitum low-fat vegan diet was associated with greater weight loss (5.8 vs. 3.8 kg) compared with an NCEP control diet.

50. *(1A)* **Pirozzo S** et al. Advice on low-fat diets for obesity (Cochrane Review): The Cochrane Library, 2005; Issue 2. http://www.cochrane.org/cochrane/revabstr/AB003640.htm (accessed 11/8/2005).

In this meta-analysis of four PRCTs with 6-month follow-up, five with 12-month follow-up, and three with 18-month follow-up, no significant differences in weight loss or other clinical parameters were noted between those overweight/obese patients treated with a low-fat diet compared with other weight-reducing calorically restricted diets.

51. *(2B)* **Nickols-Richardson SM** et al. Perceived hunger is lower and weight loss is greater in overweight premenopausal women consuming a low-carbohydrate/high-protein vs high-carbohydrate/low-fat diet. J Am Diet Assoc 2005;105:1433–1437.

In this small 6-week PRCT involving 28 overweight premenopausal women, a low-carbohydrate/high-protein diet was associated with decreased hunger perception and greater percentage of body weight loss.

52. *(2B)* **Schoeller DA** et al. Energetics of obesity and weight control: Does diet composition matter? J Am Diet Assoc 2005;105(suppl 1):S24–S28.

This is a review of the clinical literature and a commentary drawing the following conclusions: (1) that prior studies demonstrating an advantage of low-carbohydrate diets by virtue of decreased calorie intake are flawed, and studies involving 24-hour energy expenditures are not supportive of this claim; (2) that it is speculated that it is the high-protein content of a therapeutic diet that suppresses appetite and leads to weight loss, rather than a low-carbohydrate component; and (3) that hypocaloric weight-loss diets should contain 35% to 50% carbohydrate, 25% to 35% fat, and 25% to 30% protein, based on total daily energy needs.

53. *(1B)* **Moran LJ** et al. The satiating effect of dietary protein is unrelated to postprandial ghrelin secretion. J Clin Endocrinol Metab 2005;90:5205–5211.

In this 12-week randomized, parallel-design controlled study of 57 overweight, hyperinsulinemic men and women, comparable effects of high-protein (34%)/low-fat (29%) and standard protein (18%)/high-fat (45%) diets were seen: both were associated with decreased appetite, increased ghrelin, and decreased weight.

54. *(1B)* **Noakes M** et al. Effect of an energy-restricted, high-protein, low-fat diet relative to a conventional high-carbohydrate, low-fat diet on weight loss, body composition, nutritional status, and markers of cardiovascular health in obese women. Am J Clin Nutr 2005;81:1298–1306.

In this randomized controlled study of 100 obese or overweight women over a 12-week period, an energy-restricted high-protein, low-fat diet was associated with greater fat-mass loss and improvements in glycemic and lipid status compared with a high-carbohydrate diet, despite no differences in weight loss.

55. *(1B)* **Dansinger ML** et al. Comparison of the Atkins, Ornish, Weight Watchers, and Zone Diets for weight loss and heart disease risk reduction. JAMA 2005;293:43–53.

Randomized study of 160 patients finding that it is adherence to a diet that has the greater effect on success. The caloric reduction among the four groups, which had comparable weight loss overall, were 138 kcal/day (Atkins), 251 kcal/day (Zone), 244 kcal/day (Weight Watchers), and 192 kcal/day (Ornish) ($p < 0.05$).

56. *(1C)* **Zahouani A** et al. Short- and long-term evolution of body composition in 1389 obese outpatients following a very low calorie diet (Pro'gram18 VLCD). Acta Diabetol 2003;40(suppl 1):S149–S150.

In this large observational study, a VLCD was associated with weight-loss maintenance and improved obesity-associated risk factors for up to 2 years.

57. *(1A)* **Heymsfield SB** et al. Weight management using a meal replacement strategy: Meta- and pooling analysis from six studies. Int J Obes Relat Metab Disord 2003;27:537–549.

These meta-analyses of PRCTs for more than 3 months of adult subjects with BMI of 25 kg/m^2 or more demonstrate safety and efficacy of partial meal replacements on weight loss and reduction of obesity-associated risk factors.

58. *(1C)* **Reddy ST** et al. Effect of low-carbohydrate high-protein diets on acid-base balance, stone-forming propensity, and calcium metabolism. Am J Kidney Dis 2002;40:265–274.

In 10 healthy subjects, adherence to the Atkins' induction diet for 2 weeks (1,930 mean kcal/d, 164 mean g protein/d, 133 mean g fat/d, and 19 mean g carbohydrate/d) followed by the Atkins' maintenance diet (2,034 mean kcal/d, 170 mean g protein/d, 136 mean g fat/d, and 33 mean g carbohydrate/d) was associated with increased urinary acid and calcium excretion, decreased urinary citrate levels, and a trend toward increased bone resorption and decreased bone formation.

59. **Amanzadeh J** et al. Effect of high protein diet on stone-forming propensity and bone loss in rats. Kidney Int 2003;64:2142–2149.

This is a rat study demonstrating the hypocitraturic and bone hyperresorptive effects of a high-protein 60 diet.

60. *(1B)* **Bowen J** et al. A high dairy protein, high-calcium diet minimizes bone turnover in overweight adults during weight loss. J Nutr 2004;134:568–573.

In this randomized study, 50 subjects received 12 weeks of a high-protein, energy-restricted diet, with either 2,400 mg/d calcium (using dairy protein sources) or 500 mg/d calcium (using mixed protein sources), followed by a 4-week period of energy balance. Weight loss (10% initial body weight) was comparable between the two groups, but the dairy protein group had less bone hyperresorption than the mixed-protein group.

61. *(1C+)* **Friedman AN** et al. High-protein diets: Potential effects on the kidney in renal health and disease. Am J Kidney Dis 2004;44:950–962.

In this review of the clinical literature represented by human interventional studies, all but one being randomized, high-protein diets were found to pose significant harm in patients with chronic kidney disease: increased proteinuria, diuresis, natriuresis, kaliuresis, blood pressure changes, and nephrolithiasis.

62. *(1C)* **Arunabh S** et al. Body fat content and 25-hydroxyvitamin D levels in healthy women. J Clin Endocrinol Metab 2003;88:157–161.

In this cross-sectional study of 410 healthy women with BMIs ranging from 17 to 30 kg/m^2, an inverse correlation was found between percentage body fat (determined by DEXA) and 25-hydroxyvitamin D levels. This relation is thought to be due to an increased tissue distribution of vitamin D with increased adiposity.

63. *(1C)* **Buffington C** et al. Vitamin D deficiency in the morbidly obese. Obes Surg 1993;3:421–424.

In this cross-sectional study of 60 obese women being considered for bariatric surgery, 25-hydroxyvitamin D levels were negatively correlated with obesity.

64. *(2C)* **Dwyer JT** et al. Dietary supplements in weight reduction. J Am Diet Assoc 2005;105: S80–S86.

A review of weak clinical trials involving dietary supplements and obesity demonstrates inconclusive evidence for any benefit.

65. **Department of Health and Human Services and the U.S. Department of Agriculture.** Dietary guidelines for Americans, 2005. http://www.health.gov/dietaryguidelines/dga2005/document/pdf/dga2005.pdf. Accessed on October 30, 2005.

This is an extremely comprehensive and evidence-based review with specific recommendations on healthy eating and life style, including physical activity.

66. *(1B)* **Ross R** et al. Reduction in obesity and related comorbid conditions after diet-induced weight loss or exercise-induced weight loss in men: A randomized, controlled trial. Ann Intern Med 2000;133:92–103.

In this randomized controlled trial of 52 obese men over a 3-month period, daily physical activity without calorie restriction reduced abdominal obesity and insulin resistance.

67. *(1B)* **Slentz** et al. Effects of the amount of exercise on body weight, body composition, and measures of central obesity: STRRIDE: a randomized controlled study. Arch Intern Med 2004;164:31–39.

In this randomized controlled trial of 120 subjects over an 8-month period, a dose-dependent effect of physical activity on weight loss was found, independent of diet.

68. *(1A)* **Lindstrom J** et al. The Finnish Diabetes Prevention Study (DPS): Lifestyle intervention and 3-year results on diet and physical activity. Diabetes Care 2003;26:3230–3236.

This is a randomized controlled trial over a 3-year period of 522 middle-aged overweight subjects with impaired glucose tolerance, demonstrating that intensive life-style intervention for the first year followed by a maintenance period (diet and exercise) produces greater weight loss and reduced diabetes risk compared with usual care.

69. *(1B)* **Jeffery RW** et al. Physical activity and weight loss: Does prescribing higher physical activity goals improve outcome? Am J Clin Nutr 2003;78:684–689.

This is a randomized controlled trial of 202 overweight men and women found to have greater long-term (18 months) weight loss with more exercise (2,500 kcal/week) compared with less exercise (1,000 kcal/week).

70. *(1B)* **Jakicic JM** et al. Effect of exercise duration and intensity on weight loss in overweight, sedentary women: a randomized trial. JAMA 2003;290:1323–1330.

In this randomized controlled trial of 201 sedentary women followed up for 12 months, a dose–response effect of exercise with weight loss was noted.

71. *(1A)* **Padwal R** et al. Long-term pharmacotherapy for obesity and overweight. The Cochrane Database Syst Rev 2005; Issue 3. http://www.cochrane.org/reviews/en/ab004094.html (accessed on 11/8/2005).

This is a meta-analysis demonstrating weight loss with orlistat (11 PRCTs >1 year; 2.7-kg loss, 2.9% more weight loss than controls; 12% patients with >10% weight loss) and sibutramine (five PRCTs >1 year; 4.3-kg loss, 4.6% more weight loss than controls; 15% patients with >10% weight loss). Attrition rates were high: 33% for orlistat and 43% for sibutramine.

72. *(1A)* **Arterburn DE** et al. The efficacy and safety of sibutramine for weight loss: A systematic review. Arch Intern Med 2004; 164: 994–1003.

In this meta-analysis of 29 randomized placebo-controlled clinical trials and unpublished data from 10 authors, sibutramine was associated with 3- and 12-month weight losses of 2.78 kg and 4.45 kg compared with placebo. Insufficient evidence was provided regarding obesity-associated morbidity or mortality, or a long-term risk–benefit profile.

73. *(1A)* **Li Z** et al. Meta-analysis: Pharmacologic treatment of obesity. Ann Intern Med 2005;142: 532–546.

The authors performed meta-analyses based on information from electronic databases, experts in the field, and unpublished reports on sibutramine, phentermine, diethylpropion, orlistat, fluoxetine, bupropion, topiramate, sertraline, and zonisamide.

74. *(1A)* **Cavaliere H** et al. Gastrointestinal side effects of orlistat may be prevented by concomitant prescription of natural fibers (psyllium mucilloid). Int J Obes Relat Metab Disord 2001;25: 1095–1099.

This is a randomized, placebo-controlled study of 60 obese women in which 6 g of psyllium mucilloid decreased gastrointestinal symptoms associated with orlistat (120 mg PO t.i.d.) use.

75. *(1A)* **Wilding J** et al. A randomized double-blind placebo-controlled study of the long-term efficacy and safety of topiramate in the treatment of obese subjects. Int J Obes Relat Metab Disord 2004;28:1399–1410.

This is a randomized controlled trial of 1,289 overweight or obese subjects with 6-week run-in, 8-week titration, and 2-year maintenance phases. After 1 year, improvements were seen in weight loss, blood pressure, and glycemic control.

76. *(1A)* **Astrup A** et al. Topiramate: Long-term maintenance of weight loss induced by a low-calorie diet in obese subjects. Obes Res 2004;12:1658–1669.

This is a randomized controlled trial of 701 obese subjects who had already lost weight on a low-calorie diet for 8 weeks and continued with life-style changes and topiramate or placebo. Topiramate was associated with increased weight loss and was well tolerated.

77. *(1A)* **Bray GA** et al. A 6-month randomized, placebo-controlled, dose-ranging trial of topiramate for weight loss in obesity. Obes Res 2003;11:722–733.

This is a randomized controlled trial of 385 healthy obese patients found to have greater weight loss with topiramate, compared with placebo, at 64-, 96-, 192-, and 384-mg daily doses.

78. *(1B)* **McElroy SL** et al. Topiramate in the treatment of binge eating disorder associated with obesity: A randomized, placebo-controlled trial. Am J Psychiatry 203;160:255–261.

This randomized controlled study of 61 obese patients with binge-eating disorder over a 14-week period demonstrated decreased weight and binge frequency compared with placebo.

79. *(2C)* **Guerdjikova AI** et al. Response of recurrent binge eating and weight gain to topiramate in patients with binge eating disorder after bariatric surgery. Obes Surg 2005;15:273–277.

This is a report of three patients treated successfully with topiramate for an average of 10 months.

80. *(1A)* **Van Gaal** et al. Effects of the cannabinoid-1 receptor blocker rimonabant on weight reduction and cardiovascular risk factors in overweight patients: 1-year experience from the RIO-Europe study. Lancet 2005;365:1389–1397.

This is a randomized controlled trial of 920 patients followed up for 1 year on either 5 or 20 mg daily. A dose-dependent beneficial effect was seen on weight loss and features of the metabolic syndrome with minimal adverse effects.

81. *(1A)* **Colquitt J** et al. Surgery for morbid obesity: The Cochrane Database Syst Rev 2005; Issue 3. http://www.cochrane.org/reviews/en/ab003641.html (accessed 11/8/2005).

This metareview of 18 trials, of variable quality, involving 1,891 subjects, led the authors to conclude that only limited evidence existed but that surgical management of class III obesity was more effective than nonsurgical methods.

82. *(1A)* **Nguyen NT** et al. Laparoscopic versus open gastric bypass: A randomized study of outcomes, quality of life, and costs. Ann Surg 2001;234:279–289.

This randomized controlled study compares open versus laparoscopic RGB in 155 patients with BMIs of 40–60 kg/m² found longer operative time, less blood loss, shorter hospital stay, more anastomotic strictures, and fewer wound-related complications with the laparoscopic approach. Weight loss was similar between the two groups.

83. *(1A)* **Jones DB** et al. Optimal management of the morbidly obese patient. Surg Endosc 2004;18: 1029–1037.

In this evidence-based report, 1,500 clinical trials were rated, and conclusions were drawn regarding the relative merits of various bariatric surgery procedures. Strong recommendations are made, based on level 1A data.

84. *(1C)* **O'Brien PE** et al. Prospective study of a laparoscopically placed, adjustable gastric band in the treatment of morbid obesity. Br J Surg 1999;86:113–118.

Prospective, single-arm study of 302 patients receiving a LAP-BAND with 4-year follow-up. Early complications occurred in 4%, mean length of stay was 3.9 days, and late complications (prolapse of stomach through band) occurred in 9%. Mean loss of excess weight was 51% at 12 months, 58.3% at 24 months, 61.6% at 36 months, and 68.2% at 48 months.

85. *(1C)* **DeMaria EJ** et al. High failure rate after laparoscopic adjustable silicone gastric banding for treatment of morbid obesity. Ann Surg 2001;233:809–818.

This is an observational study of 36 patients receiving LAP-BAND and followed up for more than 4 years. Only four achieved a BMI less than 35 kg/m² or more than 50% loss of excess weight. More than 50% required band removal or conversion to RGB.

86. *(1C)* **Favretti F** et al. Laparoscopic banding: Selection and technique in 830 patients. Obes Surg 2002;12:385–390.

In this observational study of 830 patients receiving a LAP-BAND, mortality was 0, conversion 2.7%, major complications requiring reoperation 3.9%, minor complications requiring reoperation 11%, and failure to lose more than 30% of excess weight occurred in 20%.

87. *(1A)* **Lee WJ** et al. Laparoscopic vertical banded gastroplasty and laparoscopic gastric bypass: A comparison. Obes Surg 2004;14:626–634.

In this randomized controlled study, 80 patients with class III obesity were found to have greater loss of excess weight with RGB compared with the purely restricted vertical banded gastroplasty procedure.

88. *(1C)* **Biertho L** et al. Laparoscopic gastric bypass versus laparoscopic adjustable gastric banding: A comparative study of 1,200 cases. J Am Coll Surg 2003;197:536–544.

This is a comparison of two case series.

89. *(1C)* **Parikh MS** et al. Laparoscopic bariatric surgery in super-obese patients (BMI >50) is safe and effective: A review of 332 patients. Obes Surg 2005;15:858–863.

This retrospective study of superobese patients compares the three types of laparoscopic bariatric surgeries: LAP-BAND (n = 192) was associated with 35% loss of excess weight at 1 year, 46% at 2 years, and 50% at 3 years, with a 0.5% conversion rate, 60-minute operative time, 24-hour median length of stay, 4.7% morbidity, and no mortality; RGB (n = 97) was associated with 58% loss of excess weight at 1 year, 55% at 2 years, and 57% at 3 years, with a 2.1% conversion rate, 130-minute operative time, 72-hour median length of stay, 11.3% morbidity, and no mortality; BPD (with and without duodenal switch; n = 43) was associated with 61% loss of excess weight at 1 year, 69% at 2 years, and 77% at 3 years, with a 7.0% conversion rate, 255-minute operative time, 96-hour median length of stay, 16.3% morbidity rate, and no mortality.

90. *(1C)* **Bloomberg RD** et al. Nutritional deficiencies following bariatric surgery: What have we learned? Obes Surg 2005;15:145–154.

In this review of the literature, details of nutritional deficiencies with the common bariatric procedures are provided. Malabsorptive procedures, particularly BPD > RGB, are associated with several deficiencies, with hypoproteinemia being the most significant.

Multiple Endocrine Neoplasia

Glen W. Sizemore

DEFINITION

Two sets of multiple endocrine neoplasia (MEN) syndromes and tumor associations are well characterized after the initial proposal of Steiner and associates [1]. Table 9.1 lists the syndrome components and their penetrance. MEN 1 describes a combination of two or more tumors of pituitary, enteropancreatic, and parathyroid origin. Wermer [2] confirmed genetic origin by reporting disease in successive generations of one family. MEN 2, originally described by Sipple [3], refers to the combination of medullary thyroid carcinoma (MTC), pheochromocytoma (P), and parathyroid tumors. MEN 2 has three variants: MEN 2A patients have a normal phenotype; MEN 2B patients have a distinct phenotype (*vide infra*) with oral ganglioneuromas, marfanoid habitus, prominent corneal nerves, and general lack of parathyroid disease; familial MTC (FMTC) describes families in which patients have MTC only.

EPIDEMIOLOGY

The MEN syndromes are rare. Prevalence estimates range from 0.2 to 2.0/100,000 for MEN 1 and 2.0 to 10/100,000 for MEN 2. Initially, cases were thought to be more common in people of northern European ancestry; with time, more cases are being reported from southern and eastern Europe, Asia and, less commonly, from Africa and South America. Because the patients with these diseases are limited and spread among multiple institutions, there are few, if any, randomized double-blind studies of means to confirm diagnosis, results of different therapies, or cost-effectiveness.

ETIOLOGY

Both MEN syndromes are inherited with an autosomal dominant pattern of transmission. MEN 1 derives from mutations of a gene at chromosome 11q13. This gene encodes a 613 amino acid intranuclear protein called menin, which is considered a putative tumor suppressor. About 80% of MEN 1 patients have inherited one of more than 320 germline codon mutations that are "inactivating" and remove tumor suppression [4]. If loss of the second suppressor allele occurs, tumor development starts in a manner consistent with the Knudson and Strong "two-hit" mutational model [5]. No genotype-phenotype correlation exists in MEN 1.

In MEN 2 patients, at least 12 germline, missense, codon mutations may exist of the RET (rearranged during transfection) protooncogene at chromosome 10q11.2. More than 95% of MEN 2 cases have been found to have such mutations. This "activating" gene encodes receptor tyrosine kinases that signal cell growth and differentiation, and

Table 9.1.   Multiple Endocrine Neoplasia: Organ Involvement and Estimated Tumor Penetrance in Adults

Organ Involved	Estimated Tumor Penetrance
MEN 1	
Parathyroid	90%
Enteropancreatic	30%–75%
Functioning	
Gastrin[a]	40%–50%
Insulin[a]	10%–29%
Glucagon[a]	1%
Nonfunctioning	
Pancreatic polypeptide	17%–20%
Glucagon	2%–8%
Vasoactive intestinal polypeptide	2%
Somatostatin	2%
Other: calcitonin, serotonin, chromogranin, neurotensin, growth hormone	
Foregut carcinoid (nonfunctional)	16%
Thymic[a]	2%
Bronchial[a]	2%–8%
Gastric enterochromaffin-like[a]	7%–10%
Anterior pituitary	18%–47%
Prolactin	20%–30%, 60%
Growth hormone and prolactin	5%
Growth hormone	5%
Adrenocorticotropic	2%
Thyrotropin	1%
Nonfunctional	5%–10%
Thyroid	12%
Adrenal cortex	16%–40%
Nonendocrine tumors	
Lipoma	30%
Facial angiofibroma	88%
Collagenoma	72%
Leiomyoma	10%
MEN 2A	43%
Medullary thyroid carcinoma[a]	100%
Pheochromocytoma[a]	19%–50%
Parathyroid	15%–30%
Cutaneous lichen amyloidosis	Rare
Hirschsprung disease	Rare
MEN 2B	17%
Medullary thyroid carcinoma[a]	100%
Pheochromocytoma[a]	25%
Parathyroid	Rare
Ganglioneuroma phenotype	100%
FAMILIAL MEDULLARY CARCINOMA	
Medullary thyroid carcinoma[a]	7%

[a]Tumor with malignant potential.

it starts tumor genesis. First, a germinal mutation occurs that increases cell susceptibility to malignant transformation; the second event is a somatic mutation that transforms the mutant cell into a tumor cell. In MEN 2, a strong genotype–phenotype correlation exists.

The heritable MEN tumors have important characteristics that contrast with those of sporadic endocrine tumors: genetic origin and transmission; precursor hyperplasias that predispose to younger clinical presentations and earlier diagnosis; multiplicity and multicentricity of tumor involvement (90%, 70%, and 100% of insulin, gastrin, and calcitonin-secreting tumors, respectively, vs. 10%, 40%, and 10% in their sporadic counterparts are multicentric); a clinicopathologic spectrum with early, occult hyperplasia developing into later, symptomatic tumor; and, to some extent, a more malignant biologic behavior of some of the tumors—MTC in some families, enteropancreatic, and carcinoid.

No overlap exists between MEN 1 and MEN 2. However, Frank-Raue et al. (6) have reported a family with the coexistence of these syndromes and mutations of an MEN 1 and MEN 2 gene, each inherited from opposite family sides.

MULTIPLE ENDOCRINE NEOPLASIA TYPE 1

This is a syndrome of the three Ps: pituitary, parathyroid, and pancreas. The principal organ involvement is outlined in Table 9.1. The ranges in penetrance are thought due to characteristics of different families, their ages, and the years when the studies were done. MEN 1 typically presents after the first decade, with most symptoms developing in the third (women) and fourth (men) decades. The presenting features in 52 patients were ulcer in 40%, hypoglycemia in 31%, hyperparathyroidism in 15%, and diarrhea and pituitary disease in 6% [7].

Screening

A comprehensive family history (an inexpensive process) and DNA analysis for the MEN 1 mutation (expensive) should be pursued in patients having, suspected of having (because of the presence of two or more of its tumors), or having heritable risk for MEN 1. Sources and costs of mutation analyses can be found at www.geneclinics.org. Several benefits accrue to mutation-positive patients: clinical surveillance and care will intensify; operations for components such as multiglandular parathyroid disease and multifocal enteropancreatic tumors will differ from those in sporadic patients; and the mandatory case finding in at-risk primary relatives will be simplified (i.e., need to check for one known mutation only). Mutation-negative patients gain emotional reassurance as well as economic benefit because further clinical testing is not needed. Unfortunately, a mutation is not found in up to 30% of probands in known MEN 1 families [8]. Screening in these families must revert to annual measurement of ionized calcium, parathyroid hormone, gastrin, and prolactin [9], and the recommended abdominal MRI every 2 years. Although clinical expression generally occurs after age 10 years, the author recommends that screening begin at age 5 years because of reports of a prolactinoma in a 5-year-old [10] and an insulinoma in a 6-year-old [8].

False-negative mutation screening test results may occur in individual patients within mutation-known families at "guesstimated" frequencies [8]. Analysis of a second separate sample is recommended to reduce the risk of missing an affected to 0.25%. Thus far, false-positive mutation test results have not been reported, and the author is aware of no estimates of administrative, sampling, or reference laboratory errors.

Patients with three other diseases generally considered to be sporadic deserve mutation testing. They are the Zollinger-Ellison syndrome (ZES) because approximately 33% have MEN 1; familial hyperparathyroidism as 14% to 16% have MEN 1; and insulinoma, where 4% to 10% have the syndrome [11–13].

Enteropancreatic Disease

Enteropancreatic tumors are present in up to 75% of patients with MEN 1. They are generally multicentric and found in the gastric antrum, pancreas, and duodenal submucosa (particularly gastrinomas). Occult malignant disease is present in half of these patients by middle age [14]. Most secrete one hormone (see Table 9.1) that produces a distinct clinical syndrome; occasionally, multiple hormones are secreted. Chromogranin A and pancreatic polypeptide are other hormones that may be secreted by these tumors and produce sufficient concentrations to be useful markers for the enteropancreatic tumors.

Gastrin-Secreting Tumors

Gastrin-secreting tumors are the most common functioning tumors with the greatest malignant potential. About 90% have duodenal components. Half have metastasized before the diagnosis is made [14]. Most are small, multiple, and within the pancreas and duodenum. The clinical syndrome caused by excess gastrin secretion—ZES—does not differ between MEN 1 and sporadic tumors [7,15]. In early, clinical series multifocal peptic ulcer and esophagitis causing pain, pyloric obstruction, perforation, or hemorrhage were reported in 50% of patients; watery diarrhea occurred in 13% [7].

Diagnosis

Measurement of basal gastrin and hourly gastric acid output are mandatory. High gastrin (generally >200 pg/ml) and gastric acid secretion are the hallmarks of ZES in patients with no history of acid-reducing medications or operations. Gastric acid secretion that exceeds 15 mEq/hr is found in 68% to 97%. These tests will exclude 88% to 96% of patients who have ordinary duodenal ulcers [16]. To distinguish patients with ZES symptoms and minimally elevated basal gastrin values, a secretin test using 2 U/kg is advised. Gastrin increases of 200 mg/ml or more are diagnostic for ZES, with no false-positive responses and only occasional false-negative responses reported [17,18]. History is an inexpensive way to exclude other causes of high gastrin such as retained gastric antrum, gastric outlet obstruction, and renal failure.

If operation is planned, what localization studies should be done? More favored localization studies are somatostatin-receptor scintigraphy with octreotide (SRS) and endoscopic ultrasound (EUS). Both have sensitivities in the 80% to 90% range, with the warning that SRS may not reveal many tumors smaller than 1.5 cm [19,20]. Some also use magnetic resonance imaging (MRI) and computed tomography (CT) to exclude metastatic disease that would preclude surgical intervention; however, these modalities are insensitive for the detection of smaller tumors, localizing only 26% and 31% of insulinomas and gastrinomas, respectively [21,22]. In one case–control study of gastrinoma patients, EUS was 83% accurate, missing tumors in four and predicting nonexistent tumors in two of 36 patients (i.e., false-positive result) [23]. It was cost-effective, reducing localization costs by 50%. If these procedures are not successful, comparable sensitivity is possible with the more expensive and time-consuming percutaneous transhepatic transvenous sampling or arterial injection of a secretagogue with venous sampling for hormone measurement.

Treatment

In most patients, proton-pump inhibitors, H_2-receptor blockers, and somatostatin analogues for hormones other than gastrin effectively prevent morbidity [14].

When an operation is done, it usually includes distal pancreatectomy, intraoperative ultrasonography and palpation (to delineate additional tumors to be removed from the head of the pancreas and duodenal submucosa), and lymphadenectomy about the celiac trunk and hepatic ligament. Indications for operation in MEN 1 are evolving. We do not know if earlier surgery will reduce the symptoms and death from cancer without increasing morbidity. Long-term randomized studies of patients treated with no operation compared with a standardized operation that focuses on survival as well as operative morbidity are not available. All clinicians agree with surgery for failed medical treatment or palliation of advanced disease. Those with a more conservative bent cite a 100% survivorship over 15-years in patients with tumors smaller than 1.5 cm who have not undergone surgery [24]. Another study shows no operative cure for gastrinomas larger than 2.5 cm [25]. This weakens arguments for removal of tumors larger than 3 cm, which are further refuted by findings of no correlation between size of the primary tumor and the incidence of regional or distant metastases and the isolated discovery of metastasis associated with a 3-mm primary tumor [26].

Less-conservative clinicians argue that patients should have operation because of the difficulty in predicting which primary tumors will metastasize and when they will do so. The University of Michigan group has operated on about 15 presymptomatic patients. Their intervention includes distal pancreatectomy, intraoperative ultrasonography, palpation and removal of tumors localized in the pancreatic head, duodenal submucosa, and antrum, as well as dissection of lymph nodes along the celiac axis and hepatic ligament. All 15 patients continue to have normal gastrin levels, and in only one patient has diabetes mellitus developed [27]. Skogseid and colleagues have complementary results [28]. The follow-up is short in both studies, but the early results suggest need for a larger, longer, randomized study.

Insulin-Secreting and Other Tumor Types

Between 10% and 30% of enteropancreatic tumors secrete insulin. The youngest patient studied was age 6 years. Most tumors are pure insulin secretors; some produce both insulin and gastrin [29]. Both types cause hypoglycemia.

Diagnosis

The diagnosis is based on finding simultaneous fasting serum glucose values below 45 mg/dl and inappropriately high insulin concentrations (>10 mU/ml). Typical requirements for this study are a 72-hour fast with measurement of plasma glucose and insulin every 6 hours or measurement of C-peptide before and during induced hypoglycemia [29,30].

Treatment

Operation is recommended in all patients. The initial therapy for insulinoma is a distal pancreatectomy, which should remove about 85% of the gland [13,31]. This procedure is favored for three reasons. First, multicentric insulin-secreting tissue is present in more than 90% of patients. Second, 5% to 15% of the tumors are malignant. Third, endocrine and exocrine insufficiency is reduced significantly with distal compared with total pancreatectomy. Intraoperative monitoring of glucose is helpful in determining the degree of pancreatectomy. After operation, if hypoglycemia persists, diazoxide may be used; if metastatic disease is present, streptozocin, dacarbazine, or somatostatin analogues may be effective [32].

A glucagon-secreting tumor without the necrolysis syndrome has been reported in a euglycemic woman, and hyperglucagonemia has been reported in five of six hyperglycemic patients who had necrolysis [10,33]. Vasoactive intestinal polypeptide and other hormones have been found (see Table 9.1). Malignant behavior is rare. These tumors are resected when not controlled by medication.

Parathyroid Disease

Multigland, hyperplastic parathyroid disease is the most penetrant and generally earliest manifestation of MEN 1; it affects 87% to 97% of patients and is detected in the second and third decades [14]. Ectopic gland locations such as thymus, thyroid, and paraesophageal are common, and supernumerary glands are not unusual. MEN 1 is rare among cases of hyperparathyroidism. The differential diagnosis includes familial hyperparathyroidism alone, benign familial hypocalciuric hypercalcemia, and the more-common causes. Although it is commonly asymptomatic, the usual symptoms or signs of hyperparathyroidism may occur including severe osteopenia in 40% [34]. Thus bone mineral density measurements are very important for the assessment and follow-up of patients.

Diagnosis

Diagnosis is established by finding high concentrations of serum calcium and parathyroid hormone (PTH). Because of possible benign familial hypocalciuric hypercalcemia, calcium/creatinine clearance ratios should be calculated. General agreement exists that multiple parathyroid glands are affected with a disease spectrum from hyperplasia of all glands through combinations of hyperplasic, adenomatous, and ectopically located disease. Such multiplicity requires that all glands be identified at initial surgery; therefore before initial operation, parathyroid imaging studies are unnecessary and not cost-effective. The author thinks that: MEN 1 parathyroid operations should be done only by very experienced endocrine surgeons; intra-operative PTH measurement is important in this syndrome; patients must understand before operation that recurrence is common and reoperation possible; and hypoparathyroidism is possible even after autotransplantation.

Treatment

Indications for operation are somewhat more complex, but similar to those in sporadic disease. The favored operation is subtotal parathyroidectomy with preservation of 30 to 50 mg of identified tissue (even though this carries a high rate of recurrence requiring secondary operation). Total parathyroidectomy with autotransplantation of removed tissue is also possible. Infrequent autograft failure leads to hypoparathyroidism, or the autograft may hyperfunction and cause recurrent hypercalcemia with need for revision. In either case, cryopreservation of parathyroid tissue is advised because of increased rates of hypoparathyroidism [35,36]. In selected cases, alcohol ablation of parathyroid tissue may be used to treat recurrence when additional glands are successfully localized. Potentially troublesome recurrences with hypercalcemia and osteoporosis may be treated with bisphosphonates.

The author agrees with the recent suggestion by Ferolla et al. [37] that prophylactic thymectomy be done during parathyroidectomy in MEN 1 patients. They reported that 3.1% of (eight of 180) MEN 1 cases in the Italian registry had malignant thymic carcinoid tumors, with death or metastases in 50%. Because of this and the fact that the thymus is a common site for supernumerary parathyroid glands, it seems reasonable to remove the thymus whenever possible.

Pituitary Disease

The prevalence of pituitary disease in MEN 1 ranges from 18% (clinical findings) to 94% (autopsy results), and it is a presenting complaint in 4% of cases [7,38,39]. Tumor types are shown in Table 9.1. The pathologic spectrum ranges from hyperplasia through adenoma to carcinoma (rare). Most tumors are small microadenomas, and prolactin-secreting tumors are most common—up to 60%. A prolactin-secreting macroadenoma has been reported in a 5-year-old child [10]. A rare phenotype, the Burin variant, manifests with prolactinoma and hyperparathyroidism [40]. The symptoms, signs, diagnosis, and treatment of the pituitary tumors are similar to those of sporadic disease. Long-term follow-up for the pituitary should include examination, prolactin and insulin-like growth factor (IGF-1) measurement, and a pituitary MRI beginning at age 20 and continuing every 2 years.

Associated Diseases

Carcinoid tumors occur in up to 10% of patients [41,42]. The natural history of such lesions in MEN 1 is sparse. Most tumors do not hypersecrete, so symptoms are rare and late. CT and MRI are used for screening and follow-up. Because of the increased malignant behavior of thymic carcinoids, prophylactic thymectomy is recommended when parathyroidectomy is done [37,41]. Gastric enterochromaffin-like cell carcinoids are common. When tumors are found at the time of endoscopy for ZES, they should be removed. Multiple facial angiofibromas are present in 88% and collagenomas in 72% [43]. Within affected families, they provide an excellent marker of MEN 1. Adrenocortical abnormalities occur in up to 40%. Most are benign adenomas, but a variable pathologic and clinical spectrum exists. Cutaneous and visceral lipomas and uterine leiomyomas occur in about 10% of patients and are treated symptomatically.

MULTIPLE ENDOCRINE NEOPLASIA TYPE 2

The glands involved and the penetrance of disease in patients with MEN 2 are shown in Table 9.1. Precursor stages exist for all components: C-cell hyperplasia precedes

MTC; diffuse, nonnodular adrenomedullary hyperplasia precedes pheochromocytoma; and occult, normocalcemic parathyroid hyperplasia is observed [44–46]. More than 1,000 kindreds are known. Previously, asynchronous clinical manifestations led to discovery, beginning in the third decade. Now almost instant detection of asymptomatic affected babies or presymptomatic children occurs because of identification of RET codon mutations or high concentrations of plasma calcitonin, the hormone marker for C-cell hyperplasia or MTC.

MEN 2A patients have a normal phenotype and parathyroid disease. MEN 2B patients have an abnormal phenotype; overt parathyroid disease is distinctly uncommon. We separated this component 1975 [47] because it could be recognized on physical examination and was associated with greater mortality and morbidity than was MEN 2A. The main features are well established [48,49]. Patients have a marfanoid habitus with excessive limb length, loose-jointedness, scoliosis, anterior chest deformities, and mucosal ganglioneuromas, but no ectopia lentis and cardiovascular abnormalities of the Marfan syndrome. Associated local peroneal to diffuse muscle weakness may occur. The diffuse ganglioneuromatosis may appear as yellow or white nodules of the tarsal plates of the eyes, associated with thickened corneal nerve fibers and pink, yellow, or translucent hemispherical nodules studding the tip and anterior third of the tongue, elongated projections posterior to each orolabial commissure, and nodules within the lips. Functionally, alimentary ganglioneuromatosis produces dysphagia, constipation, diarrhea, megacolon, and diverticulosis.

Screening

Testing for RET mutations in those at risk for MEN 2 is the gold standard in this syndrome. It has replaced, but not eliminated, calcitonin stimulation tests for case finding [50]. Current sources of mutation analyses can be found at www.geneclinics.org. This is cost-effective endocrinology at its finest. For less than $1,000, those with a mutation may be advised to undergo thyroidectomy because MTC will develop in more than 95%. Skinner et al. [51] just reported an 88% cure rate for 50 consecutive patients having prophylactic thyroidectomy for MEN 2A at age 19 or younger, based on identification by RET mutation testing. Most important, patients with two negative test results, as well as their successors, will be relieved and can be excused from care. However, important concerns exist about the testing. To avoid failed diagnosis, when an initial result is negative, a repeated test of a separate sample is necessary. An estimated 5% false-negative error rate, found in sample testing, is thought to be caused by mislabeled samples, or failed identification of known or unrecognized new mutations. A repeated test should reduce this "miss" rate to 0.25%. It will not eliminate the possibility that a new or unknown mutation has caused the problem. When that possibility is strong, a calcitonin stimulation test is recommended in those considered at risk. False-positive RET testing results have been reported, even with repeated samples; one group reported that 3.4% of samples gave false-positive results [52]. Perhaps the tests were wrong; more probably, some carriers need decades to develop a second mutation that causes development of MTC, and some may never develop it.

All patients with MTC should be tested. Among patients assumed to have sporadic disease, the chance of being an index case with hereditable MEN 2 is 5.8%, with a range up to 24% [53]. Among primary relatives of those with positive RET mutations, the individual risk is 50%. Among all patients with pheochromocytoma, 4% to 8% will be index cases for MEN 2 [53]. Neumann et al. [54] did mutational analysis among 271 patients presumed to have sporadic pheochromocytoma. Although 24% had mutations suggesting von Hippel–Lindau disease, the pheochromocytoma–paraganglioma syndrome, and neurofibromatosis, only 4.8% were found to have MEN 2. Among patients with Hirschsprung disease, RET mutations were found in about 50% [14]. No evidence suggests that screening patients with familial hyperparathyroidism is cost-effective.

Tests based on calcitonin measurement continue to have a role, particularly in three populations. First is the 2% to 5% of known MEN 2 kindreds in which a mutation has not been identified [55]. Second is the cases which familial MTC is possible, based on family history, but RET analysis is negative. Third is the patients who are being followed up after thyroidectomy. The author favors stimulation studies with pentagastrin or short calcium infusion, with the warning that samples should be sent to reference laboratories having very sensitive assays that have been standardized in normal persons for the secretagogue being used. Stimulation should not be used when the basal calcitonin concentration is known to be high because calcitonin is a potent vasodilator, and shock might result.

Medullary Thyroid Carcinoma

MTC in MEN originates in parafollicular or C cells (so-called because of their synthesis and secretion of calcitonin). The tumor has a solid pattern with amyloid in the stroma and a high incidence of lymph node metastases—particularly in the central compartment of the neck. The MTC is bilateral, multicentric, associated with C-cell hyperplasia and is found in the lateral, upper, and middle lobe portions. When detected in young patients by mutation or calcitonin screening, it is generally occult. When detected clinically, generally after the second decade, the tumor occurs as a mass with or without cervical metastases.

Diagnosis

Detection of a RET mutation establishes that the patient has the potential to develop tumor, has C-cell hyperplasia, or may have MTC. If suspicion is strong and RET mutation studies are negative, the disease may be confirmed by finding high basal or secretagogue-stimulated calcitonin concentrations.

Treatment

Patients with an MEN 2 mutation, C-cell hyperplasia, or MTC require total capsular thyroidectomy, central neck nodal dissection, and functional lateral neck nodal dissection at early ages [9,56,57]. The latter reference elegantly outlines why cervical lymphadenectomy is mandatory; metastatic tumor was missed more than 50% of the time when the procedure was done electively and if nodes were palpable. The authors showed that patients having unilateral/bilateral MTC had positive nodes as follows: central, 88/78%; ipsilateral, 81/71%; and contralateral, 44/49%. When operated on by a skilled surgical team, the incidence of vocal cord paralysis, hypoparathyroidism, and anesthetic and esthetic complications is low.

Recommended ages for initial thyroidectomy in RET-positive individuals have been based on recent genotype–phenotype correlations: estimates of tumor virulence or malignant transformation linked to a known mutation, survivorship data, and the pathologic stage of tumor and metastasis [56,58]. MEN 2B patients with RET codon mutations 833, 918, and 922 have the most aggressive forms of MTC. Ten-year survivorship is 40% to 50%. Microscopic MTC is common within the first year of life, and metastasis has also been found by age 1 year [59,60]. Thyroidectomy is recommended by age 6 months. The author thinks sporadic MTC is second in virulence, with 10-year survivorship of 55% to 69%; some would disagree [61]. Virulence is less in patients with MEN 2A who have RET codon mutations 611, 618, and 634, who have a 10-year survivorship of 90% to 95%. These survival rates are a bit biased because many patients had operations at early ages, and the rate of recurrence is greater or survivorship is worse in those operated on when older. The incidence of persistence increases rapidly and correlates with the decade of operation [62,66]. Two patients with the 634 mutation deserve note because of atypical malignant transformation; one had MTC by age 2 years, and one had metastases by age 5 years [63,64]. The author disagrees with recommendations for thyroidectomy after age 5 based on genotype–phenotype data and suggests that it be done by age 2 years. However, it should be done by experienced pediatric endocrine surgeons. The lowest risk for early MTC and decreased survivorship is in those with 609, 620, 768, 790, 791, 804, and 891 mutations. Nodal metastases are "extremely uncommon" before age 20, so the author agrees that operation may be deferred until then [61].

Early thyroidectomy has reduced the mortality in hereditary MTC to less than 5%, with reported rates of 1.5% for patients operated on because of calcitonin-screening detection versus 24% for those with symptomatic tumor [14,65]. None of the author's patients who had a total thyroidectomy in the first decade of life had residual tumor. This early observation has been extended by Skinner et al. [51], who reported 50 consecutive operations in MEN 2A patients operated on by age 19 because of positive RET mutation status; 88% were cured, with mean follow-up of 7 years, and the authors reported a "lower incidence of persistent recurrent disease in children who underwent thyroidectomy before age eight."

All patients will require levothyroxine replacement. After operation, when patients have stable normal calcium concentrations, a calcitonin stimulation test should be done to evaluate outcome.

The major unsolved problem is what is to be done for patients who continue to have high calcitonin concentrations after primary surgery or in whom defined metastatic disease develops. The author thinks that those patients with demonstrated aggressive tumor and probably those with RET genotypes known to be associated with increased tumor virulence and progressively increasing calcitonin concentrations should have aggressive attempts at tumor control. Those most in need would be patients with rapid calcitonin-doubling times. In 2005 Barbet et al. [67] enlarged and extended the 1984 work of Miyauchi et al. [68] when they demonstrated that postoperative patients who had serially measured calcitonin-doubling times of less than 6 months had a 10-year survival of 8% compared with doubling times of 6 to 24 months with a survival of 37%, and 100% survival in those with doubling times longer than 24 months.

For such patients who have no evidence of distant or directly visualized hepatic metastasis (93% of which are missed by conventional radiographic procedures), the Tissell extensive cervical microdissection operation, done with curative intent, is recommended. Moley [69] showed that 38% of patients having this secondary operation had negative secretagogue-stimulated calcitonin values after 5 years.

Radiation treatment has been disappointing. Treatment with radioiodine has not decreased the recurrence of MTC or increased survivorship. External beam radiation may prolong survival briefly and give some objective tumor decrement [70]. Standard chemotherapy, as with doxorubicin or other combination protocols, has not produced complete remissions and has difficult side effects. Recent trials suggest that better therapies are coming soon. MTCs store [^{131}I]metaiodobenzylguanidine (MIBG) in catecholamine vesicles, and they also have multiple somatostatin receptors. Gao [71] reported treatments with MIBG or a somatostatin analogue, coupled with a β-radiation–emitting radioisotope, [^{90}Y]-DOTATOC, have antitumor benefits. Cuccuru [72] reported antitumor activity induced by the RET inhibitor RPI in mice bearing xenograft MTC tumors.

Pheochromocytoma

The prevalence of pheochromocytoma (P) in MEN 2 ranges from 12% in the young, through 42% in mature kindreds, to 100% [73]. Nguyen et al. [74] reported the prevalence to be 16% in a French population of nonindex MEN 2 gene mutation carriers younger than 30 years who were screened with urinary catecholamine measurements. The pathologic spectrum extends from bilateral adrenal medullary hyperplasia to large, multilobular P with accessory adrenal gland involvement. Malignant P is rare but did occur in 24% of patients in our early experience [45]. Unilateral adrenal ganglioneuromas have been reported in MEN 2A and 2B [75]. Asynchrony is common with a large ipsilateral tumor and contralateral impalpable hyperplasia or small tumor. Detection at earlier stages commonly yields low-volume chromaffin disease in asymptomatic, normotensive patients. In the MEN syndromes, P is certainly established as life threatening. Modigliani et al. [76], studying the EROMEN population of 300 MEN 2 patients, reported 25 (65%) of 39 deaths were due to P, and in 40% of those deaths, the P was undiagnosed.

Diagnosis

MEN 2 patients (RET codon mutation positive, previous unilateral adrenalectomy for P, those with metastatic P) should have screening at annual intervals and perhaps before having of general anesthesia or other stressful procedures. Machen et al. [77] suggested that routine screening for P in those with genetically encoded risk be based on the youngest age-related development of the tumor. They recommended that screening start at age 10 for patients carrying RET mutations 630, 634, and 918. The author recommends age 5 in those with the 918 mutation because two MEN 2B children, ages 5 and 8, have been reported with bilateral adrenal medullary hyperplasia [78].

The currently favored test in MEN 2 is measurement of plasma free metanephrine [79], which has greater sensitivity and specificity than plasma catecholamines and urinary catecholamines [80,81]. Before this, the diagnosis was confirmed by finding high contents of epinephrine in 24-hour urinary collections or a high epinephrine/norepinephrine ratio [82]. CT and MRI are stated to have 98% and 100% sensitivity for localization of P. The less-expensive CT is more cost-effective. MIBG scans are helpful when seeking functional metastatic disease or when bilateral tumors are assumed to be present and CT reveals only unilateral enlargement. MIBG imaging will detect the 25% of tumors missed by CT [78].

Treatment

Once diagnosis is established, blockade with appropriate α- and β-adrenergic blocking agents and glucocorticoid replacement therapy should be started. For bilateral disease, bilateral laparoscopic or open adrenalectomy has been the preferred operation. For "unilateral" disease, laparoscopic adrenalectomy is favored. The decision about initial bilateral compared with unilateral adrenalectomy is complex and should be thoroughly discussed with each patient before proceeding. Although the chromaffin disease is truly bilateral, it may be diagnostically asynchronous. Thus initial unilateral adrenalectomy leaves patients with continued risk of hypertension or crisis (particularly with pregnancy), a low risk of cancer, and with need for sequential urinary and radiographic follow-up (perhaps mutagenic if CT is used). A review of results of initial surgery in 72 patients indicated that 88% required total adrenalectomy; 55% of patients who had initial unilateral adrenalectomy required completion total adrenalectomy for clinical reasons at a mean 4.8 years after the original operation [83]. The trade-off is that after bilateral adrenalectomy, the risk of adrenal insufficiency and crisis is real. Patients require daily glucocorticoid and mineralocorticoid therapy, careful instruction about care of adrenal insufficiency and the avoidance and treatment of crisis, initial close physician follow-up observation and advice, and such patients must wear notification of the need for parenteral glucocorticoid and volume expansion in emergencies. Rare deaths due to adrenal insufficiency have been reported [12]. Therefore more surgeons are using initial bilateral or unilateral laparoscopic so-called cortical-sparing operations or use them in extraordinary situations [84]. We lack long-term results about adrenal insufficiency, recurrent pheochromocytoma, or other complications for these operations. The author worries about the expense and the mutagenic potential of the radiation used in long-term follow-up of these patients.

Parathyroid Disease

Clinical or anatomic evidence of parathyroid disease is present in 29% to 64% of patients with MEN 2A. It is most commonly found in patients with the 634 codon mutation. In the patients with parathyroid disease, parathyroid hyperplasia is present in 84% and parathyroid adenoma in 16%. Overt parathyroid disease is distinctly uncommon in patients with MEN 2B.

Diagnosis

Clinically, occult parathyroid hyperplasia is found, and mild hypercalcemia is most common. Otherwise, the disease is similar to the sporadic variety. Simultaneous high ionized or total calcium and PTH concentrations confirm the diagnosis.

Treatment

The indications for and the types of parathyroidectomy are similar for patients with MEN 2A and 1. However, because the parathyroid disease is occult more commonly in younger MEN 2A patients, and because the operation increases the incidence of hypoparathyroidism, a conservative approach to parathyroidectomy in MEN 2 is recommended. Grossly enlarged glands should be removed, and the remaining glands marked for future reference.

REFERENCES

Definition and Etiology

1. *(1C+)* **Steiner AL** et al. Study of a kindred with pheochromocytoma, medullary thyroid carcinoma, hyperparathyroidism and Cushing's disease: Multiple endocrine neoplasia, type 2. Medicine (Baltimore) 1968;47:371–409.

   The first observational study of a large family with MEN 2 characteristics, as well as the first use of the terms MEN 1 and MEN 2.

2. *(1C+)* **Wermer P.** Genetic aspects of adenomatosis of endocrine glands. Am J Med 1954;16:363.

   Observational study with the first documentation of autosomal dominant transmission of MEN 1.

3. *(1C+)* **Sipple JH.** The association of pheochromocytoma with carcinoma of the thyroid gland. Am J Med 1961;31:163.

   Reports autopsy of hypertensive man with bilateral pheochromocytoma and thyroid carcinoma (later found to be MTC) and notes 14-fold increased incidence of thyroid carcinoma in patients with pheochromocytomas.

4. *(1C)* **Marx SJ, Simonds WF.** Hereditary hormone excess: Genes, molecular pathways and syndromes. Endocrine Rev 2005;26:615–661.

   An exhaustive, thorough, and insightful review of this subject.

5. *(1C+)* **Knudson AG Jr, Strong LC.** Mutation and cancer: Neuroblastomas and pheochromocytoma. Am J Hum Genet 1972;24:514–532.

   Observational study plotted the age at onset of familial compared with that of nonfamilial pheochromocytoma. Results allowed postulation that in hereditary neoplasms, a first genetic mutation makes cells susceptible to a second somatic mutation that transforms the cell into a malignant one.

6. *(1C+)* **Frank-Raue K** et al. Coincidence of multiple endocrine neoplasia types 1 and 2: Mutations in the RET protooncogene and MEN 1 tumor suppressor gene in a family presenting with recurrent primary hyperparathyroidism. J Clin Endocrinol Metab 2005;90:4063–4067.

Multiple Endocrine Neoplasia Type 1

7. *(1C+)* **Ballard HS** et al. Familial multiple endocrine adenoma–peptic ulcer complex. Medicine (Baltimore) 1964;43:481–500.

   An early observational review of the expressions of disease in MEN 1 patients and families who were diagnosed based on clinical presentations at Henry Ford Hospital.

8. *(1C)* **Marx SJ.** Multiple endocrine neoplasia type 1: Clinical and basic insights: Syllabus for the 11th Annual Meeting of the American Association of Clinical Endocrinologists, Chicago, IL, May 1–5, 2002:14.

   These syllabus notes provide information on the genetics and mutation analysis of patients with MEN 1 from the institution caring for many patients.

9. *(1C+)* **Sizemore GW.** Multiple endocrine neoplasia. In: Becker KL, ed. Principles and practice of endocrinology and metabolism. 3rd ed. Lippincott Williams & Wilkins, Philadelphia, 2000:1696.

   A text chapter on MEN diseases, including elaborated discussions of clinical screening procedures.

10. *(1C+)* **Stratakis CA** et al. Pituitary macroadenoma in a 5-year old: An early expression of MEN 1. J Clin Endocrinol Metab 2000;85:4776–4780.

    Case report of a child with growth acceleration and acromegalic features and earliest morbidity seen in the 85 kindreds with 565 MEN 1–affected members seen at the National Institutes of Health.

11. *(1C)* **Malagelada JR** et al. Medical and surgical options in the management of patients with gastrinoma. Gastroenterology 1983;84:1524–1532.

    A review of with recommendations for clinical management of patients with ZES in MEN 1.

12. *(1C)* **Marx SJ** et al. Family studies in patients with primary parathyroid hyperplasia. Am J Med 1977;62:698–706.

    A review of and recommendations for clinical management of primary parathyroid hyperplasia in patients with MEN 1.

13. *(1C)* **Rasbach DA** et al. Surgical management of hyperinsulinism in the multiple endocrine neoplasia, type 1. Arch Surg 1985;120:584–589.

    A review of 30 patients with insulinoma and MEN 1 with recommendations for surgical management.

Enteropancreatic Disease

14. *(1C+)* **Brandi ML** et al. Guidelines for diagnosis and therapy of MEN type 1 and type 2. J Clin Endocrinol Metab 2001;86:5658–5671.

    A consensus review article from an international group of physicians specializing in treatment of MEN with data about and guides for major management decisions in affected patients.

15. *(1C)* **Zollinger RM** et al. Thirty years' experience with gastrinoma. World J Surg 1984; 8:427–435.

    An observational study that outlines ZES perfectly and comments about its increased association with familial disease.

16. *(1C+)* **Jensen RT** et al. Zollinger-Ellison syndrome: Current concepts and management. Ann Intern Med 1983;98:59–75.

    An excellent review summarizing current diagnostic criteria for ZES.

17. *(1C+)* **Deveney CW** et al. The Zollinger-Ellison syndrome: 23 years later. Ann Surg 1978;88: 384–393.

    An observational study that presented gastrin values in patients with ZES and demonstrates the importance of the secretin test in the differentiation of ZES patients with normal basal gastrin from others.

18. *(1C)* **McGuigan JE, Wolfe MM.** Secretin injection test in the diagnosis of gastrinoma. Gastroenterology 1980;79:1324.

    An observational summary of results with gastrin and the secretin test in ZES patients.

19. *(1C)* **Shi W** et al. Localization of neuroendocrine tumors with (In-111) DPTA-octreotide scintigraphy (Octreoscan): A comparative study with CT and MR imaging. Q J Med 1998;91:295–301.

    An observational study that shows sensitivity and specificity of octreotide scintigraphy for pancreatic tumor localization compared with CT and MR.

20. *(1C+)* **Bansal R** et al. Cost effectiveness of EUS for preoperative localization of pancreatic endocrine tumors. Gastrointest Endosc 1999;49:19–25.

    In this case–control study of patients undergoing surgery for pancreatic neuroendocrine tumors, 36 patients who had preoperative endoscopic ultrasound were matched to 36 previous patients who did not. The diagnostic sensitivity of EUS was 83%, and accuracy was 89%. Such results allow the discontinuation more expensive angiograms.

21. *(1C)* **Vinik AI** et al. Transhepatic portal vein catheterization for localization of insulinomas: A ten-year experience. Surgery 1991;199:1–11.

    Observational comparison of angiography and CT for localization, demonstrating that angiography is more helpful for localizing insulinomas, finding 44% with angiography compared with 26% for CT.

22. *(1C)* **Vinik AI** et al. Transhepatic portal vein catheterization localization of sporadic and MEN gastrinomas: A ten-year experience. Surgery 1990;107:246–255.

    Observational comparison of angiography, CT, and transhepatic venous measurement of gastrin for localization, demonstrated that angiography and CT were equally helpful for localizing gastrinomas, finding 29% compared with 31%, respectively, and that transhepatic venous sampling with gastrin measurement was better at about 50%.

23. *(1C)* **Vitale G** et al. Slow release lanreotide in combination with interferon-alpha 2b in the treatment of symptomatic advanced medullary thyroid carcinoma. J Clin Endocrinol Metab 2000; 85:983–988.

    In this study of seven patients with metastatic MTC, combined therapy with lanreotide and interferon for 12 months reduced flushing and diarrhea significantly, as well as produced at least transient decrements in calcitonin, but it did not decrease tumor size or prolong life.

24. *(1C)* **Norton JA** et al. Comparison of surgical results in patients with advanced and limited disease with multiple endocrine neoplasia type 1 and Zollinger-Ellison syndrome. Ann Surg 2001; 234:495–505.

    Fifty-six patients with MEN 1 and ZES who had tumors larger than 2.5 cm had somewhat variable operations that did not provide a cure, perhaps suggesting that a long wait before attempting surgery is contraindicated.

25. *(1C)* **Weber HC** et al. Determinants of metastatic rate and survival in patients with Zollinger-Ellison syndrome: A prospective long-term study. Gastroenterology 1995;108:1637–1649.

    Based on longer survivorship, these authors recommend operating on patients who are afflicted with tumors larger than 3 cm.

26. *(1C)* **Lowney JK** et al. Pancreatic islet cell tumor metastasis in multiple endocrine neoplasia type 1: Correlation with primary tumor size. Surgery 1998;124:1043–1048.

    These authors conclude that the size of primary tumors in MEN 1 does not correlate with metastatic potential, so that size is not a good criterion for justifying exploration.

27. *(1C)* **Thompson NW.** Management of pancreatic endocrine tumors in patients with multiple endocrine neoplasia type 1. Surg Oncol Clin North Am 1998;7:881–891.

Dr. Thompson's study gives a complete description of intraoperative procedures for this disease.

28. *(1B)* **Skogseid B** et al. Surgery for asymptomatic pancreatic lesions in multiple endocrine neoplasia type 1. World J Surg 1996;20:872–876.

A randomized study comparing results of similar operations between eight presymptomatic and 12 symptomatic patients. Favorable results occurred in the presymptomatic (a 25% cure rate and no localized metastasis) versus the symptomatic (a 7% cure rate and metastasis in 33%).

29. *(1C)* **Service FJ.** Clinical presentation and laboratory evaluation on hypoglycemic disorders in adults. In: Service FJ, ed. Hypoglycemic disorders. Boston, GK Hall, 1983:73.

Details of evaluations for hypoglycemia.

30. *(1C)* **Service FJ** et al. C-peptide suppression test for insulinoma. J Lab Clin Med 1977;90:180.

Describes the C-peptide suppression test and shows results it provided in affected patients.

31. *(1C)* **Demeure MJ** et al. Insulinomas associated with multiple endocrine neoplasia type 1: The need for a different surgical approach. Surgery 1991;110:998–1004.

Results demonstrate favorable outcomes in patients with distal pancreatectomy.

32. *(1C)* **Osei K, O'Dorisio TM.** The effects of a potent somatostatin analogue (SMS201-995) on serum glucose and gastro-entero-pancreatic hormones in a malignant insulinoma patient. Ann Intern Med 1985;103:223–225.

Results of the study indicated reduced hypoglycemia in a patient having this treatment.

33. *(1C)* **Croughs RJ** et al. Glucagonoma as part of the polyglandular adenoma syndrome. Am J Med 1972;52:690–698.

A case report that suggests the possibility that glucagonoma does play a role in the syndrome.

Parathyroid Disease

34. *(1C)* **Burgess JR** et al. Osteoporosis in multiple endocrine neoplasia type 1: Severity, clinical significance, relationship to primary hyperparathyroidism, and response to parathyroidectomy. Arch Surg 1999;134:1119–1123.

Report of an Australian group with great experience in MEN 1. Twenty-nine patients with MEN 1 had hyperparathyroidism: osteopenia was present in 41%, and osteoporosis in 45%. In five patients with successful parathyroidectomy and sequential bone studies, the density increased 5.2% in the femoral neck and 3.9% in the lumbar spine over a period of 12 to 24 months.

35. *(1C)* **van Heerden JA** et al. Primary hyperparathyroidism in patients with multiple endocrine neoplasia syndromes. Arch Surg 1983;118:533–536.

Forty-three patients with MEN were treated by subtotal parathyroidectomy. The cure rate was 93%, but 23% eventually had hypoparathyroidism. Because of this, the authors recommended cryopreservation of tissue for subsequent transplantation.

Pituitary Disease

36. *(1B)* **Lambert LA** et al. Surgical treatment of hyperparathyroidism in patients with multiple endocrine neoplasia type 1. Arch Surg 2005;140:374–382.

A summary of results of the M.D. Anderson Cancer Center experience in 37 patients between 1973 and 2004, as well as a thoughtful review of the problem.

37. **Ferolla P** et al. Thymic neuroendocrine carcinoma (carcinoid) in multiple endocrine neoplasia type 1 syndrome: The Italian series. J Clin Endocrinol Metab 2005;90:2603–2609.

A summarized experience about Italian MEN 1 patients with malignant thymic carcinoids. Of their 180 patients with familial MEN 1, 3.1% had this cancer, which was fatal or metastatic in 50%.

38. *(1C+)* **Burgess JR** et al. Spectrum of pituitary disease in multiple endocrine neoplasia type 1: Clinical, biochemical and radiological features of pituitary disease in a large MEN 1 kindred. J Clin Endocrinol Metab 1996;81:2642–2646.

A report of the spectrum of pituitary disease in 165 members of one kindred with MEN 1: 19% were found to have pituitary disease. It was symptomatic in only 24%, suggesting that screening is needed for detection. The data supported the use of α-subunit, prolactin, and IGF-1 measurements for screening. One third of prolactinomas did not respond to therapy with bromocriptine, suggesting less responsiveness than in sporadic tumors.

39. *(1C)* **Majewski JT, Wilson SD.** The MEA-I syndrome: An all or none phenomenon? Surgery 1979;86:475–484.

This study adds more information about penetrance of MEN 1.

40. *(1C)* **Petty EM** et al. Mapping of the gene for hereditary hyperparathyroidism and prolactinoma (MEN 1 Burin) to chromosome 11q: Evidence for a founder effect in patients from Newfoundland. Am J Hum Genet 1994;54:1060–1066.

Details the Burin variant of MEN 1, which has predominant prolactinoma and hyperparathyroidism.

Associated Diseases

41. *(1C)* **Williams ED, Celestin LR.** The association of bronchial carcinoid and pluriglandular adenomatosis. Thorax 1962;17:120.

     The first report of carcinoid tumors in MEN 1.

42. **Teh BT** et al. Clinicopathologic studies of thymic carcinoids in multiple endocrine neoplasia type 1. Medicine 1997;76:21–29.

     Article offers an excellent, thorough review of this subject.

43. *(1C+)* **Darling TN** et al. Multiple facial angiofibromas and collagenomas in patients with multiple endocrine neoplasia type 1. Arch Dermatol 1997;133:853–857.

     In 32 patients with MEN 1, facial angiofibromas were found in 88% and collagenomas in 72%. The results suggest these entities are excellent indicators of affected status.

Multiple Endocrine Neoplasia Type 2

44. *(1C+)* **Wolfe HJ** et al. C-cell hyperplasia preceding medullary thyroid carcinoma. N Engl J Med 1973;289:437–441.

     First demonstration of the medullary carcinoma precursor lesion in two sisters with MEN 2, and a comparison to the inhomogeneous spacing in normal persons. This provided the realization that bilateral total thyroidectomy would be needed, even in those with nonpalpable lesions.

45. *(1C+)* **Carney JA** et al. Adrenal medullary disease in multiple endocrine neoplasia, type 2: Pheochromocytoma and its precursors. Am J Clin Pathol 1976;66:279–290.

     This study considered the bilateral adrenal disease in the first 19 patients at the Mayo Clinic who underwent adrenalectomy for MEN 2. This study outlines adrenal medullary hyperplasia and demonstrates that the disease presents asynchronously and that these tumors could be malignant.

46. *(1B)* **Heath H II** et al. Preoperative diagnosis of occult parathyroid hyperplasia by calcium infusion in patients with multiple endocrine neoplasia, type 2a. J Clin Endocrinol Metab 1976;43: 428–435.

     A study of eight unaffected people, six normocalcemic patients with MEN 2A, and seven patients with MEN 2B. During calcium infusion, failure to suppress PTH secretion occurred in patients with 2A disease, and during surgery, they were found to have parathyroid hyperplasia. Those with MEN 2B had PTH suppression and normal glands at surgery. This work established that normocalcemic parathyroid hyperplasia could be diagnosed preoperatively in MEN 2A and that MEN 2B patients have normal parathyroid function.

47. *(1C+)* **Chong GC** et al. Medullary carcinoma of the thyroid gland. Cancer 1975;35:695–704.

     This review of Mayo patients was the first to suggest that the terms MEN 2A and MEN 2B should be used to distinguish patients with MEN 2 whose findings were distinctive. The survivorship data also established that MTC in MEN 2B patients was more virulent than in patients affected by sporadic disease and, in turn, the tumors in both were more virulent than tumors in MEN 2A.

48. *(1C)* **Carney JA** et al. Multiple endocrine neoplasia, type 2b. Pathobiol Annu 1978;8:105–153.

     This review of Mayo patients with MEN 2B established the subtle phenotypic and pathologic features of the syndrome.

49. *(1C)* **Dyck PJ** et al. Multiple endocrine neoplasia, type 2b: Phenotype recognition, neurologic features and their pathologic basis. Ann Neurol 1979;6:302–314.

     This review of Mayo patients established the phenotypic, physiologic, pathologic, and neurologic features in MEN 2B.

50. *(2B)* **Lips CJM.** Clinical management of the multiple endocrine neoplasia syndrome: Results of a computerized opinion poll at the Sixth International Workshop on Multiple Endocrine Neoplasia and von Hippel-Lindau Disease. J Intern Med 1988;243:589.

     Contains the results of a survey about management of the diseases gleaned from an international group of physicians specializing in MEN.

51. *(1A)* **Skinner MA** et al. Prophylactic thyroidectomy in multiple endocrine neoplasia type 2A. N Engl J Med 2005;353:1105–1113.

     A prospective study of 50 consecutive patients aged 19 or younger with MEN 2A identified by RET mutation who underwent total thyroidectomy. Forty-four of 50 patients or 88% seem cured by objective criteria with a 5-year or greater period of follow-up.

52. *(1C)* **Kebebew E** et al. Normal thyroid pathology in patients undergoing thyroidectomy for finding of a RET gene germline mutation: A report of three cases and review of the literature. Thyroid 1999;9:127–131.

     Summarizes three false-positive determinations in MEN germline mutations and reviews the literature on both types of results.

53. *(1C)* **Neumann HPH** et al. Pheochromocytoma, multiple endocrine neoplasia type 2, and von Hippel-Lindau disease. N Engl J Med 1993;329:1531.

     A report of the incidence of pheochromocytoma in various syndromes.

54. *(12B)* **Neumann HPH** et al. Germ-line mutations in nonsyndromic pheochromocytoma. N Engl J Med 2002;346:1159–1466.

A mutation screen of 271 patients with presumed sporadic pheochromocytoma.

55. *(1C)* **Berndt J** et al. A new hot spot for mutations in the ret proto-oncogene causing familial medullary thyroid carcinoma and multiple endocrine neoplasia type 2A. J Clin Endocrinol Metab 1998;83:770.

Medullary Thyroid Carcinoma

56. *(1C)* **Russell CF** et al. The surgical management of medullary thyroid carcinoma. Ann Surg 1983;197:42–48.

A review of the operative procedures, pathology, and status of 123 Mayo Clinic patients who had operations for MTC. The results suggested the need for central lymphadenectomy at initial surgery because of a finding that, when finished, 50% of patients had metastasis. The study also showed that in patients who initially underwent surgery, no difference was noted in results from those having modified radical and radical neck procedures.

57. *(2B)* **Cohen MS, Moley JF.** Surgical treatment of medullary thyroid carcinoma. J Intern Med 2003; 253: 616-626.

A minisymposium on surgical treatment based on the authors' extensive personal experience, review of the literature, and personal opinion.

58. *(1C)* **Saad MF** et al. Medullary carcinoma of the thyroid: A study of the clinical features and prognostic factors in 161 patients. Medicine (Baltimore) 1984;63:319–342.

Reviewed the operative procedures, pathology, and survivorship of 161 patients with MTC having surgery at M.D. Anderson Hospital.

59. *(1C)* **Stjernholm MR** et al. Medullary carcinoma of the thyroid before age 2 years. J Clin Endocrinol Metab 1980;51:252–253.

Case report of a child with MEN 2B phenotype who had total thyroidectomy at 23 months with a finding of bilateral MTC.

60. *(1C)* **Smith V** et al. Intestinal ganglioneuromatosis and multiple endocrine neoplasia type 2B: Implications for treatment. Gut 1999;45:143–146.

A report of a metastasis at age 1 year. This justifies advancing surgery in MEN 2B patients by 6 months.

61. *(1C)* **Machens A** et al. Advances in the management of hereditary medullary thyroid cancer. J Intern Med 2005;257:50–59

A review of the EUROMEM group data centered about genotype–phenotype correlations in RET oncogene–diagnosed MEN patients with personal interpretations.

62. *(1B)* **Sizemore G** et al. Multiple endocrine neoplasia type 2. Clin Endocrinol Metab 1980;9:299–315.

A review of the early Mayo Clinic experience with patients having MEN 2, which cites the authors' experience. Figure 5 shows the rates of recurrence by decade of operation.

63. *(1C)* **Modigliani E** et al. Prognostic factors for survival and for biochemical cure in medullary thyroid carcinoma: Results in 899 patients: The CETC Study Group, Groupe d'Étude des Tumeurs à Calcitonine. Clin Endocrinol (Oxf) 1998;48:265–273.

A review of the screening and operative results of the national French study group in MEN.

64. *(1C+)* **Gill JR** et al. Early presentation of metastatic medullary cancer on multiple endocrine neoplasia, type IIA: Implications for therapy. J Pediatr 1996;129:459–464.

Metastasis by age 5 years in a patient with the more-benign MEN 2A codon 634 mutation. It leads to recommendation for early surgery in that group.

65. *(1C+)* **Telenius-Berg M** et al. Impact of screening on prognosis in the multiple endocrine type 2 syndromes: Natural history and treatment results in 105 patients. Henry Ford Hosp Med J 1984;32:225–231.

A large observational study of 12 Swedish families with MEN 2A, with some data extending as far back as 1730. By comparing mortality results in patients found by pentagastrin screening with those who had symptoms, they found a 5-year postsurgical mortality rate from MTC of 1.5% in 68 patients discovered by screening versus 24% in those first seen with symptoms. The index case in the largest family led to 71 affected cases.

66. *(1C)* **Sizemore GW** et al. Epidemiology of medullary carcinoma of the thyroid gland: A 5-year experience (1971–1976). Surg Clin North Am 1977;57:633–645.

An observational study of 75 Mayo Clinic patients treated in the mid 1970s. Diagnosis and treatment in the first decade caused no tumor persistence. Diagnosis thereafter showed a progressive increase in persistence from 31% in the second decade to 67% during the seventh decade.

67. *(1C)* **Barbet J** et al. Prognostic impact of serum calcitonin and carcinoembryonic antigen doubling times in patients with medullary thyroid carcinoma. J Clin Endocrinol Metab 2005;90:6077–6084.

A large, retrospective, observational study that assesses the predictive value of postoperative calcitonin doubling times on survivorship of patients with medullary thyroid carcinoma.

68. *(1C)* **Miyauchi A** et al. Relation of doubling-time of plasma calcitonin levels to prognosis and recurrence of medullary thyroid carcinoma. Ann Surg 1984;199:461–466.

A small observational study predicted that survivorship in MTC is reduced in patients with rapid calcitonin doubling time.

69. *(1C)* **Moley JF** et al. Improved results of cervical reoperation for medullary thyroid carcinoma. Ann Surg 1997;225:734–740.

Results of a prospective study of the Tisell extensive cervical microdissection technique in selected patients showed that 38% produced (and continued to produce) negative results to testing for calcitonin with 5-year follow-up. The operation had reasonable rates of morbidity and no mortality.

70. *(1C+)* **Simpson WJ** et al. Management of medullary carcinoma of the thyroid. Am J Surg 1982;144:420–422.

This study demonstrated a twofold increased survivorship period in those who underwent secondary external radiation.

71. *(1B)* **Gao Z** et al. The role of combined imaging in metastatic medullary thyroid carcinoma. J Cancer Res Clin Oncol 2004;130:649–656.

Report of imaging capabilities and treatment possibilities for ^{131}I/^{123}I-MIBG in patients with metastatic MTC.

72. *(1B)* **Cuccuru G** et al. Cellular effects and anti-tumor activity of RET inhibitor RPI-1 on MEN2A-associated medullary thyroid carcinoma. J Natl Cancer Inst 2004;96:1006–1014.

A demonstration of tumor inhibition in nice bearing subcutaneous TT or MTC xenografts.

Pheochromocytoma

73. *(1C)* **Howe JR** et al. Prevalence of pheochromocytoma and hyperparathyroidism in multiple endocrine neoplasia type 2A: Results of long-term follow-up. Surgery 1993;114:1070–1077.

These authors conclude that the penetrance of pheochromocytoma and hyperparathyroidism is variable in different kindreds with MEN 2A, but that the overall prevalence of pheochromocytoma approximates 40%, and that of hyperparathyroidism, 35%.

74. *(1C)* **Nguyen L** et al. Pheochromocytoma in multiple endocrine neoplasia type 2: A prospective study. Eur J Endocrinol 2001;144:37–44.

A prospective study of 87 French MEN RET codon mutation carriers, aged 0.8–29 years, who were screened with 24-hour urinary catecholamine determinations during a mean 7.6-year study. Fourteen (16%) of 87 had pheochromocytoma. CT failed to identify 25% of tumors, and MIBG diagnosed 10 of 11 patients correctly.

75. *(1C)* **Lora MS** et al. Adrenal ganglioneuromas in children with multiple endocrine neoplasia type 2: A report of two cases. J Clin Endocrinol Metab 2005;90:4383–4387.

Case reports of unilateral adrenal ganglioneuroma in children with MEN 2A and MEN 2B.

76. *(1B)* **Modigliani E** et al. Pheochromocytoma in multiple endocrine neoplasia type 2: European study. J Intern Med 1995;238:363–367.

A review of the European consortium experience with MEN2.

77. *(1B)* **Machens A** et al. Codon-specific development of pheochromocytoma in multiple endocrine neoplasia type 2. J Clin Endocrinol Metab 2005;90:3999–4003.

A cohort study with mean observation period of 27 years measuring time to diagnosis of pheochromocytoma in 206 consecutive with RET mutations. Earliest age at manifestation for genotypes 918, 634, 618, and 620 was 22, 18, 29, and 39 years, respectively. They concluded annual screening should start at age 10 years for those with mutations in codons 918, 634, and 630, and from age 20 in the rest.

78. *(2B)* **Decker RA** et al. Evaluation of children with multiple endocrine neoplasia type 2B following thyroidectomy. J Pediatr Surg 1990;25:939–943.

Within this report are descriptions of two cases with early pheochromocytoma.

79. *(1A)* **Pacak K** et al. Biochemical diagnosis, localization and management of pheochromocytoma: Focus on multiple endocrine neoplasia type 2 in relation to other hereditary syndromes and sporadic forms of the tumor. J Intern Med 2005;257:60–68.

Figure 1 in this minisymposium compares plasma concentrations of metanephrine and catecholamines for making the diagnosis of pheochromocytoma in MEN 2, von Hippel–Lindau, and sporadic patients. For pheochromocytoma in MEN 2, measurement of plasma metanephrine was best.

80. *(1C+)* **Lenders JW** et al. Biochemical diagnosis of pheochromocytoma: Which test is best? JAMA 2002;287:1427–1434.

A comparison of multiple types of catecholamine and metabolites for the detection of pheochromocytoma.

81. *(1C)* **Lenders JWM** et al. Phaeochromocytoma. Lancet 2005;366:665–675.

A review article on pheochromocytoma.

82. *(1C+)* **Gagel RF** et al. Natural history of the familial medullary thyroid carcinoma–pheochromocytoma syndrome and the identification of the preneoplastic stages by screening studies: A 5-year report. Trans Assoc Am Physicians 1975;88:177–191.

In this study of fractionated urinary catecholamines in 77 at-risk members of families with MEN 2, unaffected family members had epinephrine excretion below 20 mg/24 hr with a mean of 6 mg, and eight pheochromocytoma-affected members had values above normal with a mean of 108 mg/24 hr.

83. *(1C)* **van Heerden JA** et al. Surgical management of the adrenal glands in the multiple endocrine neoplasia 2 syndrome. World J Surg 1984;8:612–621.

Seventeen patients with MEN 2 had bilateral adrenalectomy for adrenomedullary disease. With a mean follow-up of 10 years, the need for adrenal replacement therapy had not caused problems; seven uneventful pregnancies occurred, and 23 surgeries requiring general anesthesia had been uneventful.

84. *(1C)* **Neumann HP** et al. Preserved adrenocortical function after laparoscopic bilateral sparing surgery for hereditary pheochromocytoma. J Clin Endocrinol Metab 1999;84:2608–2610.

Four patients with hereditary bilateral adrenal pheochromocytoma were treated with laparoscopic surgery in an organ-sparing fashion. Postoperatively, all patients had normal urinary excretion of epinephrine and norepinephrine and normal cortisol responses to intravenous ACTH.

Carcinoid Tumors

Nathan J. O'Dorisio, M. Sue O'Dorisio, and
Thomas M. O'Dorisio

DEFINITION

Neuroendocrine tumors are characterized by the production, storage, and secretion of polypeptides, biogenic amines, and hormones. Carcinoid tumors, first classified in the early 1900s by Oberndorfer, fall under this designation. Oberndorfer noted small tumors of the gastrointestinal (GI) tract that were more indolent than adenocarcinomas and similar to the multiple tumors initially found and described by Lubarsch at autopsy of two patients in 1888. Carcinoid syndrome is an uncommon constellation of symptoms (<10% of these tumors) and is associated with diarrhea, flushing (usually facial), hypotension, wheezing, edema, and nocturnal perspiration.

ETIOLOGY

Carcinoid tumors arise from neuroendocrine cells and can be classified according to where they occur in the body. The location has classically been based on the embryonic divisions of the alimentary tract and is divided into foregut (lungs, bronchi, stomach, and pancreas), midgut (small intestine, appendix, and proximal colon), and hindgut (distal colon, rectum, and genitourinary tract). Among the foregut tumors, those of the pulmonary system are thought to derive their origin from the Kulchitsky cells, located within the mucosa. Within the stomach, the tumors arise from the enterochromafin (EC) cells and have been associated with hyperplasia secondary to hypergastrinemic states. Studies in humans with proton-pump inhibitors have not as yet borne out gastrin-induced EC cell hyperplasia. An association between gastric carcinoid and Zollinger–Ellison with multiple endocrine neoplasia type 1 (MEN 1) syndrome (see later) is almost 100% [1]. Among the midgut tumors, those of the small intestine are thought to derive from hyperplasia of the serotonin-producing intraepithelial cells. Those tumors of the appendix presumptively arise from the subepithelial cells within the submucosa and lamina propria [2]. The reason for the hyperplasia is unknown. Of the hindgut tumors, colon carcinoids also arise from the serotonin-producing cells of the epithelium, whereas in the rectum, the cells contain "glicentin" (67-amino acid residue peptide) and glucagon-like peptides (GLP) [2]. The carcinoid syndrome is related to the release of those peptides and amines produced and stored within carcinoid tumors. Most symptoms are due to overproduction of tryptophan (especially the amine serotonin) or decreased elimination of the breakdown products. This is especially true of serotonin overproduction when carcinoid tumors metastasize to the liver.

EPIDEMIOLOGY

Carcinoid tumors are the most common type of neuroendocrine tumor in adults, accounting for approximately 55% of all new occurrences yearly affecting the GI tract. The overall occurrence is, however, still rare. Several studies have postulated the incidence to be one to two cases per 100,000 people [3,4]. The rate is similar for women, men, and among races, with slight variations based on the location and type of tumor expressed. Carcinoids occur across the age spectrum, with the peak incidence occurring between 50 and 70 years of age. Among carcinoid tumors, the most common site is the appendix, followed by the rectum and then the ileum. Carcinoid is the also the most common tumor of the appendix and can account for up to one third of small bowel neoplasms. In contrast, carcinoid tumors represent less than 2% of organ-specific tumors in the pulmonary, gastric, and colonic/rectal systems. Carcinoid syndrome occurs only in a minority of patients, 75% to 80% of whom have small bowel disease other than carcinoid. The incidence of carcinoid syndrome, overall, is 10% for small bowel disease (especially ileum), and less than 1% for appendiceal and rectal tumors, and usually reflects liver metastases. Because of the slow-growing nature of these tumors, the prevalence is estimated to be about 185,000 per year.

PATHOLOGY

As previously mentioned, carcinoid tumors are classified according to the different embryonic divisions of the GI tract (fore-, mid-, and hindgut). The individual cells are further divided as "typical" and "atypical," with typical cells classified as insular, trabecular, glandular, undifferentiated, and mixed [2,5]. Malignant versus benign is based on cellular histology as well as tumor size at surgery and site of primary occurrence. "Typical" pulmonary carcinoids are indolent and perihilar in location, with fewer than 15% metastasizing. In contrast, "atypical" carcinoids of the lung have a 30% to 50% incidence of metastases and are often more aggressive. They may secrete adrenocorticotropic hormone (ACTH) and occur with Cushing syndrome. Of the gastric carcinoids, up to 75% are type 1 and associated with chronic atrophic gastritis, 10% to 15% are type 2 and associated with Zollinger–Ellison syndrome, and the remainder are sporadic or type 3. Most tumors are smaller than 1 cm in diameter, and types 1 and 2 have a more benign course. Those tumors larger than 2 cm (and type 3 tumors) are more likely to have metastatic disease at the time of diagnosis. Small bowel carcinoid is most commonly found in the ileum and often has multiple local sites of involvement. Unlike gastric tumors, tumor size greater or less than 2 cm is a less-reliable predictor of metastasis [6]. It has been observed that ileal tumors larger than 2 cm at surgery will metastasize locally or regionally 100% of the time. Within the appendix, most tumors occur at the tip, and most are not associated with symptoms. Of appendiceal tumors, 95% are smaller than 1 cm; however, the 2-cm size delineation appears to correlate with both metastatic disease and the carcinoid syndrome [6]. Colonic tumors are often right-sided, with most occurring around the cecum. These tumors tend to be larger at diagnosis (5 cm) and more commonly associated with distant metastases, although fewer than 5% exhibit features of carcinoid syndrome. Rectal carcinoids occur predominantly (99%) within the zone defined as 4 cm to 13 cm above the dentate line, although the reason for this is not known. The majority (two of three) are smaller than 1 cm, but the association with metastatic disease and carcinoid syndrome is again defined by an absolute size of 2 cm.

Among all carcinoid tumors, more than 80% express somatostatin receptors. Of the five somatostatin-receptor subtypes currently known to exist, types 2, 3, and 5 have been demonstrated on carcinoid tumors, with type 2 predominating. As previously noted, carcinoid syndrome can be attributed to altered metabolism of tryptophan and subsequent conversion to serotonin or other breakdown products. Diarrhea, flushing, nocturnal perspiration, and cardiac manifestations (especially right-sided valve disease) have all been linked with this mechanism, whereas histamine from some gastric tumors may be associated with atypical flushing and pruritis as well as an increased occurrence of duodenal ulcers seen in this population.

The carcinoid syndrome usually is directly related to the ability of the tumor to secrete serotonin into the circulation system and bypass the breakdown that occurs in the liver [7]. As well, it can exceed the liver metabolism threshold, resulting in high circulating serotonin concentrations. Evidence of this can be seen in the high association with hepatic metastases and the low incidence in patients with limited or local disease. One caveat to this syndrome is ovarian carcinoids; although rare, these are more often associated with this syndrome because of their direct systemic circulation. It is thought that the episodic secretion of serotonin and vasoactive peptides is due to the non-autonomous nature of the neuroendocrine tumors and the presence of somatostatin subtype 2 receptors on them.

DIAGNOSIS

Because of the indolent nature [thought to be due, in part, to the binding of endogenous somatostatin to the tumor somatostatin receptor subtype 2 (sst2)] and mostly occult presentation of most carcinoid neoplasms, the diagnosis is commonly not made until late in the course of the disease. Pulmonary involvement often manifests as cough, recurrent pneumonia, or hemoptysis. Gastric tumors are commonly found on routine endoscopies for symptoms of abdominal pain or gastritis, whereas those in the small bowel may occur with signs of obstruction or nonspecific abdominal pain; some regrettably are labeled "psychosomatic" in origin. Appendiceal lesions commonly are found during routine appendectomies for appendicitis but may occur with obstruction if located in the base rather than the tip of the appendix. Abdominal pain without obstruction is a common complaint in colonic tumors, as well as rectal pain with associated tumors. Intestinal bleeding is an uncommon presentation for both rectal and colonic tumors and is almost nonexistent with small bowel tumors. Rectal carcinoids are often found incidentally on routine colonoscopy or sigmoidoscopy. The carcinoid syndrome is often characteristic and can be the initial presentation for the underlying tumor.

Because of the heterogeneity of the presenting symptoms and indolent course of most carcinoid, very little consensus exists on the best imaging modality. The small size of most functioning tumors (<2 cm) creates a problem for most diagnostic strategies. For carcinoid tumors with high-affinity somatostatin receptors, subtype 2, the OctreoScan has proven superior to other modalities, with a sensitivity of 89% [7]. This scan allows localization of small lesions as well as defines the extent of distant metastases. Chromogranin A is a member of the family of polypeptides stored in the secretory granules of neuronal and neuroendocrine cells and their tumors. Circulating plasma chromogranin A levels are currently thought to be the best general "marker" for neuroendocrine tumors, including carcinoids [8]. When carcinoid tumor is suspected, specific assay tests for the secretory product in question is the test of choice. Most commonly this is a 24-hour urine collection for 5-HIAA, although blood levels can sometimes be used. However, it is important to note that, unless metastasis is already present in the liver, 5-HIAA may not be appreciably elevated. The diagnosis of symptomatic carcinoid tumor may be extremely difficult, especially early, when these tumors are not autonomous and are under regulatory control (via somatostatin and its binding to the tumor membrane somatostatin receptor subtype 2). In this regard, we suggest that an OctreoScan be done at least one time early in the patient's course of diagnosis. Serial plasma serotonin may also be helpful and is considered to be very sensitive but not specific.

TREATMENT

The basis of treatment for most carcinoid tumors rests in tumor removal and symptomatic control. For pulmonary lesions, local resection has been shown to be associated with a low rate of recurrence and 5-year survival of 90%. Type 1 and 2 gastric carcinoids, smaller than 1 cm, are treated with local endoscopic resection with excellent prognosis, whereas type 3 lesions and those larger than 2 cm necessitate a radical gastrectomy. Because of the more-malignant nature and higher frequency of metastasis at diagnosis, small bowel tumors are often treated with small bowel and associated mesenteric dissection. We support extirpation of small bowel primaries, regardless of metastatic status, because they can often obstruct. Simple tumors involving the appendix may be treated with appendectomy, whereas lesions larger than 2 cm often receive a right hemicolectomy. Involvement of the colon commonly necessitates a total colectomy, whereas a rectal lesion smaller than 1 cm can receive local resection. However, rectal lesions larger than 2 cm should be referred for low anterior or abdominoperineal resection. In those patients in whom carcinoid-associated valvular heart disease develops, valve replacement can be of benefit, although it is often associated with a high morbidity and mortality rate. For metastatic carcinoid in the liver, increasing literature suggests that local resection and hepatic debulking should be offered as surgical adjuncts. Further, if active, hepatic debulking may improve symptoms and reduce the octreotide requirement.

As with the diagnosis of carcinoid tumors, the advent of somatostatin analogues (predominantly octreotide acetate, Sandostatin) has also lead to the improved treatment and life expectancy of patients with these tumors. Currently Sandostatin LAR depot (monthly) and Lanreotide SR (biweekly) are the treatments of choice for controlling symptoms associated with these neoplasms and may also reduce the incidence of carcinoid heart disease (Lanreotide SR is not presently available in the United States). These congeners have been shown to reduce symptoms (including diarrhea and flushing) in 88% of patients, as well as decrease 5-HIAA levels in up to 72%. They are also currently recommended for administration before surgery or chemotherapy to prevent the occurrence of carcinoid crisis. The specific somatostatin-receptor–targeted radionuclide antineoplastic therapy [OctreoTher Yttrium-90-DOTA-(tyr)-octreotide] is continuing to evolve and gain favor as a viable alternative therapy to chemotherapy. Recent studies have shown both improvements in symptoms and stabilization or partial tumor regression in 65% to 70% of patients thus far treated more than 3 years.

Although, to a lesser extent than the somatostatin analogues, interferon-α has been shown to reduce both symptoms and tumor size, the high incidence of side effects can be disabling and extract a significant toll. Recent studies have shown that somatostatin used in conjunction with interferon-α is superior to either used alone. Results from trials with chemotherapy have been disappointing; resulting in response rates of less than 20%. Currently, chemotherapy is recommended only when other therapies, especially surgery and octreotide, have failed. In general, a strongly positive photon emission tomography (PET) and weakly positive OctreoScan may predict better response to chemotherapy. Of symptomatic patients with hepatic involvement refractory to first-line treatments, hepatic artery chemoembolization can result in a decrease in hormone levels and tumor size. Again, this procedure can be associated with significant morbidity, including fever, nausea, and vomiting, especially when hepatic arteries are used for complete embolizations.

REFERENCES

1. **Kulke MH, Mayer RJ.** Carcinoid tumors. N Engl J Med 1999;340:858–868.

   This comprehensive review (135 references) discusses carcinoid tumors from classification to incidence through presentation, diagnosis, and treatment.

2. **Capella C et al.** Revised classification of neuroendocrine tumours of the lung, pancreas and gut. Virchows Arch 1995;1995:547–560

   This article proposes a European classification system for neuroendocrine tumors of the lung, pancreas, and gut. It is a framework proposed in an attempt to encompass the morphologic, functional, and biologic features of the tumors.

3. *(1C)* **Modlin IM, Sandor A.** An analysis of 8305 cases of carcinoid tumors. Cancer 1997;79: 813–829.

   This retrospective case review is the largest published. The 8,305 cases were taken from the data banks and surveillance programs from the National Cancer Institute. The authors looked at overall incidence as well as individual tumor occurrence and survival data. They conclude that the overall incidence of carcinoids appears to have increased in the past 20 years and is most likely due to improved surveillance, data registries, and diagnostic technologies. The study also points out a 45.3% rate of metastatic disease at the time of diagnosis and an overall disease specific 5-year survival of 50.4%.

4. *(1C)* **Godwin JD.** Carcinoid tumors: An analysis of 2837 cases. Cancer 1975;36:560–569.

This is a retrospective review of 2,837 cases from the files of the National Cancer Institute which served as the initial cases used in reference 2 above. They report tumors found in the lung, ovary, biliary, and gastrointestinal tract. Overall prevalence was highest in the appendix, rectum, and ileum. There was a low rate of concurrent or multiple neoplasms. Five year survival ranged from 99% for appendiceal tumors to 33% for sigmoid colon tumors. Findings for this study were compared with those of other studies.

5. **Arnold R.** Diagnosis and management of neuroendocrine tumors. In: 8th United European Gastroenterology Week, www.Medscape.com, 2001.

This is a review of the current pathologic classification system, a discussion of the pathology, diagnostic markers, imaging modalities, and current treatment options.

6. **Loftus JP, van Heerden JA.** Surgical management of gastrointestinal carcinoid tumors. Adv Surg 1995;28:317–336.

This review briefly discusses the history of gastrointestinal carcinoid tumors and their spectrum of disease. It is then followed by a complete discussion of the challenges surgeons face when confronted with these tumors. These challenges include accidentally discovered carcinoids, importance of size, diagnosis, and prognosis as well as management including adjuvant chemotherapy.

7. **Caplin ME** et al. Carcinoid tumour. Lancet 1998;352:799–805

This is a review of the pathology of carcinoid tumors and a comprehensive discussion of the new treatment options available including octreotide for diagnosis and management. The authors conclude that there are currently better diagnostic tools and therapeutic options for patients with carcinoid tumors. They also recommend that patients be treated with a multidisciplinary approach.

8. *(1B)* **Baudin E** et al. Neuron-specific enolase and chromogranin A as markers of neuroendocrine tumours. Br J Cancer 1998;78:1102–1107.

Chromogranin A (CgA) and circulating neuron-specific enolase (NSE) levels were measured in 128 patients with neuroendocrine tumors to compare sensitivity, specificity, and prognostic value. Elevated CgA levels were significantly associated with the presence of other secretions and a heavy tumor burden. CgA appeared to be a better marker of tumor evolution than NSE, and the authors recommend CgA as a general screening marker for patients with neuroendocrine tumors.

9. *(1C+)* **Feldman JM, O'Dorisio TM.** Role of neuropeptides and serotonin in the diagnosis of carcinoid tumors. Am J Med 1986;81(suppl 6B):41–48.

This case review looked at different markers for the diagnosis of neuroendocrine tumors. The authors conclude that serotonin is the most specific marker, but not sensitive due to its episodic secretion nature.

10. **Krenning EP** et al. Somatostatin receptor scintigraphy. Ann NY Acad Sci 1994;733:416.

This comprehensive review looks at the role of radiolabeled somatostatin in localizing and diagnosing neuroendocrine tumors. The article covers the distribution, side-effect profile, in vitro and in vivo studies with this technology. It also covers interactions between the body's natural somatostatin receptors and the radiolabeled somatostatin.

11. *(1C+)* **Nuttall KL, Pingree SS.** The incidence of elevations in urine 5-hydroxyindoleacetic acid. Ann Clin Lab Sci 1998;25:167–174.

This randomized controlled trial set out to set the reference range for urine 5-hydroxyindoleacetic acid (5-HIAA) from 947 specimens. The results showed that frequent elevations of urine 5-HIAA and an elevated test result should be used only to corroborate a suspected carcinoid in the face of other consistent findings. They also note that 5-HIAA does not usually increase until carcinoid tumors have metastasized to the liver.

12. *(1C)* **Janson ET** et al. Carcinoid tumors: Analysis of prognostic factors and survival in 301 patients from a referral center. Ann Oncol 1997;36:607–614.

Three hundred and one consecutive carcinoid patients were evaluated over a 15-year with respect to tumor distribution, hormone production, prognostic factors, and survival. They found that survival was significantly shorter with midgut carcinoid, patients with more than five liver metastases, and high levels of 5-HIAA, plasma chromogranin A or neuropeptide K.

13. **Maton PN.** The carcinoid syndrome. JAMA 1988;260:1602–1605.

This review article presents a 54-year-old woman with carcinoid syndrome as the basis for discussion of carcinoid syndrome. The author discusses the syndrome as well as its relation to carcinoid tumors and the pathology diagnosis and treatment of the various tumors and the syndrome.

14. **Dunne MJ** et al. Sandostatin® and gastroenteropancreatic endocrine tumors: Therapeutic characteristics. In: O'Dorisio TM, ed. Sandostatin® in the treatment of gastroenteropancreatic endocrine tumors: Consensus Round Table, Scottsdale (Arizona), 1987. Springer Verlag (London): Sandoz Medical Publications, 1989, 93–113.

This chapter is an in-depth review (35 references) of the therapeutic characteristics of octreotide (Sandostatin). The authors show that octreotide has a low side effect profile and is beneficial for decreasing the symptoms of carcinoid tumors, including the diarrhea, flushing and increased serum levels of 5-hydroxyindoleacetic acid. They did not find any significant tumor-size response to drug administration. These results were then assembled and used by Elton and colleagues for FDA approval in early 1989.

15. *(1C+)* **Paganelli G** et al. Receptor-mediated radiotherapy with 90Y-DOTA-D-Phe1-Tyr3-octreotide. Eur J Nucl Med 2001;28:426–434.

This study took 30 consecutive patients with somatostatin receptor–positive tumors and looked at dosage, safety profile, and therapeutic efficacy. The patients were divided into groups of five and given subsequently higher doses of radiotherapy in increments of 0.37 GBq. Total injectable dose for this study was deemed limited by the estimated toxic dose to the kidneys of 20 to 25 Gy. The authors noted a complete or partial response in 23%, stable disease in 64%, and progression in 13%. They also conclude that high doses (total 7.77 GBq) were of low risk for myelotoxicity, but cumulative dose toxicity to the kidneys was still a risk factor and should be monitored closely.

16. *(1C)* **Thompson GB** et al. Carcinoid tumors of the gastrointestinal tract: Presentation, management and prognosis. Surgery 1985;98:1054–1063.

This is a case-review study of 154 patients who were surgically treated for gastrointestinal carcinoids at the Mayo Clinic between 1972 and 1982. The most frequent sites for tumor involvement were the ileum (43%), rectum (30%), and appendix (11%). They report that preoperative studies were of limited value except for endoscopy, and the overall mortality rate was 2.6%. There was also an unusually high incidence of metastasis from ileal primary tumors smaller than 1 cm (18%).

17. **Que FG** et al. Hepatic surgery for metastatic gastrointestinal neuroendocrine tumors. Cancer Control 2002;9:67–79.

This review evaluated the role as well as the rationale for cytoreductive hepatic surgery in the management of metastatic gastrointestinal neuroendocrine malignancies.

18. *(1B)* **Arnold R** et al. Gastroenteropancreatic endocrine tumours: Effect of Sandostatin® on tumour growth. Digestion 1993;54:72–75.

One hundred fifteen gastroenteropancreatic patients with malignant endocrine tumors were entered into this prospective trial to determine the efficacy of 200 μg of octreotide (Sandostatin) on tumor growth. The study was able to show an initially favorable effect for 54% at 3 months; however, the effect was short lived, as only 38% showed response at 12 months. They also proved that the effect mirrored the suppression of serum and urine hormone levels.

19. **Plockinger U** et al. Guidelines for the diagnosis and treatment of neuroendocrine gastrointestinal tumours. Neuroendocrinology 2004;80:394–424.

A consensus guideline from the European Neuroendocrine Tumour Society. These guidelines cover the presentation, diagnosis, and treatment options for foregut, midgut, and hindgut neuroendocrine tumors.

20. **Kwekkeboom DJ** et al. Overview of results of peptide receptor radionuclide therapy with 3 radiolabeled somatatin analogs. J Nucl Med 2005;46(suppl 1):62S–66S.

This review looks at three different radiolabeled octreotide compounds and the varying efficacy in the treatment of gastroenteropancreatic tumors.

21. **Sutcliffe** et al. Management of neuroendocrine liver metastes. J of Surg 2004;187(1).

A review of concepts regarding diagnosis and treatment of neuroendocrine hepatic metastatic disease.

Paraneoplastic Endocrine Syndromes

Subhash Kukreja

Cancer cells frequently produce peptides that are not normally synthesized by the tissue of origin. In addition, peptides that are normally produced in a paracrine or autocrine manner may be produced in larger quantities by the cancer cells and released into the circulation. Cancer cells frequently lack the machinery to process peptides into mature hormones, and therefore only precursor or incomplete forms of the protein are usually released. These partial peptides or precursor forms of the hormones may either be biologically inactive or may have weak biologic activity. Therefore clinical syndromes due to ectopic production of these hormones are seen less frequently than might be predicted, based on the immunoassay studies. Ectopic production of steroid hormones by cancer cells is rare. However, steroid hormones may be present in higher concentration because of increased production of enzymes by the tumor cells (e.g., synthesis of 1α-hydroxylase by certain lymphomas allows increase in the synthesis of 1,25-dihydroxyvitamin D [1,25(OH)2D]. Another example is an increased aromatase activity in hepatocellular carcinoma with conversion of androgens to estrogens, resulting in gynecomastia.

Paraneoplastic syndrome is defined as the tumor-related clinical manifestations that occur distant from the site of the tumor and are mediated by humoral factors. Endocrine syndromes are outlined in Table 11.1 [1–12]. Hypercalcemia of malignancy is one of the most common clinical syndromes due to ectopic hormone production and is described in some detail. Other common endocrine syndromes such as Cushing syndrome and syndrome of inappropriate antidiuretic hormone secretion are described elsewhere in this volume. Moreover, many nonendocrine paraneoplastic manifestations of cancer are not covered in this chapter (e.g., polycythemia, various neuropathies, cerebellar degeneration).

HYPERCALCEMIA OF MALIGNANCY

Definition

Under physiologic conditions, serum calcium is maintained within a narrow range. Serum calcium is bound to proteins that are composed predominantly of albumin, so that under normal conditions, approximately 45% of the calcium is available in the physiologically active, ionized, or free form. In the presence of hypoalbuminemia, total serum calcium values may be low, whereas ionized calcium values may be normal or even elevated. Conversely, in some cases of multiple myeloma, abnormal globulins may bind calcium so that total serum calcium is high and ionized calcium is normal [13,14]. Various correction formulas have been devised to correct serum total calcium for serum protein/albumin concentrations. These correction formulas are derived from regression analysis of serum calcium and albumin/total proteins. None of

Table 11.1. Paraneoplastic Endocrine Syndromes

Clinical Manifestations	Hormones	Common Tumors	Diagnosis	Treatment	Comments
Hypocalcemia [1]	Osteoblast-stimulating factors that have not yet been fully characterized	Prostate cancer most common Lung and breast cancer less common	Hypocalcemia, hypomagnesemia, high serum PTH, low serum magnesium Tumor lysis or effects of chemotherapy may also cause hypocalcemia	Intravenous and oral calcium and large doses of $1,25(OH)_2D$	There is extensive bone involvement by osteoblastic lesions, and hypocalcemia is difficult to control
Oncogenic osteomalacia [2,3]	Fibroblast growth factor 23, fibroblast growth factor 7	Mesenchymal tumors, hemangiopericytomas, prostate cancer	Hypophosphatemia, normocalcemia, low $1,25(OH)_2D$ and rickets or osteomalacia	Search and removal of tumor if possible; calcitriol and phosphate	The tumors may be difficult to find and are usually benign
Syndrome of inappropriate ADH secretion [4]	Antidiuretic hormone	Small cell lung cancer, other cell type lung cancer, pancreatic cancer, thymoma, lymphoma	Hyponatremia, low serum osmolarity, increased urine osmolarity, urine sodium >20 mEq/L, low serum uric acid, low BUN	Fluid restriction, saline, furosemide, hypertonic saline in emergency situations; demeclocycline	The syndrome may occur due to stimulation of ADH secretion by chemotherapy agents or opioids
Ectopic Cushing's syndrome [5,6]	ACTH	Small cell lung cancer, bronchial carcinoid, thymoma, pancreatic cancer, pheochromocytoma, medullary thyroid cancer	High serum cortisol, no suppression with high dose dexamethasone, no stimulation with CRH or desmopressin and no gradient on inferior petrosal sinus sampling	Tumor removal if possible Ketoconazole, metyrapone, mitotane, aminoglutethamide	Syndrome due to carcinoid tumors difficult to differentiate from pituitary-dependent disease

Clinical Manifestations	Hormones	Common Tumors	Diagnosis	Treatment	Comments
Acromegaly [7]	GHRH secretion more common than GH secretion	Carcinoid, endocrine pancreatic tumors	Elevated GH and IGF, no GH response to GHRH, GHRH assay	Removal of primary tumor; somatostatin analogues, GH receptor antagonists	Rare cause of acromegaly; ectopic GH linked to hypertrophic osteoarthropathy but not proven
Hyperthyroidism [8,9]	HCG	Trophoblastic tumors Ectopic TSH secretion is rare	High T4 and T3, low TSH and lack of TSH response to TRH	Removal of tumor Thyroid ablation not usually needed	HCG stimulates TSH receptor
Hypoglycemia [10–12]	Pro-IGF-2 (big IGF-2)	Mesenchymal tumors (fibroma, mesothelioma, fibrosarcoma and rhabdomyosarcoma), hepatocellular and adrenal carcinoma	High IGF-2, Low IGF-1 and IGF-BP3, suppressed insulin level	Removal of primary-tumor, GH therapy, streptozotocin, glucagon infusion, high-dose glucocorticoids, glucose	Octreotide is not helpful

these formulas accurately predicts the state of ionized calcium [15,16]; therefore ionized calcium should be measured to assess the calcium status accurately when protein abnormalities are present.

Malignancy-associated hypercalcemia (MAH) is defined as the presence of elevated serum calcium levels in a patient with cancer (either solid tumor or hematologic) in whom the hypercalcemia is caused by factors produced by the cancer. This implies that the hypercalcemia should be reversed by the removal of the tumor. In practice, however, complete removal or cure of the tumor can rarely be achieved because the disease is often advanced by the time the diagnosis of hypercalcemia is made. Other diseases associated with hypercalcemia (e.g., primary hyperparathyroidism, sarcoidosis, excessive vitamin D intake) can occur coincidentally in patients with malignancy and should be excluded. This is particularly important because the presence of hypercalcemia in a patient with cancer indicates an extremely poor prognosis. If it can be shown that the hypercalcemia in a cancer patient is not due to malignancy, this may indicate a better prognosis.

Etiology

If bone metastases are present in a hypercalcemic cancer patient, it is traditionally assumed that the bone metastases are responsible for the hypercalcemia. In an examination of serum calcium values in patients with bone metastases, however, Ralston and colleagues [17] demonstrated that contrary to expectations, an inverse correlation existed between serum calcium levels and the number of bone metastatic lesions in patients with various malignancies. Hypercalcemia is frequently observed without significant bone metastases in certain types of tumors (e.g., squamous cell cancers), whereas in other tumors (e.g., small cell carcinoma of the lung and prostate cancer), bone metastases are frequently observed in the absence of hypercalcemia. Secretion of local osteolytic factors by certain tumors may play a significant role in the pathogenesis of both hypercalcemia and bone metastases.

Bone resorption is increased in most patients with MAH. Various osteolytic factors secreted by cancer cells have been described. In the case of solid tumors, this factor is parathyroid hormone–related protein (PTHrP) [18]. The peptide has structural homology to PTH in only eight of the first 13 amino acids, and yet a remarkable similarity exists in the biologic actions of the two peptides. Elevated levels of serum PTHrP are observed in 70% to 100% of patients with hypercalcemia resulting from solid tumors, including breast cancer [18]. Breast cancer cells derived from the bone marrow lesions produce PTHrP with greater frequency than do those derived from other metastatic sites [19].

In the case of multiple myeloma and other hematologic malignancies, various other cytokines, such as tumor necrosis factors, RANK ligand, interleukins 1 and 6 (IL-1 and IL-6), hepatocyte growth factor, and macrophage inflammatory protein-1α have been implicated in increased osteolysis [20]. However, recent studies demonstrate that even in multiple myeloma and in other hematologic malignancies, serum PTHrP levels are elevated in about one third of cases and that this peptide may be responsible in part for the increased osteolysis in these tumors as well [21].

Another factor that plays a role in the pathogenesis of hypercalcemia in Hodgkin and non-Hodgkin lymphomas is increased serum $1,25(OH)_2D$ production [22]. In these tumors, the lymphomatous tissue is able to convert $25\text{-}(OH)D$ into the active metabolite, $1,25(OH)_2D$. Serum $1,25(OH)_2D$ levels are elevated (unlike in hypercalcemia of solid tumors and multiple myeloma, where these levels are suppressed).

Therefore PTHrP is the main factor responsible for the hypercalcemia in most solid tumors and in some hematologic malignancies. Increased 1α-hydroxylase activity resulting in increased serum $1,25(OH)_2D$ is the responsible factor in many cases of Hodgkin and non-Hodgkin lymphomas, whereas various cytokines may be responsible for the hypercalcemia in multiple myeloma and certain other hematologic malignancies. The etiology of hypercalcemia associated with solid tumors, wherein serum PTHrP levels are not elevated (up to 30% of reported cases), remains to be defined. In many of these cases, hypercalcemia may be caused by secretion of local osteolytic factors by the tumor present in bone. Alternatively, the assays used for PTHrP measurement may not have been sufficiently sensitive to detect the increased production of this peptide.

Epidemiology

Hypercalcemia has been reported to affect about 10% to 40% of all patients with cancer at some time during the course of the disease. However, this may reflect a selection bias, especially if the studies are done in hospitalized patients. Hypercalcemia occurs in late stages of cancer, and such patients are more likely to be hospitalized. At the time of initial presentation, the incidence of hypercalcemia in cancer patients is about 1% [23]. Non–small cell lung cancer, renal cancer, lymphoma, multiple myeloma, and breast cancer are the malignancies most commonly associated with hypercalcemia. The highest incidence of hypercalcemia on a percentage basis is observed in renal cell carcinoma [23]. Carcinoma of prostate, colon, and small cell carcinoma of the lung are rarely associated with hypercalcemia, despite a high prevalence of bone metastases in these cancers.

Pathophysiology

PTH-related protein, despite its limited homology to PTH, appears to act through the same receptor as PTH (PTH/PTHrP type I receptor). The clinical features of hypercalcemia of malignancy due to solid tumors are similar to those of hyperparathyroidism in many respects (e.g., hypercalcemia, hypophosphatemia, relative hypocalciuria, and increased bone resorption). In other aspects, manifestations of hypercalcemia malignancy due to PTHrP overproduction are different from those of primary hyperparathyroidism, and these include relatively lower serum $1,25(OH)_2D$ and decreased bone formation observed in hypercalcemia of malignancy [24,25]. The decreased bone formation observed in MAH may be related to the secretion of other cytokines (e.g., IL-1 and IL-6), although the mechanisms remain largely unexplained. In the case of Hodgkin and non-Hodgkin lymphomas, the elevated serum $1,25(OH)_2D$ levels enhance gastrointestinal calcium absorption, and serum PTH is suppressed with increased serum phosphate and urine calcium excretion.

Diagnosis

Primary hyperparathyroidism is the most common cause of hypercalcemia in the general population. In most instances, the hypercalcemia has been present for a long time and is mild to moderate. In MAH, which is the second most common cause of hypercalcemia, the hypercalcemia is usually more severe and occurs over a relatively short time. This hypercalcemia becomes manifest late in the course of the malignancy, and the tumor is generally advanced by the time diagnosis of hypercalcemia is confirmed. A complete history and physical examination and simple laboratory and radiologic studies would generally reveal the source of malignancy (i.e., lung cancer, head and neck cancer, carcinoma of the esophagus, breast cancer, multiple myeloma, lymphomas). Retroperitoneal tumors (e.g., renal cell cancer and some lymphomas) may not be readily apparent on initial evaluation, but even in these instances, clinical signs and simple imaging studies often reveal cancer. The laboratory test with the highest yield in the differential diagnosis of hypercalcemia is measurement of serum PTH. Serum PTH level is elevated or in the high-normal range in all patients with primary hyperparathyroidism. Conversely, serum PTH levels are suppressed in almost all cases of hypercalcemia of malignancy, with the rare exception of a few reported cases of the production of native PTH by cancer [26]. In the presence of a tumor type that is commonly associated with MAH, the presence of suppressed PTH level confirms the etiology of hypercalcemia. If serum PTH levels are elevated, then the patient, in all likelihood, has concomitant hyperparathyroidism. If hypercalcemia is observed in association with a tumor type not commonly associated with hypercalcemia (e.g., small cell cancer of the lung, prostate cancer, colon cancer) and serum PTH levels are suppressed, another cause of the hypercalcemia should be sought.

Serum PTHrP levels are increased in 70% to 100% of patients with hypercalcemia due to solid tumors, and this assay may be used in patients in whom the cause of hypercalcemia is not readily apparent. Serum 1,25(OH)$_2$D measurement is of value in the diagnosis of hypercalcemia in granulomatous disease and Hodgkin and non-Hodgkin lymphomas, in which these levels are usually elevated. Serum and urine protein electrophoresis is helpful for the diagnosis of multiple myeloma. In the presence of normal renal function, serum phosphate values are low or in the low-normal range in MAH, similar to that seen in the primary hyperparathyroidism. Other tests (e.g., 24-hour urine calcium, urinary cyclic adenosine monophosphate measurements) are of limited value in the differential diagnosis.

Treatment

Patients with hypercalcemia are often volume depleted because of nausea, vomiting, and polyuria, which is a result of a decrease in urine-concentrating ability from a direct effect of hypercalcemia on the renal tubules. 0.9 % NaCl infusion of 3 to 4 L/day often reduces the serum calcium concentration by 1.0 to 1.5 mg/dl. Increased bone resorption is the major mechanism by which the tumors produce hypercalcemia; agents that inhibit osteoclast activity are highly effective in management of these patients. The agents in this class are plicamycin, calcitonin, gallium nitrate, and bisphosphonates [27]. Bisphosphonates are potent antiresorptive agents that have become the drug of choice for treatment of hypercalcemia. The first bisphosphonate to be used for this purpose was etidronate, but its use has been replaced by the second- and third-generation bisphosphonates (e.g., pamidronate, alendronate, and zoledronate). Intravenous pamidronate and zoledronate are now approved for treatment of MAH. Pamidronate, 90 mg given over a 2- to 4-hour infusion, is as effective as the dose given over 24 hours. A flulike syndrome is seen in up to 20% of patients, but this adverse effect is transient. Hypocalcaemia may occasionally occur in a small percentage of patients but is usually asymptomatic [28,29]. Zoledronate appears to be a more potent bisphosphonate than pamidronate [30]. More-rapid administration of zoledronate (i.e., over a 5-minute period) is associated with the risk of development of renal failure and therefore is not recommended. Other bisphosphonates, such as ibandronate and clodronate, are also effective. These compounds are not approved for use in the United States but are widely used in other countries [29]. The initial effects of bisphosphonates on reduction in serum calcium are observed within 12 to 24 hours, with peak effect being observed in 4 to 7 days. The effect generally lasts for 1 to 3 weeks, depending on the extent of PTHrP production by the tumor.

Hypercalcemic patients with Hodgkin and non-Hodgkin lymphomas, by a mechanism associated with increased 1,25(OH)$_2$D production, respond well to glucocorticoid therapy. They should receive 20 to 40 mg/day of prednisone. Patients with hypercalcemia resulting from multiple myeloma respond well to bisphosphonates and glucocorticoids.

In animal studies, inhibition of RANK ligand by osteoprotegrin results in potent inhibition of bone resorption and reversal of hypercalcemia in two animal models of humoral hypercalcemia of malignancy [31.]. A humanized antibody to RANK ligand (denosumab or AMG 162) has been developed and shown to increase bone mineral density and inhibit bone resorption in women with osteoporosis [32]. Future studies will determine whether these agents are safe and effective in the treatment of hypercalcemia of malignancy.

Prognosis

The prognosis is poor for cancer patients by the time hypercalcemia becomes apparent, with a median survival of only 30 to 70 days [33,34]. In breast cancer with mild hypercalcemia (i.e., ionized serum calcium, 1.36–1.48 mmol/L), the prognosis is better, with a median survival of 17.7 months. Treatment of hypercalcemia is mainly palliative, and a decrease in serum calcium levels in these patients significantly improves symptoms and quality of life [33,34].

BISPHOSPHONATES AND BONE METASTASES

Laboratory evidence suggests that after the initial seeding and attachment of tumor cells to the bone marrow, increased osteolysis plays a significant role in the establishment and growth of tumor into the bone. In animal models, administration of agents that inhibit bone resorption results in reduction in the incidence and severity of bone metastases. Therefore a strong rationale exists for antiresorptive therapy to be helpful in the prevention and treatment of bone metastasis. Newer bisphosphonates, such as zoledronate, may offer additional beneficial effects in reducing skeletal tumor growth by inhibition of angiogenesis through reduction of vascular endothelial growth factor (VEGF) levels [35]. A recent review of the available literature concluded that bisphosphonates such as pamidronate, zoledronate, ibandronate, and clodronate are effective in reducing the incidence of skeletal events such as pathologic fracture, spinal cord compression, and hypercalcemia, without a proven benefit on prolonging survival [36–38]. In the case of multiple myeloma, strong evidence has been posited that adding bisphosphonates to standard chemotherapy results in a reduction of future skeletal complications of vertebral fracture and pain without affecting survival [39].

REFERENCES

1. *(1C)* **Kukreja SC** et al. Hypocalcemia in patients with prostate cancer. Calcif Tissue Int 1988;43:340–345.

   This article describes a case of severe hypocalcemia in a patient with extensive osteoblastic metastases due to prostate cancer. Prevalence of hypocalcemia was examined in an additional 112 patients. The prevalence of true hypocalcemia based on ionized calcium measurement in patients with prostate cancer is low (<2%), even though total calcium levels decrease in up to 14%; most of these patients have bone metastasis.

2. **Shimada T** et al. Cloning and characterization of FGF23 as a causative factor of tumor-induced osteomalacia. Proc Natl Acad Sci USA 2001;98:6500–6505.

   Recent evidence has shown that missense mutations in the RXXR motif of the FGF-23 occur in autosomal dominant hypophosphatemic rickets resulting in its decreased degradation. In X-linked hypophosphatemic rickets, mutations in the protease, PHEX, which degrades FGF-23, have been demonstrated. In this study, the authors identified that FGF-23 is the hypophosphatemic factor synthesized and secreted by a tumor associated with oncogenic osteomalacia. FGF-23 administration reproduced the clinical features of the disease in mice including low 1,25(OH)D levels. The increased production of FGF-23 in oncogenic osteomalacia and decreased degradation in hypophosphatemic rickets appears to be the link that explains phosphate wasting in these diseases.

3. *(1C)* **Carpenter TO** et al. Fibroblast growth factor 7: An inhibitor of phosphate transport derived from oncogenic osteomalacia-causing tumor. J Clin Endocrinol Metab 2005;90:1012–1020.

   In this study, the authors demonstrate that in two patients with oncogenic osteomalacia, excessive production of FGF7 rather than that of FGF23 was responsible for the renal phosphate wasting and hypophosphatemia. Therefore members of the FGF family (other than FGF23) are expressed by oncogenic osteomalacia–associated tumors and may play a role in mediating this syndrome.

4. *(1C)* **Berghmans T** et al. A prospective study on hyponatremia in medical cancer patients: Epidemiology, aetiology and differential diagnosis. Support Care Cancer 2000;8:192–197.

   The incidence of hyponatremia (serum Na <130 mEq/L) was determined prospectively in all patients admitted to a cancer hospital over an 11-month period. The observed incidence was 3.7%. Sodium depletion and syndrome of inappropriate secretion of antidiuretic hormone each explained hyponatremia in about one third of the total cases. Blood urea nitrogen, serum uric acid, and fractional sodium excretion values were most helpful in the differential diagnosis. The mortality rate in the hyponatremic patients was higher (19.5%) than that in the group as a whole (6.3%).

5. *(1C)* **Ilias I** et al. Cushing's syndrome due to ectopic corticotropin secretion: Twenty years experience at the National Institutes of Health. J Clin Endocrinol Metab 2005;90:4955–4962.

   The authors report their experience in diagnosing and treating 90 patients with ectopic Cushing syndrome at a tertiary care clinical research center. Eighty-six percent to 94% of patients did not respond to CRH or dexamethasone suppression, whereas 66 of 67 had negative inferior petrosal sinus sampling (IPSS). To control hypercortisolism, 62 patients received medical treatment, and 33 had bilateral adrenalectomy. Imaging localized tumors in 67 of 90 patients. Surgery confirmed an ACTH-secreting tumor in 59 of 66 patients and cured 65%. The authors concluded that a negative IPSS is the best test in identifying ectopic ACTH syndrome. Although only 47% achieved cure, survival is good, except in patients with small cell lung cancer, medullary thyroid cancer, and gastrinoma.

6. *(1C)* **Kaltsas GA** et al. A critical analysis of the value of simultaneous inferior petrosal sinus sampling in Cushing's disease and the occult ectopic adrenocorticotropin syndrome. J Clin Endocrinol Metab 1999;84:487–492.

In this study, the frequency of occult ectopic Cushing syndrome was found to be 5.5% (six cases compared with 107 cases for Cushing disease). Inferior petrosal sinus sampling after CRH showed an inferior petrosal sinus/peripheral gradient less than 2 in all cases of ectopic ACTH syndrome. A bilateral inferior petrosal sinus/peripheral ratio that exceeded 2, obtained 5 minutes after CRH stimulation, had a sensitivity of 97% and a specificity of 100% in diagnosing Cushing disease.

7. *(1C)* **Thorner MO** et al. Extrahypothalamic growth-hormone–releasing factor (GRF) secretion is a rare cause of acromegaly: Plasma GRF levels in 177 acromegalic patients. J Clin Endocrinol Metab 1984;59:846–849.

Ectopic growth-hormone releasing hormone (GHRH) secretion is a proven cause of acromegaly. In this study, plasma levels of GHRH were in the normal range in all of 177 acromegalic patients. Based on the results of the study, it appears that ectopic GHRH secretion is a rare cause of acromegaly.

8. *(1C)* **Morley JE** et al. Choriocarcinoma as a cause of thyrotoxicosis. Am J Med 1976;60: 1036–1040.

Three patients with hyperthyroidism associated with choriocarcinoma are described. The decrease in severity of hyperthyroidism paralleled the decline in serum HCG levels. The serum from these patients contained TSH bioactivity that was related to HCG.

9. *(1C)* **Hershman JM.** Human chorionic gonadotropin and the thyroid: Hyperemesis gravidarum and trophoblastic tumors. Thyroid 1999;9:653–657.

This review describes that trophoblastic tumors, hydatidiform mole, and choriocarcinoma secrete very large amounts of HCG and cause hyperthyroidism when the serum hCG exceeds about 200 IU/ml. There is a correlation between the biochemical severity of hyperthyroidism and the serum HCG in these patients. Removal of the mole or effective chemotherapy of the choriocarcinoma cures the hyperthyroidism.

10. *(1C)* **Hizuka N** et al. Serum insulin-like growth factor II in 44 patients with non-islet cell tumor hypoglycemia. Endocr J 1998;45(suppl):S61–S65.

Serum levels of pro–IGF II ("big" IGF) were elevated in 31 of the 44 patients with non–islet cell tumor hypoglycemia. Elevated IGF II levels were found in only 13 of the 31 patients. Serum IGF I levels were low in all patients, including 11 patients who did not have elevated IGF II levels. It is suggested that both a high IGF II level and low IGF I level play a role in the pathogenesis of the syndrome.

11. *(1C)* **Drake WM** et al. Dose-related effects of growth hormone on IGF-I and IGF-binding protein-3 levels in non-islet cell tumour hypoglycaemia. Eur J Endocrinol 1998;139:532–536.

The authors treated two patients with non–islet cell tumor hypoglycemia by using recombinant growth hormone. This treatment resulted in an increased serum IGF I and IGF-binding protein 3 (IGF BP3) levels and an amelioration of hypoglycemia. The mechanism of the beneficial effect appears partly related to the increased IGF BP 3 levels with resultant decrease in free serum IGF II levels. The IGF BP 3 levels, however, did not completely normalize despite high-dose growth hormone therapy, suggesting that other mechanism may be involved in explaining the beneficial effects of growth hormone therapy in this syndrome.

12. *(1C)* **Bourcigaux N** et al. Treatment of hypoglycemia using combined glucocorticoid and recombinant human growth hormone in a patient with a metastatic non-islet cell tumor hypoglycemia. Clin Ther 2005;27:246–251.

In a patient with inoperable non–islet cell tumor hypoglycemia, fasting plasma glucose level was normalized with a combination of low-dose prednisone and recombinant hGH. This combination was more effective than high-dose monotherapy with either drug in reestablishing the IGF system and in long-term management for hypoglycemia, and did not cause any adverse events.

Hypercalcemia of Malignancy

13. *(1C)* **Pearce CJ** et al. Hypercalcaemia due to calcium binding by a polymeric IgA kappa-paraprotein. Ann Clin Biochem 1991;28:229–234.

A patient with multiple myeloma and elevation in total serum calcium and normal ionized calcium is described. In vitro studies demonstrated that there was abnormal binding of calcium to the paraprotein IgA κ, thus explaining the false finding of hypercalcemia.

14. *(1C)* **Smith BJ** et al. Frequency of calcium binding by monoclonal immunoglobulins in multiple myeloma. Ann Clin Lab Sci 1984;14:261–264.

To examine the frequency with which abnormal binding to paraprotein may result in elevated serum total with normal ionized calcium values, those authors studied 34 patients with multiple myeloma. Both total and ionized calcium were elevated in three patients. In this series, no abnormal binding between the paraproteins and calcium was observed. This suggests that falsely elevated serum calcium levels are not common in patients with multiple myeloma.

15. *(1C)* **Ladenson JH** et al. Failure of total calcium corrected for protein, albumin, and pH to correctly assess free calcium status. J Clin Endocrinol Metab 1978;46:986–993.

The authors used various published formulas to correct observed calcium for serum protein and albumin abnormalities in 2,454 samples sent for calcium analysis and correlated these values to the measured ionized calcium levels. None of the formulas produced substantially better agreement than that observed between the uncorrected calcium and ionized calcium. The studies concluded that correction of measured serum calcium does not seem to adequately predict calcium status as measured by free calcium.

16. *(1C)* **Shemerdiak WP** et al. Evaluation of routine ionized calcium determination in cancer patients. Clin Chem 1981;27:1621–1622.

In this study, serum total and ionized calcium levels were determined in 59 controls and 95 cancer patients. Various correction formulas were used to determine whether these would predict the calcium status better than that predicted from measurement of total calcium alone. Of the 95 cancer patients, 12 were judged to be hypercalcemic by both total and ionized calcium measurement. An additional 11 patients were found to have elevated ionized with normal total calcium values; the serum calcium elevation in these patients, however, was mild. Application of various correction formulas did not aid significantly in identifying these patients. The study concluded that for most cancer patients, total calcium measurement is adequate. In the presence of protein abnormalities, correction formulas do not aid in correct classification of the calcium status. In these patients, ionized calcium should be determined to assess calcium status accurately.

17. *(1C)* **Ralston S** et al. Hypercalcaemia and metastatic bone disease: Is there a causal link? Lancet 1982;2:903–905.

Bone scans in 725 unselected cancer patients at the Glasgow Royal Infirmary were reviewed. Further analysis was performed in 160 patients with definite metastatic bone disease and 35 hypercalcemic patients without bone metastasis. Bronchogenic and breast cancer were the two most common diagnoses (48% and 31%, respectively). Of the total of 87 hypercalcemic patients, 40% had no evidence of bone metastases, and only 32.5% of the patients with bone metastases had hypercalcemia. The adjusted total serum calcium levels were significantly lower in patients with extensive metastatic disease (>6 lesions on bone scan) compared with those with milder disease (<6 lesions on bone scan). The authors concluded that a causal link does not appear to exist between bone metastasis and hypercalcemia.

18. **Rankin W** et al. Parathyroid hormone-related protein and hypercalcemia. Cancer 1997; 80(suppl):1564–71.

An excellent review of the discovery and physiology of PTH-related protein and of the evidence linking it to the pathogenesis of hypercalcemia of malignancy including that observed in breast cancer.

19. **Martin TJ** et al. Mechanisms in the skeletal complications of breast cancer. Endocr Relat Cancer 2000;7:271–284.

About 70% of patients with advanced breast cancer will have metastatic bone disease, and about 30% of patients will experience hypercalcemia. The review describes that various osteolytic factors such as PTHrP may be involved in the pathogenesis of both of these manifestations of cancer.

20. **Callander NS** et al. Myeloma bone disease. Semin Hematol 2001;38:276–285.

Bone destruction occurs in 70% to 80% of patients with multiple myeloma. This is an excellent review of the various osteoclast-activating factors implicated in the pathogenesis of myeloma bone disease. These include tumor necrosis factors, RANK ligand, IL-1 and IL-6, hepatocyte growth factor, and macrophage inflammatory protein-1a. Bone cytokines (e.g., IL-6) are released as a result of the osteolysis and may in turn play a role in the stimulation of myeloma cell growth. This provides the rationale for the use of antiresorptive therapy in the management of multiple myeloma.

21. *(1C)* **Firkin F** et al. Parathyroid hormone-related protein in hypercalcaemia associated with haematological malignancy. Br J Haematol 1996;94:486–492.

In this prospective study of patients admitted to a clinical hematology unit, hypercalcemia was detected in 18 of 165 patients. Of the 17 patients who were investigated further, hypercalcemia was ascribed to primary hyperparathyroidism in three patients. The other cases of hypercalcemia occurred as follows: nine with multiple myeloma, five with B-cell non-Hodgkin lymphoma, and one with myeloid hyperplasia. PTHrP levels were elevated and correlated with serum calcium level elevation in three of nine myeloma cases and two of four lymphoma patients. Therefore PTHrP appears to be involved in the pathogenesis of hypercalcemia in hematologic malignancies.

22. *(1C)* **Seymour JF** et al. Calcitriol production in hypercalcemic and normocalcemic patients with non-Hodgkin lymphoma. Ann Intern Med 1994;121:633–640.

In this prospective study performed at a referral medical center, serum $1,25(OH)_2D$ levels were elevated in 12 of the 22 hypercalcemic patients using a reference range developed by using hypercalcemic myeloma patients as the control population. If the reference range from normocalcemic subjects were used, only half the patients would be classified as having elevated $1,25(OH)_2D$ levels.

23. *(1C+)* **Vassilopoulou-Sellin R** et al. Incidence of hypercalcemia in patients with malignancy referred to a comprehensive cancer center. Cancer 1993;71:1309–1312.

In this retrospective analysis of laboratory data from 7,667 patients registered at a referral cancer center, the incidence of hypercalcemia within the first 2 months of the registration was determined. Severe hypercalcemia, defined as serum calcium level above 12 mg/dl, was present in 40 (0.52%), and moderate hypercalcemia, defined as serum calcium levels of 10.8 to 12 mg/dl, was present in an additional 48 patients (0.63%) with a total incidence of 1.05%. Non–small cell lung cancer, renal cancer, lymphoma, multiple myeloma, and breast cancer were the malignancies most commonly associated with hypercalcemia. The highest incidence of hypercalcemia on a percentage basis was observed in renal cell carcinoma. Carcinoma of the prostate, colon, and small cell carcinoma of the lung are rarely associated with hypercalcemia, despite a high prevalence of bone metastases in these cancers.

24. *(1C)* **Stewart AF** et al. Biochemical evaluation of patients with cancer-associated hypercalcemia: Evidence for humoral and nonhumoral groups. N Engl J Med 1980;303:1377–1383.

   In this prospective study of 50 consecutive hypercalcemic cancer patients seen at a university hospital, urine cAMP, serum calcium, PTH, and 1,25(OH)$_2$D levels were determined. Urine nephrogenous cAMP levels (a marker of PTH action on kidney) were elevated in 41 patients with hypercalcemia of malignancy and in patients with primary hyperparathyroidism. Serum PTH levels were elevated in patients with primary hyperparathyroidism and low in cancer patients. The studies provided strong evidence that the humoral factor or factors responsible for hypercalcemia have strong similarity of biologic action to that of PTH and yet are different immunologically. This and other similar studies laid the foundation for later discovery of the PTHrP. The study also described that serum 1,25(OH)$_2$D levels are lower in hypercalcemia of malignancy, as compared with those seen in primary hyperparathyroidism.

25. **Stewart AF.** Clinical practice: Hypercalcemia associated with cancer. N Engl J Med 2005;352: 373–379.

   This review offers practical updated information on the diagnosis and treatment for patients with hypercalcemia associated with malignancy

26. *(1C+)* **Nussbaum SR** et al. Highly sensitive two-site immunoradiometric assay of parathyrin, and its clinical utility in evaluating patients with hypercalcemia. Clin Chem 1987;33:1364–1367.

   A highly sensitive and specific two-site immunoradiometric for serum PTH is described. There was a complete separation of serum PTH values between 37 patients with surgically proven primary hyperparathyroidism and 23 patients with hypercalcemia of cancer. In hypercalcemia of malignancy, PTH levels were at or below the lower limits of normal. Subsequent studies performed in several hundreds of patients with both syndromes have confirmed these findings.

27. *(1B)* **Ralston SH** et al. Comparison of aminohydroxypropylidene diphosphonate, mithramycin, and corticosteroids/calcitonin in treatment of cancer-associated hypercalcaemia. Lancet 1985;2: 907–910.

   Thirty-nine patients with hypercalcemia due to cancer were randomly assigned to receive aminohydroxypropylidene diphosphonate (pamidronate, 15 mg daily in saline until serum calcium normalized); mithramycin (plicamycin, 25 mg/kg and repeated 48 hours later if serum calcium was still elevated); or calcitonin plus corticosteroids (salmon calcitonin, 400 MRC units every 8 hours, and prednisolone, 40 mg/day). Calcitonin/corticosteroids had the fastest onset of action (<24 hours), but the effects were short-lived, with most patients remaining hypercalcemic during days 6 to 9 after start of treatment. Plicamycin's effect was seen within 48 hours, and it lasted for 6 to 9 days. Pamidronate's effect was at 72 hours, but it lasted for longer than 9 days.

28. *(1A)* **Nussbaum SR** et al. Single-dose intravenous therapy with pamidronate for the treatment of hypercalcemia of malignancy: Comparison of 30-, 60-, and 90-mg dosages. Am J Med 1993; 95:297–304.

   In this double-blind, randomized, multicenter clinical trial, 50 cancer patients with corrected serum calcium above 12 mg/dl were treated with pamidronate, 30, 60, or 90 mg given as a 24-hour infusion. Serum calcium corrected in 40%, 61%, and 100% of patients receiving the 30-, 60-, and 90-mg doses, respectively. The median duration of action was 4, 5, and 6 days in the three groups, respectively.

29. **Body JJ.** Current and future directions in medical therapy: Hypercalcemia. Cancer 2000; 88(suppl):3054–3058.

   This is a review of the current management of hypercalcemia of cancer, including a comparison of the newer second- and third-generation bisphosphonates (e.g., clodronate, pamidronate, ibandronate, zoledronate). After initial hydration, bisphosphonates are the most effective treatments available. Control of the hypercalcemia can be obtained in more than 90% of cases with the use of bisphosphonates.

30. *(1A)* **Major P** et al. Zoledronic acid is superior to pamidronate in the treatment of hypercalcemia of malignancy: A pooled analysis of two randomized, controlled clinical trials. J Clin Oncol 2001;19:558–567.

   In this pooled analysis of two parallel multicenter randomized trials, 275 patients were evaluated for efficacy of 4- or 8-mg zoledronate given as a 5-minute infusion or 90-mg pamidronate given as a 2-hour infusion. The complete response rates by day 10 were 88.4%, 86.7%, and 69.7% for 4-mg zoledronate, 8-mg zoledronate, and 90-mg pamidronate, respectively. The median duration of complete response was 32, 43, and 18 days, respectively. The study indicates that zoledronate, 4 or 8 mg, is superior to pamidronate in the management of hypercalcemia of cancer.

31. *(1A)* **Morony S** et al. The inhibition of RANKL causes greater suppression of bone resorption and hypercalcemia compared with bisphosphonates in two models of humoral hypercalcemia of malignancy. Endocrinology 2005;146:3235–3243.

   The authors used the RANKL inhibitor osteoprotegerin (OPG) to evaluate the role of osteoclast-mediated hypercalcemia in two murine models of HHM. In both models, OPG (0.2–5 mg/kg) caused rapid reversal of established hypercalcemia, and the speed and duration of hypercalcemia suppression were significantly greater with OPG (5 mg/kg) than with high-dose bisphosphonates (pamidronate or zoledronic acid, 5 mg/kg). OPG also caused greater reductions in osteoclast surface and biochemical markers of bone resorption compared with either bisphosphonate. Antiresorptive therapy with a RANKL inhibitor might be a rational approach to controlling HHM.

32. *(1A)* McClung M et al. Denosumab in postmenopausal women with low bone mineral density. N Engl J Med 2006;354:821–831.

In this study, the effects of a fully human monoclonal antibody denosumab (formerly known as AMG 162), which binds RANKL with high affinity and specificity and inhibits RANKL action, on bone mineral density and bone resorption markers in 412 postmenopausal women were tested. Denosumab treatment for 12 months resulted in an increase in bone mineral density and inhibition of bone resorption in a dose-dependent manner, and these effects were greater than those seen with alendronate.

33. *(1C)* **Ralston SH** et al. Cancer-associated hypercalcemia morbidity and mortality: Clinical experience in 126 treated patients. Ann Intern Med 1990;112:499–504.

This was a retrospective analysis of 126 consecutive patients with cancer-associated hypercalcemia in a teaching hospital in the United Kingdom. The study examined the effects of medical calcium-lowering treatment on symptom relief and survival in 126 patients with various cancers (squamous cell lung cancer was the most common with 43 cases and breast cancer the second most common with 22 cases). The survival rate depended on whether specific anticancer therapy was possible (26 patients) in whom the median survival was 135 days compared with a survival of 30 days for those who did not receive anticancer treatment. There were significant palliative benefits from antihypercalcemic therapy. The symptoms of polyuria, constipation, anorexia, nausea/vomiting, and lethargy improved significantly after serum calcium levels were controlled. In many cases, symptoms improved enough to allow patients to be discharged from the hospital.

34. *(1C)* Kristensen B et al. Survival in breast cancer patients after the first episode of hypercalcaemia. J Intern Med 1998;244:189–198.

The study was conducted in a cancer center in Denmark. A consecutive cohort of 212 hypercalcemic breast cancer patients was observed during follow-up to determine survival. Of these, 193 patients had bone metastases and were further analyzed based on serum calcium levels. The patients continued to receive other treatments for cancer. The median survival for the overall group was 6.7 months. The median survival in patients with mild hypercalcemia (ionized calcium, 1.36–1.48 mmol/L; n = 102), moderate hypercalcemia (1.49–1.60 mmol/L; n = 41) and severe hypercalcemia (.1.6 mmol/L; n = 50) were 17.7, 2.8, and 1.4 months, respectively. A second group of 51 hypercalcemic patients who received bisphosphonates was also studied. Survival in this group was not significantly different than in those who did not receive these agents. Survival in breast cancer is decreased significantly in patients with moderate to severe hypercalcemia. It was also shown that bisphosphonate treatment does not prolong survival.

Bisphosphonate Use in Bone Metastasis and Bone Pain

35. *(1C)* Vincenzi B et al. Zoledronic acid-related angiogenesis modifications and survival in advanced breast cancer patients. J Interferon Cytokine Res 2005;25:144–151.

Forty-two consecutive breast cancer patients with scintigraphic and radiographic evidence of bone metastases were treated with a single infusion of 4 mg zoledronic acid before anticancer chemotherapy. There was a significant reduction in circulating levels of VEGF after 21 days in 60% of patients. The analysis of survival showed that patients with a reduction in the circulating VEGF levels had a longer time to first skeletal-related event (p = 0.0002), time to bone progression disease (p = 0.0024), and time to performance status worsening (p = 0.0352) than those without the VEGF reduction.

36. (1A) **Hillner BE** et al. American Society of Clinical Oncology guideline on the role of bisphosphonates in breast cancer: American Society of Clinical Oncology Bisphosphonates Expert Panel. J Clin Oncol 2000;18:1378–1391.

A review of the current literature on the use of bisphosphonates shows no impact on overall survival. The review indicates there are benefits, such as reductions in skeletal complications (i.e., pathologic fractures), surgery for fracture or impending fracture, radiation, spinal cord compression, and hypercalcemia. Intravenous pamidronate, 90 mg delivered over 1 to 2 hours every 3 to 4 weeks, is recommended in patients with metastatic breast cancer who have imaging-confirmed evidence of lytic destruction of bone and who are concurrently receiving systemic therapy with hormonal therapy or chemotherapy. For women with abnormal bone scan results but with no bony destruction revealed by imaging studies and no localized pain, insufficient exists to suggest use of bisphosphonates. Starting bisphosphonate therapy in patients without evidence of bony metastasis, even in the presence of other extraskeletal metastases, is not recommended.

37. *(1A)* Wong R et al. Bisphosphonates for the relief of pain secondary to bone metastases. Cochrane Database Syst Rev 2002;2:CD002068.

This review included 30 randomized controlled studies (21 blinded, four open, and five actively controlled) with a total of 3,682 subjects. In the eight studies in which pain could be evaluated, pooled data showed benefits for the treatment group, with an NNT at 4 weeks of 11 (95% CI, 6–36) and at 12 weeks of 7 (95% CI, 5–12). One study showed a small improvement in quality of life for the treatment group at 4 weeks. Bisphosphonates should be considered as a second-line therapy.

38. *(1A)* **Pavlakis N** et al. Bisphosphonates for breast cancer. Cochrane Database Syst Rev 2005;3: CD003474.

This is an update of the previous review (Cochrane Database Syst Rev. 2002;(1):CD003474.) Twenty-one randomized studies were included. All studies in advanced breast cancer included women with clinically evident bone metastases (osteolytic and/or mixed osteolytic/osteoblastic) by plain radiograph and/or radionucleotide bone scans. Overall, intravenous bisphosphonates reduced the risk of developing a skeletal event by 17% (95% CI, 0.78–0.89) compared with oral bisphosphonates, which reduce the risk of developing a skeletal event by 16% (95% CI, 0.76–0.93). Of the currently available bisphosphonates, 4-mg IV zolendronate reduces the risk of developing a skeletal event by 41% (RR, 0.59; 95% CI, 0.42–0.82), compared with 33% by 90 mg IV pamidronate (RR, 0.77; 95% CI, 0.69–0.87), 18% by 6 mg IV ibandronate (RR, 0.82; 95% CI, 0.67–1.00), 14% by 50 mg oral ibandronate (RR, 0.86; 95% CI, 0.73–1.02) and 16% by 1,600 mg oral clodronate (RR, 0.84; 95% CI, 0.72–0.98). Overall conclusion of the analysis revealed that in women with advanced breast cancer and clinically evident bone metastases, the use of bisphosphonates (oral or intravenous) in addition to hormone therapy or chemotherapy, when compared with placebo or no bisphosphonates, reduces the risk of developing a skeletal event and the skeletal event rate, as well as increasing the time to skeletal event. Some bisphosphonates may also reduce bone pain in women with advanced breast cancer and clinically evident bone metastases and may improve global quality of life. The optimal timing of initiation of bisphosphonate therapy and duration of treatment is uncertain. In women with early breast cancer, the effectiveness of bisphosphonates remains an open question for research.

39. *(1A)* **Djulbegovic B** et al. Bisphosphonates in multiple myeloma. Cochrane Database Syst Rev 2001;4:CD003188.

This systemic review was done to determine whether adding bisphosphonates to standard therapy in multiple myeloma decreases skeletal-related morbidity (i.e., pathologic fractures), skeletal-related mortality, and overall mortality. In addition, the effects of bisphosphonates on pain, quality of life, and incidence of hypercalcemia were examined. Eleven randomized trials with 1,113 patients analyzed as bisphosphonates groups and 1,070 analyzed as control groups were included. The treatment with bisphosphonates resulted in a decrease in the incidence of new vertebral fractures (NNT = 10) and in amelioration of pain (NNT = 11). There was no effect on survival.

Genetics

Peter Kopp

DEFINITION

Genetic components contribute to virtually all disorders, with the exception of simple trauma. Many chromosomal and monogenic disorders can now be explained at the molecular level, permitting us to establish the diagnosis by mutational analysis (Tables 12.1 and 12.2) [1–4]. It is important to recognize that genetic and environmental *modifiers* may also strongly influence the phenotype in monogenic disorders, which simply present the least complex form in a continuum of complex disorders [5]. For example, siblings with identical mutations in the transcription factor PROP1, which lead to combined pituitary hormone deficiency (CPHD) [6], may have variable constellations of anterior pituitary hormone deficiencies, and the onset of the hormonal defects may differ [7]. In phenylketonuria (PKU), the development of the neurologic defects is dependent on the amount of phenylalanine in the diet. In *complex disorders*, also referred to as *polygenic* or *multifactorial* disorders, several or multiple genes contribute to the pathogenesis, typically in conjunction with environmental and life-style factors such as in diabetes mellitus type 2 (see Chapter 6) [5,8–11].

The information about the human genome sequence through the *Human Genome Project* (HGP) is facilitating genetic analyses substantially [5,9,12], and the ongoing advances in the functional characterization of the human genome, transcriptome, and proteome are fundamentally changing our understanding of the molecular mechanisms underlying (patho)physiologic processes [12]. Ongoing efforts such as the *HapMap* project will facilitate the understanding of complex disorders [13]. The HapMap project has determined single-nucleotide polymorphisms (SNPs), variants that occur on average every 300 base pairs (bp) throughout the genome, in DNA samples from multiple individuals from four different ethnic backgrounds. Adjacent SNPs are inherited together as blocks, referred to as haplotypes; hence the name HapMap. These blocks can be identified by selected marker SNPs, so called Tag SNPs. The availability of this information permits characterizing a limited number of SNPs to determine the set of haplotypes present in an individual (e.g., in cases and controls). This, in turn, will now permit performing genome-wide association studies by searching for associations of certain haplotypes with a disease phenotype of interest, an essential step for unraveling the genetic factors contributing to complex disorders.

Table 12.1.   Chromosomal Disorders with Endocrine Manifestations

Disorder	Phenotype	Chromosomal Defect	OMIM
Turner syndrome	Ovarian failure, short stature, autoimmune thyroid disease	45,XO	
Klinefelter syndrome	Hypogonadism, tall stature	47,XXY	
Prader-Willi syndrome	Short stature, obesity, hypogonadism	del15 q11–13 (paternal copy) Maternal uniparental disomy	176270

Because *somatic* mutations in genes controlling cell growth, survival, and differentiation are key elements in the pathogenesis of neoplasia, benign and malignant tumors can also be viewed as genetic disorders [5,10,14]. Moreover, many cancers are associated with a predisposition conferred by hereditary *germline* mutations. The multiple endocrine neoplasia syndromes 1 and 2 (MEN 1 and MEN 2) are excellent examples to illustrate this (see Table 12.2) [15]. MEN 2 also highlights the impact of genetic analysis for carrier detection in the clinical management of families with this tumor syndrome (Chapter 9) [15]. A thorough understanding of the molecular pathogenesis of cancer also is of paramount importance for the development of novel therapeutic modalities. The mutations in the tyrosine kinase RET causing MEN 2 [15], or the serine-threonine kinase B-Raf found frequently in papillary thyroid cancers [16], make them attractive targets for therapy with kinase inhibitors [17], a paradigm shown to be successful in chronic myelogenous leukemia by the specific inhibition of the Bcr-Abl tyrosine kinase through imatinib [18].

Numerous endocrine disorders have been elucidated at the molecular level [2–5,19]. For comprehensive overviews, and for the discussion of the principles of human genetics, DNA structure and molecular biology analyses, which are beyond the scope of this chapter, the reader is referred to several comprehensive reviews and textbooks [5,8,10,20].

ETIOLOGY

Mutations in DNA cause alterations and abnormal function in the encoded RNA and protein products, thereby leading to disease [21]. Mutations can occur randomly or through factors such as radiation and chemicals. Mutations occurring in the germline (sperm or oocytes) can be transmitted to progeny. If the germline is mosaic, a mutation can be transmitted to some offspring but not to others [5]. Mutations occurring during early development lead to somatic *mosaicism*, as illustrated by the McCune–Albright syndrome [22]. Somatic mutations conferring a growth advantage to cells, or a decrease in apoptosis, can be associated with neoplasia [14]. Epigenetic alterations (e.g., altered DNA methylation) is also frequently found in malignancies and can result in altered gene expression [14]. With the exception of triplet nucleotide repeats [5], which can progressively expand, mutations are usually stable.

Structurally, mutations are extremely diverse [21]. They can involve the entire genome, as in triploidy, or gross numeric or structural alterations in chromosomes or individual genes [8,19]. Large deletions may affect a part of a gene, an entire gene, or several genes (*contiguous gene syndrome*). Mutations affecting single nucleotides are referred to as *point mutations*. A mutation in the coding region leading to an amino acid substitution is referred to as *missense mutation*, and a mutation resulting in a stop codon is a *nonsense mutation*. Small nucleotide deletions or insertions cause a shift of the reading frame (*frameshift*), and this typically results in an abnormal protein of variable length after the deletion. It is not sufficiently appreciated that mutations also occur in noncoding regions. Mutations in intronic sequences may destroy or create splice-donor or splice-acceptor sites, and mutations in regulatory sequences result in altered gene transcription.

EPIDEMIOLOGY

The frequency of monogenic disorders is highly variable [21]. Some monogenic disorders are extremely rare. Many recessive disorders occur in only inbred populations or consanguineous matings. In many dominant and X-linked disorders, *de novo* mutations account for a significant fraction of cases [5,8,10]. The rates for new mutations for autosomal dominant and X-linked disorders are estimated to be about 10^{-5} to 10^{-6}/locus per generation. Other monogenic disorders are, however, relatively frequent. The classic examples include cystic fibrosis (Northern European populations), the thalassemias (Mediterranean, Southeast Asia), and sickle cell trait/disease (West Africa) [1]. It is generally thought that accumulation of these deleterious alleles in a population is due to a selective advantage in heterozygotes. For example, heterozygotes for the sickle cell mutation have a reduced morbidity and mortality from malaria because their erythrocytes provide a less-favorable environment for *Plasmodium* parasites.

The distribution patterns of different genotypes in a population is the focus of population genetics [8,10]. If the frequency of an allele is known, and assuming that the population is in a state of equilibrium, the frequency of the genotypes can be determined (*Hardy–Weinberg theorem*). This is useful for the calculations of carrier frequencies, disease prevalence, and estimates of penetrance. The equilibrium can be modified by migration, new mutation(s), and genetic drift (i.e., random fluctuations in allele frequencies in small populations).

The genetic epidemiology of complex disorders is challenging because several or multiple loci may contribute to the phenotype, and that it is influenced by multiple gene–gene and gene–environment interactions. In the endocrine field, this is impressively illustrated by our current understanding of the genetics of diabetes mellitus (Chapter 6) (11). The monogenic autosomal-dominant forms of diabetes (MODY 1 to 6; maturity-onset diabetes of the young) have been elucidated at the molecular level and are caused by severe mutations in genes that are essential for development and/or function of the pancreatic beta cell [23]. These mutations are rare in the population. In contrast, our knowledge about the genetic basis of diabetes mellitus type 2 remains relatively modest [11]. This may be explained by the difficulty in detecting alleles that contribute only mildly to the phenotype, and the fact that these alleles are frequent in the general population. Moreover, one should recognize that the clinical diagnosis of diabetes mellitus type 2 may encompass various entities of impaired insulin action and secretion, and that the elucidation of the genetic components will require more homogeneous collections of patients.

PATHOPHYSIOLOGY

Very broadly, endocrine disorders can be categorized into four major types of conditions: (a) hormone excess, (b) hormone deficiency, (c) hormone resistance, and (d) tumors of endocrine glands without alterations of hormone secretion [2]. Numerous conditions in these categories have recently been explained by mutations in genes involved in growth or function of endocrine tissues, thereby leading to a better understanding of the pathophysiology at the molecular level, and often providing a means for accurate diagnosis [2–4,24].

The functional consequences of mutations can be broadly classified as gain-of-function and loss-of-function mutations [5]. Gain-of-function mutations are typically dominant. In contrast, inactivating mutations are usually recessive, and affected individuals are homozygous or compound heterozygous (i.e., carrying two different mutant alleles in the same gene) for the disease-causing mutations. Alternatively, a mutation in a single allele can result in *haploinsufficiency*, a situation in which one

Table 12.2. Molecular Basis of Selected Endocrine Disorders

Disorder/Phenotype[a]	Gene	Inheritance	OMIM
Hypothalamic and pituitary disorders			
CPHD (GH, PRL, TSH, LH, FSH)	PROP1	AR	601538
Short stature	GH	AR, AD	139250
Neurohypophyseal diabetes insipidus	AVP-NPII	AD, AR	192340
Obesity	Leptin receptor	AR	601007
Thyroid			
Congenital hypothyroidism with thyroid hypoplasia	PAX8	AD	167415
Bamforth–Lazarus syndrome: congenital hypothyroidism, cleft palate, spiky hair	TTF2 (FOXE1)	AR	602617
Pendred syndrome: sensorineural deafness, impaired iodide organification	PDS (SLC26A4)	AR	274600
Congenital hypothyroidism, thyroglobulin defects	TG	AR	188450
Resistance to thyroid hormone	THRB	AD, (AR)	190160
Parathyroid and bone disorders			
Familial benign hypocalciuric hypercalcemia	CASR	AD	601199
Familial hypoparathyroidism	CASR	AD	601199
Albright hereditary osteodystrophy	GNAS1	AD	103580
Adrenal gland			
Congenital adrenal hyperplasia, 21-hydroxlyase	CYP21	AR	201910
Glucocorticoid-remediable aldosteronism	CYP11B2-CYP11B1 fusion gene	AD	103900
Adrenal hypoplasia, congenital hypogonadism	DAX1 (NROB1)	X	300473

Disorder/Phenotype[a]	Gene	Inheritance	OMIM
Pancreas			
MODY 1	HNF4α	AD	125850
MODY 2	GCK	AD (inactivating mutations)	125851
MODY 3	HNF1α	AD	600496
MODY 4, renal cysts	IPF1	AD	606392
MODY 5	HNF1β	AD	604284
MODY 6	NEUROD1	AD	606394
Pancreas agenesis	IPF1	AR	600733
Gonads			
Androgen insensitivity, androgen-receptor inactivation	AR	AR	300068
Androgen insensitivity, 5α-reductase deficiency	SRD5A2	AR	607306
Aromatase deficiency, female genitalia with masculinization during puberty	CYP19A1	AR	107910
Water and salt metabolism			
Nephrogenic diabetes insipidus (X-linked form)	AVPR2	X	304800
Nephrogenic diabetes insipidus	AQP2	AR, AD	107777
Liddle syndrome: hypokalemic metabolic acidosis, hypertension	SCNN1B or SCNN1G	AD	177200

continued

Table 12.2. *Continued*

Disorder/Phenotype[a]	Gene	Inheritance	OMIM
Lipid metabolism			
Obesity	LEP	Leptin	164160
Familial hypercholesterinemia	LDLR	AD	606945
Tumor syndromes			
Multiple endocrine neoplasia 1	MEN 1	AD	131100
Parathyroid adenoma, pituitary adenoma, pancreas tumors			
Multiple endocrine neoplasia 2	RET	AD	171400
A. Medullary thyroid cancer, pheochromocytoma, parathyroid hyperplasia. B. + ganglioneuromas			
Von Hippel–Lindau disease	VHL	AD	193300
Renal carcinomas, pheochromocytomas, other tumors			
Somatic mosaicism			
McCune–Albright syndrome: precocious puberty, fibrous dysplasia, café-au-lait spots, hyperthyroidism	GNAS1	Mosaic somatic mutation acquired in early development	174800
Complex syndromes			
Autoimmune polyglandular syndrome type 1: adrenal insufficiency, hypoparathyroidism, candidiasis	AIRE	AR	240300

Disorder/Phenotype[a]	Gene	Inheritance	OMIM
Complex disorders			
Diabetes mellitus type 1	HLA DR3/4-DQ201/0302, HLA DR4/4-DQ0300/03022, HLA DR3/3-DQ0201/0201		222100
	Insulin VNTR, NEUROD, CTLA4		
	Multiple others		
Diabetes mellitus type 2	CPN10, PPAR···INS, SUR1, IPF1, IRS-1		125853
	Multiple others		

[a]This list contains only selected examples. In addition, the reader should be aware that the same or similar phenotype can be caused by mutations in other genes.
AD, autosomal dominant; AR autosomal recessive; X, X-chromosomal; CPHD, combined pituitary hormone deficiency.
Modified from Kopp P. Genetics, genomics, proteomics, and bioinformatics. In: Brook GD, Brown R (eds). Clinical pediatric endocrinology, 5th ed. Blackwell Science, Oxford, 2005, pp. 18–44.

normal allele is not sufficient to maintain a normal phenotype, and this may result in dominant inheritance [5]. Haploinsufficiency is a frequently observed mechanism in diseases associated with mutations in transcription factors or rate-limiting enzymes [25–27]. Mutation in a single allele can also result in loss of function through a dominant-negative effect [28,29]. In this case, the mutated allele interferes with the function of the normal gene product by one of several different mechanisms: a) the mutant protein may interfere with other members of a multimeric protein complex, as illustrated by mutations in aquaporin 2 in the autosomal dominant form of nephrogenic diabetes insipidus [29,30]; b) the mutant protein may occupy binding sites on proteins or promoter response elements, as illustrated by thyroid hormone resistance [28]; or c) the mutant protein can be cytotoxic, as, for example, in autosomal dominant neuro-hypophyseal diabetes insipidus [31], in which the abnormally folded proteins are trapped within the endoplasmic reticulum, thereby leading to progressive destruction of vasopressin-secreting neurons.

DIAGNOSIS

Approach to the Patient

It cannot be emphasized enough that a careful clinical examination with thorough phenotyping, using appropriate biochemical and ancillary tests, is absolutely essential [32]. One should always be aware of the possibility of *phenocopies,* i.e., a phenotype that is identical or similar to the suspected disorder, but that has a distinct genetic or nongenetic pathogenesis [33]. For example, obesity may be simply the consequence of life-style factors, but it can also be caused by several Mendelian defects (Chapter 34) [34]. The presence of phenocopies in a family can be problematic because it can confound linkage studies and genetic testing.

The family history is of great importance for the recognition of a hereditary component. It should include the establishment of a pedigree of the nuclear or the extended family [5,8,10]. The history, in combination with the pedigree, may become of practical relevance for genetic counseling, carrier detection, quantitative risk estimation for individuals within the kindred, or early intervention and prevention of a disease in relatives of the index patient(s). However, a precise risk estimate is often possible only after genetic testing. The ethnic background is relevant because certain alleles are more common in certain populations.

When evaluating relatives of an index patient with a genetic disorder, the phenomena of variable *expressivity* and *incomplete penetrance* should always be considered [5]. Penetrance is complete if all carriers of a given mutation express the phenotype, and *incomplete* if some individuals do not express the phenotype. Incomplete penetrance is characterized by a disease phenotype skipping generations, with unaffected carriers transmitting the mutant gene. Expressivity describes the degree to which a phenotype is expressed, the *phenotypic spectrum.* The mechanisms resulting in variable expressivity and incomplete penetrance include the need for modifiers such as *genetic background*, gender, and environmental factors, emphasizing again that these factors play a prominent role not only in complex disorders, but also in Mendelian traits.

Phenotypic heterogeneity may also arise from differences in the effect of mutations at different sites within the same gene. This is well illustrated by mutations in the androgen receptor; mild mutations may cause epispadias, whereas severe inactivation of the receptor results in complete resistance to testosterone with testicular feminization [35].

Information about Genetic Disorders

If a clinician seeks information about a genetic disorder, or a particular nonsyndromic or syndromic phenotype, consultation of the continuously updated *Online Mendelian Inheritance in Man* (OMIM) catalogue (http://www.ncbi.nlm.nih.gov/omim/) is an excellent starting point (Table 12.3). OMIM lists several thousand genetic disorders, and it provides information about the clinical phenotype, the molecular basis, allelic variants, relevant animal models, and pertinent references. Embedded links to other electronic resources (e.g., PubMed for literature searches, GenBank for sequence in-

Table 12.3. Selected Genetics Databases

Site	Content	URL
OMIM Online Mendelian Inheritance in Man	Catalog of human genetic disorders	http://www.ncbi.nlm.nih.gov/omim/
National Center for Biotechnology Information (NCBI)	Portal with links to genomic databases, PubMed, OMIM, and educational on-line resources	http://www.ncbi.nlm.nih.gov/
GeneTests	Directory of laboratories offering genetic testing	http://www.genetests.org/
GeneCards	A database of human genes and their role in disease	http://bioinformatics.weizmann.ac.il/cards/
American College of Medical Genetics	Portal with databases relevant for the diagnosis, treatment, and prevention of genetic diseases	http://www.acmg.net/
Chromosomal Variation in Man	Catalog of chromosomal disorders	http://www.wiley.com/legacy/products/subject/life/borgaonkar/access.html
Mitochondrial Disorders	Catalog of disorders associated with mitochondrial DNA mutations	http://www.neuro.wustl.edu/neuromuscular/mitosyn.html
DNA Repeat Sequences & Disease	Catalog of disorders associated with DNA repeats	http://www.neuro.wustl.edu/neuromuscular/mother/dnarep.htm
National Organization for Rare Disorders	Catalog of rare disorders including clinical presentation, diagnostic evaluation, and treatment	http://www.rarediseases.org/
HapMap Project Web	Portal to the International Haplotype Map Project	http://www.hapmap.org

formation, databases compiling gene mutations) provide relevant information for both clinicians and basic researchers. Selected additional databases that provide relevant information are listed in Table 12.3, and several recent textbook chapters discuss the genetic etiology and mechanisms underlying endocrine disorders [2–4].

Genetic Counseling

Consultation with a medical geneticist and/or medical counselor is often indicated for the management of patients with a sporadic or inherited genetic disorder [36,37]. This is helpful for diagnostic purposes, the identification of management issues, and determination of genetic risk in relatives and offspring. It may also be of importance for appropriate psychological support.

Genetic Testing

Genetic testing aims at detecting (molecular) alterations associated with inherited or sporadic disorders. Depending on the test, it will be performed with sources such as metaphase chromosomes, genomic or mitochondrial DNA, RNA, chromosomes, proteins, or metabolites [5,8,10,20]. Different clinically relevant forms of genetic testing include preimplantation testing, prenatal testing, newborn screening, carrier screening, diagnostic testing, paternity/maternity tests, and zygosity tests. Research and investigational tests are important for improving the understanding of rare conditions or developing clinical tests, but the results may not always be available to the patient and the physician.

Diagnostic molecular testing should be performed to confirm, or exclude, a diagnosis relying on clinical evaluation and biochemical testing. Information of the exact genetic defect can be of value because it can provide certainty about the diagnosis; it may allow prediction about the clinical course and serve as a basis for genetic counseling and molecular diagnosis in other family members or future pregnancies.

Predictive testing or carrier screening permits the identification of individuals who are carriers of a mutation, and similarly to determine who is not at risk because of absence of the mutation. This is exemplified by the analysis of children of families with MEN 2 (Chapter 9) [15].

If genetic testing is considered, the proband and the family should be carefully informed about the potential consequences of positive results, including psychological distress and the possibility of discrimination. Equally important is the discussion of the meaning of negative results. This should also include a discussion of false-negative or inconclusive results, and technical limitations of the tests. For these reasons, genetic testing should be performed only after obtaining informed consent. Genetic testing in children poses additional ethical issues. Ethical guidelines published by the American Society of Human Genetics and the American Academy of Pediatrics address aspects that should be considered when testing children and adolescents [38,39]. Unless the analysis may provide relevant insights into the molecular pathogenesis of a disorder, it should be limited to situations in which the results may have an impact on the medical management, and it requires informed consent by the parents. If no apparent benefit is possible, testing should usually be deferred until the patient can consent independently. This is, for example, of relevance in devastating disorders such as Huntington disease.

Sample Collection

Sample collection is dependent on the nature of the test and must be performed according to instructions by the laboratory performing the analysis [40]. If a disease-causing mutation is expected because of germline transmission, DNA is most commonly collected from nucleated blood cells, and typically 5 ml of EDTA is sufficient for this purpose. In the case of somatic mutations, which are limited to the affected tissue, an adequate sample of the lesion will serve for the extraction of DNA or RNA. RNA degrades very quickly, and the sample serving for its extraction has to be frozen or immersed in special solutions immediately. For cytogenetic analyses, cells are often collected from peripheral blood or buccal smears, but other tissues can also serve as source. Biochemical tests continue to play an important role in the analysis of metabolic disorders and will require appropriate collection of plasma, serum, or urine. For the detection of pathogens, the material to be analyzed will vary and may include blood, cerebrospinal fluid, solid tissues, sputum, or fluid obtained through bronchioalveolar lavage.

Laboratories Performing Genetic Tests

Genetic testing is becoming more readily available through commercial laboratories for a number of endocrine disorders [e.g., MEN 2, congenital adrenal hyperplasia (CAH), the various forms of MODY, or nephrogenic and autosomal dominant neurohypophyseal diabetes insipidus]. For rare disorders, the test may be performed only in a specialized laboratory. The *GeneTests* web site (http://www.genetests.org/servlet/access), a publicly funded medical genetics information resource, contains a Laboratory Directory that is useful for identifying CLIA (Clinical Laboratory Improvement Amendments)-approved laboratories offering testing for inherited disorders (Table 12-3). For other rare disorders, the test may be available only through research laboratories.

Practical Limitations of Genetic Testing

The public, as well as many physicians, are not aware of certain conceptual and technical challenges that may be associated with genetic testing. Aside from issues related to sample management and technical errors, they include, among others, the possibility of *locus heterogeneity, allelic heterogeneity,* and the possibility of *polymorphisms* [2,5,8,10].

Locus heterogeneity, also referred to as nonallelic heterogeneity, designates the fact that an identical or highly similar phenotype may result from mutations in different genes located at different loci within the genome. Congenital hypothyroidism due to defects in thyroid hormone synthesis within the thyrocyte can be caused by mutations in several genes encoding proteins that exert key steps in this process (*NIS,* sodium/iodide symporter; *PDS/SLC26A4,* pendrin; *TPO,* thyroid peroxidase; *TG,* thyroglobulin; *THOX2,* thyroid oxidase 2) [41]. In such a situation, genetic testing is complex and expensive because several different genes must be analyzed. Locus heterogeneity can also cause a problem for linkage studies because it can reduce the ability to identify disease loci.

Allelic heterogeneity indicates that different mutations in the same gene can cause an identical or similar phenotype. For example, more than 1,420 mutations are known in the CFTR gene (Cystic Fibrosis Mutation Database: http://www.genet.sickkids. on.ca/cftr/). Although an initial analysis will focus on mutations that are particularly frequent, a negative result does not exclude the presence of a mutation elsewhere in the gene. One should also be aware that mutational analyses are usually focusing on the coding region of a gene without considering regulatory and intronic regions. Given that disease-causing mutations may be located outside the coding regions, any negative results may have to be interpreted with caution. The development of novel and cheaper sequencing technologies is therefore necessary.

Polymorphisms are sequence variations that may occur more or less frequently in the genome of the general population. Many of them do not have any functional consequences, but others may lead to subtle functional alterations in the gene product (mRNA or protein). Whereas frequently occurring polymorphisms can be detected relatively easily by assessing their presence in a cohort of unrelated normal individuals, rare polymorphisms require rigorous functional analyses in vitro to distinguish them from disease-causing mutations.

TREATMENT

Given the broad spectrum of disorders with a genetic component or a genetic basis, a discussion of the appropriate treatments is beyond the scope of this chapter. Similarly, a discussion of gene therapy, the transfer of genetic material into a patient [42], which is still in early experimental stages, cannot be discussed here. It should be recognized that molecular genetics already has a significant impact on the treatment of human disease. Peptide hormones (*insulin, growth hormone, erythropoietin, thyrotropin, parathyroid hormone*), growth factors (*colony-stimulating factors*), cytokines (*interferons*), or vaccines (*hepatitis B*) can now be produced in large amounts by using recombinant DNA technology. Targeted modification of these peptides provides the practitioner with improved therapies, as illustrated by genetically modified insulin analogues with altered kinetics [54]. The targeted design of specific inhibitors, best illustrated by imatinib as inhibitor of the Bcr-Abl tyrosine kinase [18], serves as proof of principle that the elucidation of the molecular pathogenesis is of great importance for the development of novel therapeutic modalities.

ACKNOWLEDGMENTS

This work has been supported by 1R01 DK63024-01 from NIDDK/National Institutes of Health.

REFERENCES

1. **Scriver CR** et al., eds. The metabolic and molecular bases of inherited disease. 8th ed. McGraw-Hill, New York, 2000.

   A comprehensive textbook with outstanding chapters about inherited disorders.

2. **Jameson JL, Kopp P.** Applications of molecular biology and genetics in endocrinology. In: DeGroot LD, Jameson JL eds. Endocrinology. 5th ed. WB Saunders, Philadelphia, 2006, pp. 83–108.

   A review presenting important principles of molecular biology together with a detailed discussion of the molecular basis of many endocrine disorders.

3. **Kopp P.** Genetics, genomics, proteomics, and bioinformatics. In: Brook GD, Brown R, eds. Clinical pediatric endocrinology. 5th ed. Blackwell Science, Oxford, 2005, pp. 18–44.

   A detailed review containing multiple tables summarizing the molecular basis of endocrine disorders.

4. **Potter AE, Phillips JA.** Genetic disorders in pediatric endocrinology. In: Pescovitz OH, Eugster EA, eds. Pediatric endocrinology: Mechanisms and management. Lippincott Williams & Wilkins, Philadelphia, 2004, pp. 1–23.

   A review with a discussion of the molecular basis of many important pediatric disorders and useful tables.

5. **Kopp P, Jameson JL.** Principles of human genetics. In: Braunwald E et al., eds. Harrison's principles of internal medicine. 16th ed. McGraw-Hill, New York, 2004, pp. 359–379.

   A chapter covering the essential elements necessary for the understanding of principles of molecular biology and inherited disease.

6. **Moseley CT, Phillips JA.** Pituitary gene mutations and the growth hormone pathway. Semin Reprod Med 2000;18:21–29.

   A review on dwarfism discussing isolated growth hormone deficiency (IGHD), combined pituitary hormone deficiency (CPHD), and resistance to growth hormone (GH) due to GH receptor and insulin-like growth factor 1 (IGF1) defects.

7. *(1C1)* **Fluck C** et al. Phenotypic variability in familial combined pituitary hormone deficiency caused by a PROP1 gene mutation resulting in the substitution of Arg→Cys at codon 120 (R120C). J Clin Endocrinol Metab 1998;83:3727–3734.

   In this study, five subjects with combined pituitary hormone deficiency (CPHD) caused by the same mutation in the transcription factor PROP1 (R120C) from two consanguineous families were followed longitudinally. The study highlights that there is variability in the phenotype in terms of hormone deficiencies, and that the temporal onset of the defects is also variable.

8. **Gelehrter TD** et al., eds. Principles of medical genetics. 2nd ed. Lippincott Williams & Wilkins, Philadelphia, 1998.

   An excellent and balanced introduction into principles of medical genetics.

9. **Guttmacher AE, Collins FS.** Genomic medicine: A primer. N Engl J Med 2002;347:1512–1520.

   A short summary and outlook about the impact of genomic medicine.

10. **Nussbaum RL** et al., ed. Thompson and Thompson genetics in medicine. 6th ed. Elsevier Science, New York, 2001.

    An excellent introduction to principles of medical genetics.

11. **Florez JC** et al. The inherited basis of diabetes mellitus: Implications for the genetic analysis of complex traits. Annu Rev Genomics Hum Genet 2003;4:257–291.

    A detailed discussion of the genetics of monogenic forms of diabetes mellitus, as well as of diabetes mellitus type 1 and type 2. The discussion highlights challenges associated with the elucidation of complex disorders.

12. **Collins FS** et al. A vision for the future of genomics research. Nature 2003;422:835–847.

An excellent overview about landmarks in genetics and genomics, and a vision of the impacts of genomics on biology, health, and society.

13. *(1C1)* **Altshuler D** et al. A haplotype map of the human genome. Nature 2005;437:1299–1320.

This study presents the HapMap database of common variation in the human genome. More than one million single nucleotide polymorphisms (SNPs) were obtained in 269 DNA samples from four populations. These data document the generality of recombination hotspots, a block-like structure of linkage disequilibrium and low haplotype diversity, leading to substantial correlations of SNPs with many of their neighbors. The study shows how the HapMap resource can guide the design and analysis of genetic association studies, shed light on structural variation and recombination, and identify loci that may have been subject to natural selection during human evolution.

14. **Balmain A** et al. The genetics and genomics of cancer. Nat Genet 2003;33:238–244.

A good review of principles of cancer genetics.

15. *(1C1)* **Brandi ML** et al. Guidelines for diagnosis and therapy of MEN type 1 and type 2. J Clin Endocrinol Metab 2001;86:5658–5671.

This is a consensus statement from an international group summarizing current recommendations for the diagnosis, management, and surveillance of patients with MEN 1 and MEN 2.

16. *(1C)* **Kimura ET** et al. High prevalence of BRAF mutations in thyroid cancer: Genetic evidence for constitutive activation of the RET/PTC-RAS-BRAF signaling pathway in papillary thyroid carcinoma. Cancer Res 2003;63:1454–1457.

This study demonstrated somatic mutations in B-RAF (V599E) in 35.8% of papillary thyroid cancers. Moreover, the study demonstrated that cancers harboring B-RAF mutations do not contain mutations in other proteins of the same signaling pathway such as RET/PTC and RAS.

17. **Fagin JA.** How thyroid tumors start and why it matters: Kinase mutants as targets for solid cancer pharmacotherapy. J Endocrinol 2004;183:249–256.

An excellent review about molecular alterations found in thyroid cancers and their potential impact for the development of novel therapeutic modalities.

18. **Druker BJ** et al. Effects of a selective inhibitor of the Abl tyrosine kinase on the growth of Bcr-Abl positive cells. Nat Med 1996;2:561–566.

This important study showed that imatinib, an inhibitor of the Abl protein tyrosine kinase, decreases cellular proliferation and tumor formation by Bcr-Abl–expressing cells. In colony-forming assays of cells obtained from patients with chronic myelogenous leukemia, colony formation could be inhibited in 92%–98%. The authors concluded that "this compound may be useful in the treatment of bcr-abl–positive leukemias," a prediction that has been fulfilled.

19. **Fechner PY.** Genetic syndromes with endocrinopathies. In: Pescovitz OH, Eugster EA, eds. Pediatric endocrinology: Mechanisms and management. Lippincott Williams & Wilkins, Philadelphia, 2004, pp. 24–34.

A short overview on genetic syndromes with endocrine components.

20. **Jameson JL.** Application of molecular biology and genetics in endocrinology. In: DeGroot L, Jameson J, eds. Endocrinology. 4th ed. Saunders, Philadelphia, 2001, pp. 143–166.

An overview on the principles of molecular biology and selected techniques.

21. **Antonarakis SE** et al. The nature and mechanisms of human gene mutations. In: Scriver CR et al., eds. The metabolic and molecular bases of inherited disease. 8th ed. McGraw-Hill, New York, 2000, pp. 343–377.

A detailed discussion of the mechanisms and consequences of DNA mutations.

22. *(1C1)* **Weinstein LS** et al. Activating mutations of the stimulatory G protein in the McCune-Albright syndrome. N Engl J Med 1991;325:1688–1695.

This study reported the molecular basis of McCune-Albright syndrome (MAS) (i.e., somatic mutations in the GNAS1 gene, which encodes the stimulatory G a subunit). These patients are mosaic for these mutations, which occur early in development. The mosaicism explains the highly variable phenotype in MAS patients.

23. **Hattersley AT.** Molecular genetics goes to the diabetes clinic. Clin Med 2005;5:476–481.

This review discusses how molecular genetic testing can be used to make a diagnosis of the 1% to 2% of all diabetic patients with monogenic diabetes. Making a diagnosis of monogenic diabetes is relevant because it may have therapeutic consequences. Glucokinase MODY patients need no treatment, HNF1a MODY patients are very sensitive to low-dose sulfonylureas, and patients with neonatal diabetes due to Kir6.2 mutations, despite being insulin dependent, can discontinue insulin and be well controlled on high-dose sulfonylurea tablets.

24. **Marx SJ, Simonds WF.** Hereditary hormone excess: Genes, molecular pathways, and syndromes. Endocr Rev 2005;26:615–661.

A good discussion of genetic disorders resulting in syndromes of hormone excess.

25. **Seidman JG, Seidman C**. Transcription factor haploinsufficiency: When half a loaf is not enough. J Clin Invest 2002;109:451–455.

   This short overview highlights the importance of mutations in transcription factors leading to haploinsufficiency as a cause of genetic disorders.

26. **De Felice M, Di Lauro R**. Thyroid development and its disorders: Genetics and molecular mechanisms. Endocr Rev 2004;25:722–746.

   This review discusses the molecular basis of thyroid development and the developmental defects associated with congenital hypothyroidism.

27. **New MI**. An update of congenital adrenal hyperplasia. Ann N Y Acad Sci 2004;1038:14–43.

   A comprehensive review of clinical, genetic, epidemiologic, and therapeutic aspects of congenital adrenal hyperplasia (CAH).

28. **Refetoff S** et al. The syndromes of resistance to thyroid hormone. Endocr Rev 1993;14:348–399.

   A comprehensive review of resistance to thyroid hormone.

29. *(1C1)* **Mulders SM** et al. An aquaporin-2 water channel mutant which causes autosomal dominant nephrogenic diabetes insipidus is retained in the Golgi complex. J Clin Invest 1998;102:57–66.

   Mutations in the aquaporin-2 (AQP2) water channel gene cause autosomal recessive nephrogenic diabetes insipidus (NDI). In this study, a mutation in the carboxyterminal tail of AQP2 (E258K) was found to cause an autosomal dominant form of NDI. The mutant had a dominant-negative effect on the water permeability conferred by wild-type AQP2. Immunoblot and microscopic analyses revealed that AQP2-E258K was, in contrast to AQP2 mutants in recessive NDI, not retarded in the endoplasmic reticulum, but retained in the Golgi compartment. Because AQPs are thought to tetramerize, the dominant inheritance of NDI in this patient appears to be caused by the retention of the wild type through the mutant. The study illustrates that different mutations in the same protein may have variable functional consequences, thereby resulting in different patterns of inheritance.

30. **Morello JP, Bichet DG**. Nephrogenic diabetes insipidus. Annu Rev Physiol 2001;63:607–630.

   A comprehensive review of clinical, genetic, epidemiologic, and therapeutic aspects of the various forms of nephrogenic diabetes insipidus (NDI).

31. *(1C1)* **Ito M** et al. Molecular basis of autosomal dominant neurohypophyseal diabetes insipidus: Cellular toxicity caused by the accumulation of mutant vasopressin precursors within the endoplasmic reticulum. J Clin Invest 1997;99:1897–1905.

   Mutations in the arginine vasopressin (AVP) gene cause autosomal dominant familial neurohypophyseal diabetes insipidus (FNDI). In this study, wild-type or several different mutant AVP genes were stably expressed in neuro2A neuroblastoma cells. Each of the mutants caused exhibited diminished intracellular trafficking of mutant AVP precursors, resulting in inefficient secretion of immunoreactive AVP. Immunofluorescence studies demonstrated marked accumulation of mutant AVP precursors within the endoplasmic reticulum, and the cells showed reduced viability. The study provides evidence that the dominant inheritance is caused by neuronal toxicity of the mutant proteins.

32. **Aylsworth AS**. Defining disease phenotypes. In: Haines JL, Pericak-Vance MA, eds. Gene mapping in complex human diseases. Wiley-Liss, New York, 1998, pp. 53–76.

   A practical overview discussing the approach to the patient and phenotype definition.

33. *(1C1)* **Kopp P** et al. Phenocopies for deafness and goiter development in a large inbred Brazilian kindred with Pendred's syndrome associated with a novel mutation in the PDS gene. J Clin Endocrinol Metab 1999;84:336–341.

   In this study, 41 individuals from a large, highly inbred pedigree from Northeastern Brazil were examined for features of Pendred syndrome (goiter, impaired iodide organification, and congenital sensorineural deafness). Linkage studies and sequence analysis of the coding region of the PDS gene were performed with DNA from 36 individuals. The index patient, with the classical triad of deafness, positive perchlorate test, and goiter, was found to be homozygous for a mutation resulting in a frameshift and a premature stop codon. Two other patients with deafness were found to be homozygous for this mutation; 19 were heterozygous and 14 were homozygous for the wild type allele. Surprisingly, six deaf individuals in this kindred were not homozygous for the PDS gene mutation; three were heterozygous and three were homozygous for the wild-type allele, suggesting a probable distinct genetic cause for their deafness. All three homozygous individuals for the PDS mutation had goiters. However, goiters were also found in 10 heterozygous individuals and in six individuals without the PDS mutation and are most likely caused by iodine deficiency. The comparison of phenotype and genotype revealed that phenocopies generated by distinct environmental and/or genetic causes are present in this kindred and that the diagnosis of Pendred syndrome may be difficult without molecular analysis.

34. **Farooqi IS, O'Rahilly S**. Monogenic obesity in humans. Annu Rev Med 2005;56:443–458.

   This review discusses the monogenic forms of obesity, in particular the disorders that result from genetic disruption of the leptin–melanocortin pathway, but also other syndromic forms of obesity. The review contains pictures illustrating the dramatic consequences of these mutations.

35. **McPhaul MJ** et al. Genetic basis of endocrine disease, 4: The spectrum of mutations in the androgen receptor gene that causes androgen resistance. J Clin Endocrinol Metab 1993;76:17–23.

This older review illustrates that mutations in the androgen receptor (AR) gene cause a wide spectrum of phenotypic abnormalities ranging from a female phenotype (i.e., complete testicular feminization) to that of undervirilized or infertile men.

36. **Fine BA**. Genetic counseling. In: Jameson JL, ed. Principles of molecular medicine. Humana Press, Totowa, 1998, pp. 89–95.

A short overview on the profession of genetic counselor, the counseling process, and aspects of training.

37. **Harper P**. Practical genetic counseling. 5th ed. Oxford University Press, New York, 2004.

A handbook covering all aspects of genetic counseling.

38. *(1C1)* **American Society of Human Genetics Board of Directors, American College of Medical Genetics Board of Directors**. Points to consider: ethical, legal, and psychosocial implications of genetic testing in children and adolescents. Am J Hum Genet 1995;57:1233–1241.

Consensus guidelines for genetic testing in children and adolescents.

39. *(1C1)* **Nelson RM** et al. Ethical issues with genetic testing in pediatrics. Pediatrics 2001;107: 1451–1455.

Consensus guidelines for genetic testing in pediatrics including newborn screening, carrier testing, and testing for susceptibility to late-onset conditions.

40. **Vance JM**. The collection of biological samples for DNA analysis. In: Haines JL, Pericak-Vance MA, eds. Gene mapping in complex human diseases. Wiley-Liss, New York, 1998:201–211.

A practical guideline discussing all aspects of sample collection.

41. **Kopp P**. Perspective: genetic defects in the etiology of congenital hypothyroidism. Endocrinology 2002;143:2019–2024.

A review of genetic defects causing congenital hypothyroidism.

42. **Pfeifer A, Verma IM**. Gene therapy: Promises and problems. Annu Rev Genom Hum Genet 2001;2:177–211.

A review of techniques used for gene transfer and potential problems and risks.

43. **Brown EM** et al. Disorders with increased or decreased responsiveness to extracellular Ca^{21} owing to mutations in the Ca^{21}-sensing receptor. In: Spiegel AM, ed. G proteins, receptors and disease. Humana Press, Totowa, 1998, pp. 181–204

This review presents the physiology of the calcium-sensing receptor (CASR) and the consequences of activating and inactivating mutations. Monoallelic inactivating mutations in the CASR cause familial hypercalcemic hypocalciuria (FHH), biallelic inactivating mutations result in neonatal severe primary hyperparathyroidism (NSHPT). At the other end of the spectrum, activating mutations in the CASR cause autosomal dominant hypocalcemia (ADH).

44. *(1C1)* **Neumann HP** et al. Germ-line mutations in nonsyndromic pheochromocytoma. N Engl J Med 2002;346:1459–1466.

In this study, 271 patients who presented with nonsyndromic pheochromocytomas and without a family history of the disease, were analyzed for mutations in genes that are associated with familial forms of pheochromocytomas: the proto-oncogene RET (associated with multiple endocrine neoplasia type 2 (MEN-2)], and the tumor-suppressor gene VHL (associated with von Hippel–Lindau disease), and succinate dehydrogenase subunit D (SDHD) and succinate dehydrogenase subunit B (SDHB). Sixty-six (24%) were found to have mutations. Of these 66, 30 had mutations of VHL, 13 of RET, 11 of SDHD, and 12 of SDHB. Younger age, multifocal tumors, and extraadrenal tumors were significantly associated with the presence of a mutation. Because almost one fourth of patients with apparently sporadic pheochromocytoma may be carriers of mutations, the authors concluded routine analysis for mutations of RET, VHL, SDHD, and SDHB is indicated to identify pheochromocytoma-associated syndromes that would otherwise be missed.

45. **Phelan JK, McCabe ER**. Mutations in NR0B1 (DAX1) and NR5A1 (SF1) responsible for adrenal hypoplasia congenita. Hum Mutat 2001;18:472–487.

Mutations in the transcription factor DAX1 (NR0B1) cause X-linked adrenal hypoplasia congenita (AHC) and can result in hypogonadotropic hypogonadism. This review provides an excellent overview about DAX1 mutations and their consequences. It also discusses the role of SF1 mutations, which result also in AHC and abnormal gonadal development in males.

46. **Achermann JC** et al. Genetic causes of human reproductive disease. J Clin Endocrinol Metab 2002;87:2447–2454.

An excellent overview of genetic defects resulting in hypothalamic–pituitary or gonadal dysfunction.

47. **Lifton RP** et al. Molecular mechanisms of human hypertension. Cell 2001;104:545–556.

An excellent review discussing the molecular basis of hypertension including mendelian disorders resulting in altered net renal salt reabsorption and elevated blood pressure.

48. **Rader DJ** et al. Monogenic hypercholesterolemia: New insights in pathogenesis and treatment. J Clin Invest 2003;111:1795–1803.

This review summarizes the molecular pathogenesis and treatment of monogenic forms of severe hypercholesterolemia, as well as implications for the management of common forms of hypercholesterolemia.

49. **Garg A.** Acquired and inherited lipodystrophies. N Engl J Med 2004;350:1220–1234.

An excellent review of the various forms of lipodystrophies.

50. *(1C)* **Hegele R.** LMNA mutation position predicts organ system involvement in laminopathies. Clin Genet 2005;68:31–34.

Laminopathies are a family of monogenic multisystem disorders that result from mutation in lamin A *LMNA* (MIM 150330). To date, 16 distinct disease phenotypes have been shown to result from scores of various *LMNA* mutations, including 12 autosomal dominant (AD) and four autosomal recessive (AR) phenotypes. They include, among others, familial partial lipodystrophy (Dunnigan) and Emery-Dreifuss muscular dystrophy. In this study, 91 reported causative lamina A (LMNA) mutations associated with laminopathies were then classified according to their position and analyzed by hierarchic cluster analysis (HCA) for assembling 16 laminopathies into two classes based on organ system involvement. HCA laminopathy class and LMNA mutation position were strongly associated, and the findings support the hypothesis that laminopathy phenotype and LMNA genotype are nonrandomly associated. HCA may be a tool to help with the study of phenotype–genotype associations or "phenomics."

51. **Weinstein LS** et al. Endocrine manifestations of stimulatory G protein alpha-subunit mutations and the role of genomic imprinting. Endocr Rev 2001;22:675–705.

A thorough review of the complexities of the GNAS1 gene and the role of imprinting in gene expression. Monoallelic loss-of-function mutations in the *GNAS1* gene lead to Albright hereditary osteodystrophy (AHO). Paternal transmission of *GNAS1* mutations leads to an isolated AHO phenotype (*pseudo*pseudohypoparathyroidism), whereas maternal transmission leads to AHO in combination with hormone resistance to PTH, TSH, and gonadotropins (pseudohypoparathyroidism type IA). These phenotypic differences are explained by tissue-specific imprinting of the *GNAS1* gene, which is expressed primarily from the maternal allele in the thyroid, gonadotropes, and proximal renal tubule. In most other tissues, the *GNAS1* gene is expressed biallelically. In patients with isolated renal resistance to PTH (pseudohypoparathyroidism type IB), defective imprinting of the *GNAS1* gene results in decreased Gs·⋅·expression in the proximal renal tubules.

52. **Betterle C** et al. Autoimmune adrenal insufficiency and autoimmune polyendocrine syndromes: Autoantibodies, autoantigens, and their applicability in diagnosis and disease prediction. Endocr Rev 2002;23:327–364.

A comprehensive review of clinical, genetic, epidemiologic, and therapeutic aspects of autoimmune adrenal insufficiency and autoimmune polyglandular syndromes.

53. **Clayton EW.** Ethical, legal, and social implications of genomic medicine. N Engl J Med 2003; 349:562–569.

An excellent short overview about ethical, legal, and social concerns associated with genetic testing and genomics.

54. **Hirsch IB.** Insulin analogues. N Engl J Med 2005;352:174–183.

This excellent review highlights the evolution from insulin obtained from animals, to its recombinant production and its targeted modification.

Subject Index

A

Abdominal adiposity, in obesity, 211

Acarbose
  in complications of diabetes, 169
  in type 2 diabetes, 159, 161, 176

ACE inhibitors
  cardiovascular disease complications
    of diabetes, 170
  renal disease complications from
    diabetes, use of, 175

Acetone breath, in diabetic
    ketoacidosis, 163

Acquired male hypogonadism, 137

Acromegaly, 14–16
  clinical presentation of, 14
  definition of, 14
  diagnosis of, 14–15
  dopamine agonist treatments, 16
  epidemiology of, 14
  etiology of, 14
  growth hormone receptor antagonist
    treatments, 16
  neurosurgery on, 15
  pathophysiology of, 14
  radiation therapy for, 15–16
  somatostatin analogue treatments, 15
  treatment of, 15–16

Addison disease, 68. *See also* Adrenal
    insufficiency

Adenomas
  adrenal adenomas, cause of primary
    hyperaldosteronism, 62
  pituitary tumors, 4–6
  thyroid nodules, 38–40

Adolescents, diabetes in, type 1
  clinical manifestations, 155
  diet, 157
  hypoglycemia, epidemiology of, 167

Adrenal adenomas, cause of primary
    hyperaldosteronism, 62

Adrenal androgen production,
    evaluation of, 58

Adrenal androgen replacement therapy,
    in adrenal insufficiency, 72

Adrenal cortical scintigraphy, 60

Adrenal disorders, 57–75. *See also*
    specific disorders
  adrenal androgen production,
    evaluation of, 58
  adrenal cortical scintigraphy, 60
  adrenal medulla, evaluation of, 58
  adrenal medullary scintigraphy, 60
  adrenal vein sampling, 61, 63

adrenocorticotropic hormone
    measurements, 57–58
  computed tomography scanning, 59
  congenital adrenal hyperplasia,
    evaluation of, 58
  cortisol evaluations, 57
  Cushing syndrome, 64–66
  dynamic adrenal tests, 58
  function evaluations, 57–58
  genetic basis for, 264t
  glucocorticoid function, evaluation of,
    57–58
  imaging, 58–61, 63, 66, 67, 71
  incidentaloma as, 66–68
  insufficiency as, 68–72
  magnetic resonance imaging, 59–60
  mineralocorticoid function,
    evaluation of, 58
  pheochromocytoma as, 72–75,
    233–234
  positron emission tomography, 60–61
  primary hyperaldosteronism as, 61–64

Adrenal hyperplasia
  amenorrhea treatments, 129
  primary hyperaldosteronism,
    cause of, 62

Adrenal incidentaloma, 66–68
  computed tomography scans, 68
  definition of, 66
  diagnosis of, 67, 68t
  etiology of, 66–67
  follow-up, 68
  history and physical examination, 67
  imaging, 67
  surgery for, 67
  treatment, 67–68

Adrenal insufficiency, 68–72
  adrenal androgen replacement
    therapy, 72
  adrenocorticotropic hormone
    measurements, 71
  adrenocorticotropic hormone
    stimulation test, 70–71
  aldosterone production, 70, 71
  clinical symptoms of, 70
  corticotropin-releasing hormone
    test, 71
  cortisol production, 70
  cosyntropin stimulation test, 70–71
  definition of, 68
  diagnosis of, 70–71
  electrolyte abnormality correction, 71
  epidemiology of, 68–70